GLOBAL FERTILITY TRANSITION

GLOBAL FERTILITY TRANSITION

Rodolfo A. Bulatao
John B. Casterline
Editors

POPULATION AND DEVELOPMENT REVIEW
A Supplement to Volume 27, 2001

POPULATION COUNCIL
New York

Library of Congress Cataloging-in-Publication Data

Global fertility transition / Rodolfo A. Bulatao, John B. Casterline.
p. cm.
Includes bibliographical references and index.
ISBN 0-87834-103-X (pbk. : alk. paper)
1. Demographic transition. 2. Fertility, Human. I. Bulatao, Rodolfo A., 1944- II. Casterline, J. B.

HB887 .G57 2001
304.6'32--dc21 2001045840

ISSN 0098-7921
ISBN 0-87834-103-X

Printed in the United States of America.

CONTENTS

FOREWORD

Few concepts have defined a scientific discipline as distinctly as the demographic transition has defined demography. As a way of describing demographic history, it enjoys universal acceptance. All societies, at one time or another, move from a near-equilibrium condition of high mortality and high fertility toward a presumed low-fertility and low-mortality equilibrium. While many variations have been identified in how this transition occurs, few demographers question the basic fact of its existence.

Notwithstanding the virtual consensus on the *fact* of the demographic transition, there has been considerable debate about what causes it to happen and how it actually operates. While no paradigmatic "theory of the demographic transition" has emerged from research, certain central propositions have carried great weight with scholars and policymakers alike over the years, especially those drawn from microeconomic theories of household decisionmaking. Among the most widely cited of these propositions is one that holds that parents make decisions about family size on the basis of the present and future contribution of children to family well-being, particularly economic well-being. As development occurs in a society through industrialization, urbanization, vocational specialization—and reduced child mortality—and as the value of children declines relative to the cost of rearing them, fertility, too, will decline. This proposition appeared for many years to fit the historical experience of most of today's industrialized countries, although the influential Princeton study of the demographic transition in Europe cast serious doubt on how well it actually conformed to patterns of demographic change in eighteenth- and nineteenth-century Europe.

In any case, classical "structuralist" propositions about the demographic transition—propositions that posit the necessity of fundamental changes in the structure of a society and economy—have come to seem less and less useful in explaining the extraordinarily rapid fertility transitions being experienced by many developing countries today. Two features of classical theory, in particular, appear increasingly questionable: that basic changes in social and economic relationships must occur before fertility will change, and that the process is a gradual one that requires many decades to complete. There are simply too many examples of countries that have passed rapidly through the transition, and without many of the structural transformations assumed to be necessary, for the structuralist model to remain credible. Yet, for many people, scholars and policymakers alike, this model remains a central tenet of population theory and policy.

It was with this anomaly in mind that in 1998 the Rockefeller Foundation convened at its Bellagio Study and Conference Center a meeting of some of the best and most active scholars of demographic change, to examine the state of theories of the global fertility transition and eventually to produce a volume of papers that both assess the current state of affairs and challenge researchers to explore new theoretical leads. I believe this supplement to *Population and Development Review* succeeds admirably on both counts, moving our understanding of the fertility transition from its structuralist past to a much more sophisticated understanding of the contributions of communication and ideational change, public policy, and gender relations to contemporary fertility change.

Steven W. Sinding
New York
May 2001

ACKNOWLEDGMENTS

Earlier versions of these chapters were presented at a Conference on Global Fertility Transition, held in Bellagio, Italy, on 18–22 May 1998. Steven W. Sinding, then at the Rockefeller Foundation, initiated planning for such a conference. Rodolfo A. Bulatao, serving as a consultant to the Foundation, helped organize the conference with Sinding and Sara E. Seims. The Rockefeller Foundation provided financial support.

A number of participants in the conference are not represented in this volume but contributed to it through their comments and observations, both during the conference and subsequently. These include Pat Caldwell, Ethel Churchill, Joel Cohen, Paul Demeny, Sonalde Desai, Parfait Eloundou-Enyegue, Ronald Lee, Carolyn Makinson, Cheikh Mbacké, Mark Montgomery, Michael Teitelbaum, Noriko Tsuya, Susan Watkins, Robert Willis, and Chris Wilson.

Publication of this volume was supported by the Rockefeller Foundation and the Andrew W. Mellon Foundation. Janet O'Connell provided essential support in organizing the conference, and Doreen Totaram provided valuable assistance in assembling the volume.

Rodolfo A. Bulatao

John B. Casterline

Introduction

RODOLFO A. BULATAO

WORLD FERTILITY IS declining steadily. In 1970–75, about 60 percent of all countries had total fertility of 4.5 births per woman or higher. A decade later, this figure had fallen to 50 percent, and by 1990–95 it had fallen further to 40 percent. Over these two decades, the proportion with total fertility under 2.5 rose from one-sixth to one-third of all countries.

That fertility would fall worldwide for decades has long been expected. But notable declines have also appeared in the least-advanced developing countries, as well as in advanced industrial countries. And between 1985–90 and 1990–95, fertility decline worldwide accelerated beyond its previous pace, faster than anticipated by any preceding projections for that period (National Research Council 2000: 295–296). Is there a common theoretical explanation for widespread declines? Does fertility theory need to be rethought? Can anything be inferred about future fertility trends? These questions originally motivated this collection of articles.

Massive shifts in fertility in the late twentieth century went along with sweeping societal changes. This relationship is at the root of many theoretical explanations for fertility decline, seen as part of a broad demographic transition to lower birth and death rates. Some explanations of decline did appeal to the effectiveness of family planning programs, but since some modicum of government intervention is now typically part of the development process, these programs can be treated in the same context—as a part of development. Whether development-based theoretical explanations still apply in a period in which decline accelerated, and whether they continue to apply to fertility declines in industrial countries (often considered post-transitional or as involved in a second-stage transition: van de Kaa 1987), are the central issues for this volume. The contributors provide various answers, generally organized around particular disciplinary or subdisciplinary perspectives. Before reviewing these different accounts, this introduction identifies some basic explanations that underlie them. These explanations refer to fertility transition broadly, generally without much distinction between such features of transition as initial onset, the process of transitional decline (with its stages, starts and stops, and general pace), the end of transition, and post-transitional trends (or the "second fertility transition"). While distinguishing such features and relating them to theoretical explanations would be illuminating and would help situate the various approaches to be discussed, we do not have the opportunity to consider that here.

Eight explanations

Eight basic explanations for fertility transition link the chapters in this volume to the classic statement of transition by Notestein (1953) and subsequent theoretical work by Davis (1963), Coale (1973), Becker (1960), Carlsson (1966), Caldwell (1977), Easterlin (1978), Cleland and Wilson (1987), Hirschman (1994), and Mason (1997), among others.

1 Mortality reduction. Long-run declines in birth and death rates have always appeared closely related, giving rise to speculation about a possible equilibrium between the two. Davis (1963) extended the idea of such an equilibrium to incorporate the effects of migration in his concept of "multiphasic" demographic response. The specific mechanisms of linkage between reductions in death rates and birth rates are complex and do not necessarily involve couples' directly calculating the balance, although their actions may produce one.

2 Reduced economic contributions from children. Children contribute less if they cannot work while young, have to spend many hours and years in school, and are less committed to supporting aging parents. The reduction in such economic contributions in the course of socioeconomic development provides a possible reason why couples might want fewer children. The financial costs of rearing children are also an economic factor. These costs rise in the course of development, although whether they rise as a proportion of income is less clear.

3 Opportunity costs of childbearing. Rearing children interferes with adult activities. It can make it difficult for the mother to work, and her income forgone is a cost to the family. It limits parents' social activities and other consumption. One might combine these opportunity costs with the preceding economic factors, but they are worth distinguishing because the dynamics of and emphasis on opportunity costs can differ over time.

4 Family transformation. The shift to fewer births accompanies a transformation in the institution of the family from a multigenerational concern with clear lines of authority to a small, conjugal unit focused on the individual needs of the members. This family transformation, and the changes in values accompanying it, may itself be responsible for preferences for having fewer children. Gender-specific roles within the family

may also change, affecting the joint preferences of the couple as well as the ability of women to realize their preferences.

5 Vanishing cultural props for childbearing. From religious injunctions to the encouragement of tribal and village elders, high fertility often receives support and even celebration in traditional societies. These normative props lose their force as societies modernize. Weakening normative control may empower individuals to make their own choices, often for smaller families.

6 Improved access to effective fertility regulation. Better methods of contraception and abortion, and less-fettered access to such methods, should make it easier to control fertility. Assuming some initial at least latent desire to do so, greater access should give an impetus to fertility decline.

7 Marriage delay. While each of the preceding explanations may account for fertility decline within marriage, marriage delay has often added to overall fertility decline. Unlike the universal declines in marital fertility, marriage delay appears neither inevitable nor universal, but nevertheless must also be taken into account.

8 Diffusion. Diffusion refers to the spread of ideas and practices that lead to lower fertility. In a sense, it is not an independent explanation. What diffuses must be ideas or practices connected with one or more of the preceding explanations, or with some other substantive explanation that may have been overlooked. The diffusion explanation appears to address only the process of, rather than a fundamental reason for, fertility change. Nevertheless, it directs attention to the fact that individuals and couples do not act in isolation: they interact and influence each other, giving the process of fertility change its particular dynamics.

These eight basic explanations might be seen as separate, potentially disjoint insights about the reasons for fertility transition. They have been expressed here without reference to specific empirical indicators that might operationalize them. The variable of education, for instance, could reflect all of these explanations simultaneously: educated individuals expect lower child mortality, feel more restricted by children, have easier access to reproductive health care, are more open to the media, and are more likely to influence others. What the explanations are meant to reflect rather than empirical variables are fundamental reasons for lower fertility that are posited in one theory after another.

Theoretical approaches

One could assess the evidence for each explanation and evaluate its role in different fertility theories (see, e.g., Bulatao 1979). Instead, for each theoretical approach represented in this volume, this introduction tries to identify which basic explanations are stressed. It also asks what the approach says, if anything, about acceleration or deceleration in the course of fertility transition, and how the approach accounts for changes in pace. And it considers what predictions flow from the arguments about future fertility. For theorists who may be concerned with providing broad insights, the latter questions may well surpass their ambitions. However, if our concern is with theorizing about recent fertility trends, such questions need to be asked.

Demographic approach

John Cleland (this volume) provides a demographic approach to explaining fertility transition. He focuses on mortality, essentially explaining one demographic phenomenon with another. Restating Davis's (1963) position, he assumes that societies inevitably respond to lower mortality by lowering fertility, thereby bringing population growth rates back close to zero.

Cleland makes all other explanations for fertility transition subsidiary to the impact of mortality reduction. With the variety of settings and conditions under which fertility transition occurred in the last two centuries, he argues, the only true common factor that can be identified is preceding large mortality reductions. In particular, he criticizes as insufficient—though not entirely irrelevant—"demand" explanations for fertility transition (in our terms, explanations related to reduced economic contributions from children, increased restrictions exerted by them, family transformation, and vanishing cultural props for childbearing). Favoring the view that pretransitional fertility was largely in equilibrium with mortality, he sees demand for large numbers of surviving children as never having been strong, and therefore the disappearance of this demand as being at best a subsidiary force in fertility transition.

Past arguments for the primacy in fertility transition of mortality reductions have foundered on the difficulty of substantiating the empirical link. Researchers have suggested many ways mortality decline—in particular rising child survival probabilities—could produce lower fertility (see, e.g., Cohen and Montgomery 1998). All of these paths depend on individual perceptions and expectations of mortality risks, however, and such perceptions and expectations appear not to change sufficiently in a timely manner to produce observed fertility changes. Some fertility decline can be expected when infecundability increases, as more children survive and breastfeeding durations lengthen. Some fertility decline could also result when couples no longer need to replace lost children or bear "extra" children as insurance against child deaths. But these and related explanations cannot account for more than a portion of observed fertility declines (Montgomery 1998; Palloni and Rafalimanana 1999).

Cleland provides two types of response to this problem. First, he argues that the mortality–fertility link is not dependent on perceptions of child survival. Instead, the larger families resulting from higher levels of child survival exert economic pressure on families, which leads to fertility decline (see also Davis 1963). Second, he argues that this link and all other links are in any case too complex for empirical verification in specific historical cases.

As an overarching approach to explaining fertility transition, Cleland does not elaborate this demographic approach (which in any event may not be capable of elaboration) to allow for prediction of when or where fertility will decline. What lag exists between mortality reduction and fertility decline is left deliberately vague, with the links between the two being multiple and not necessarily similar from case to case. This approach therefore does not imply and cannot account for decade-to-decade unevenness in the pace of global or even national fertility decline. It attempts to account only for fertility transition in a general sense, particularly for its inevitability.

From the focus on the mortality–fertility balance, one might draw the implication that long-run fertility is likely to be close to replacement. This assumes that fertility sufficiently low to lead to population decline is as societally stressful as too-high fertility. Cleland does not make such a prediction, although, provided extraneous factors such as migration are excluded, his central argument may lead to it.

Historical approach

In contrast to Cleland, John Caldwell (this volume) pays scant attention to mortality reduction. He provides instead a multilayered interpretation of global fertility decline, both in developing and industrial countries, since the 1960s. Socioeconomic development is part of his interpretation, to the extent that insufficient socioeconomic change is his explanation for why some social groups were excluded from the global fertility decline. A second and more interesting part of the interpretation involves the development of new, more efficient contraceptives, which he argues facilitated fertility decline in both industrial and developing regions. This was further facilitated by a third factor: the diffusion of concern about the population explosion, leading in industrial countries to increased legitimation of smaller families and in developing countries to elite support for family planning programs.

This multilayered interpretation is arguably a vast improvement on Caldwell's (1976) unified theoretical vision that posited a "great divide" between pretransitional and transitional regimes characterized by a change in the direction of the wealth flows from children to parents. (Elegantly simple ideas such as this can take on an afterlife of their own, even when they are wrong.) His current chapter attempts to interpret the historical record from broad social trends and forces, rather than appealing to the dynamics of household decisions about fertility. It can be characterized, for lack of a more precise label, as an essentially historical approach.

At the core of Caldwell's argument is a belief that fertility trends since the 1960s, in both developing and industrial countries, must have parallel historical explanations. By blurring the distinction between forces affecting fertility in these two settings, Caldwell effectively abandons the idea that fertility transition has some terminus. Presumably, then, continued economic growth and social development and continually improving methods of fertility regulation could lead to endlessly declining fertility. However, Caldwell also recognizes the impact on fertility of widely diffused ideas about societal and global imperatives. And presumably, at some point in the twenty-first century, global opinion could become pronatalist. What this approach implies, therefore, about future fertility is uncertain.

Sociological approach

John Casterline (this volume) draws on all the explanations simultaneously. These are organized into three clusters, pertaining to mortality reduction, falling demand for children, and increasing ability to regulate fertility (cf. Bulatao and Lee 1983). Mortality reduction receives less attention than the other two clusters. Although Casterline stresses the role of fertility-regulation methods and their diffusion, he also takes pains to rescue demand explanations from the criticism that typical indicators of demand, particularly socioeconomic variables, do not correlate strongly with fertility trends.

Focusing on determinants of the pace of fertility decline during transition, Casterline argues that one should not expect a straightforward relationship between determinants and fertility levels. Effects are path-dependent, affected by the particular history of each setting. For instance, the choice of a contraceptive method by a few active innovators in one community can "lock in" the community to future dependence primarily on this method, even if other methods would be safer, cheaper, or more convenient (Potter 1999). Effects also depend not on objective conditions but on individual perceptions of these conditions (an observation that links this approach to the psychological approach discussed next). Perceptions can be modified by social influence, producing a web of causal influences that can be difficult to disentangle.

No single explanation can be said to be central to Casterline's argument, which attempts to be comprehensive. Nonetheless, his argument implies that many explanations for fertility transition can be rescued from unfavorable evidence. In opening the door to the analysis of historical and psychosocial causality in fertility behavior, Casterline offers the hope of a comprehensive theory but also in effect, until this is attained, provides a means to account for a wide range of empirical results unfavorable to particular hypotheses.

The focus on perceptions and social influence provides possible explanations for the timing of the onset of fertility decline and sudden accelerations and decelerations in the tempo of fertility decline. Even if objective conditions show a stable trend, perceptions can change suddenly, leading to rapid changes in fertility (John Haaga, this volume). Social influence can initially suppress individual reactions to changes in objective conditions and eventually magnify the response, producing sharp fluctuations in fertility trends unpredictable from more stable patterns of socioeconomic indicators.

In attempting to account for the pace at which fertility declines, Casterline provides few leads to when and at what point decline may end. Nor can arguments be made by analogy with more demographically advanced countries. The reliance on the idea of path dependence suggests that fertility in each country will follow its own distinctive trajectory.

Psychological approach

One variant of a psychological approach to fertility transition has been offered by Lesthaeghe and Vanderhoeft (1997), who argue that individual fertility change requires that the individual be ready, willing, and able to change. To be willing is to recognize the practical benefits of having fewer children; to be able is to have access to methods for fertility regulation; and to be ready—the most difficult of the concepts to ascertain—is to be open to considering the prospect of family limitation. These three conditions, parallelling an earlier statement by Coale (1973), also resemble factors distinguished in the sociological approach.

An alternative psychological approach focuses on shifts in the values underlying fertility decisions. Dirk van de Kaa (this volume) exemplifies this approach (see also Lesthaeghe and Surkyn 1988). Focusing on post-transition societies, he treats as central to fertility change the values related to postmodernity and postmaterialism. These values center on individualism: freedom, self-expression, and the personal search for a better quality of life represent a radical departure from traditional values, institutional authority, and group ethics enshrined in religion. The spread of individualistic values suppresses altruistic childbearing.

The approach is applied mainly to post-transition fertility, not to the process of fertility transition, though it should be relevant at least to the late stages. The vanishing of cultural props to high fertility is emphasized, as are the restrictions on parents' freedom inherent in childbearing and childrearing. The individualistic tendencies that replace the cultural props seem to favor smaller families, though not unambiguously (see Christine

Bachrach, this volume). Van de Kaa's evidence on this point, from large European surveys, is not clearcut. He does suggest that postmodern values—particularly the increase in cohabitation—may have less influence on birth limitation than on the postponement of births.

Why do postmodern values develop and spread? The one social structural factor van de Kaa identifies is increasing affluence, which frees individuals from immediate concern with basic human needs. Aside from that, postmodernism appears to be mostly a matter of fashion, rooted in changes in the socialization of younger generations. Although values related to children and childbearing could be formulated in a much more specific fashion and related to changes in social structure (e.g., Bulatao 1982; Bachrach, this volume), van de Kaa opts for a global perspective that may explain much more than fertility change but is not intended to provide a precise accounting of fertility trends.

Predicting the spread of particular values is difficult, and predicting the fertility change that may result is still more so. Anticipating when fertility change may accelerate or decelerate is clearly not an objective of the psychological approach. Nor is it clear from the approach what the long-run prediction for fertility should be. Speaking of postmodernity implies that a return to earlier values is not likely, but whether postmodernity will persist and what values might be part of the new "modernity" that succeeds it are indeterminate.

Economic approach

This volume does not provide examples of a strict economic approach. Willis (1998) discusses fertility theory as embedded in work on the economics of the family and human capital theory. These two areas of economics, developed since the 1960s, as well as microeconomic theory generally, provide a framework, more fully integrated and elaborated than in other disciplines, within which fertility models have been proposed.

In economic models the cost of children is central, both the opportunity cost related to labor force participation mothers must forgo to care for children and other costs that limit the investment in "child quality," mainly schooling. Parents' optimal investment in child quality (and therefore optimal child quantity, which is simultaneously determined under an income constraint) is affected by assumed intergenerational transfers, particularly expected support in old age. Desired child quantity changes in the course of economic development for several reasons, including the rising returns to female employment. Willis especially emphasizes the increasing demand for skilled labor, which raises the premium on child quality.

Economic models are sufficiently diverse and detailed to provide explanations for variations in the pace of fertility transition. With the links that they draw between changes in economic circumstances and household calculations of optimal childbearing, faster or slower fertility decline can be traced to changes in economic structure. For the long term, however, the economic approach provides conflicting predictions. On the one hand, the continually rising cost of time and increasing demands for schooling seem to imply a continuing fall in fertility. On the other hand, Willis recognizes the substantial contributions that younger generations make to older generations, especially in modern welfare societies, through public-sector transfers. The gains accruing to their own children, if captured by parents, would presumably help set a floor on future fertility in advanced industrial societies.

Gender perspective

In contrast to the broad sweep of the preceding approaches to explaining fertility transition, the gender perspective, as represented in this volume by Karen Oppenheim Mason, involves a collection of indirect influences on fertility. The family and gender explanation, naturally central in this perspective, is itself a secondary explanation of transition. Family and gender systems make a difference because of their relationship to all the other explanations, modifying the influence of other factors on fertility.

For instance, Mason accepts the importance of the diffusion of information and attitudes about fertility regulation—but argues that women's freedom of movement and control over resources facilitate the diffusion process, whereas rigid gender stratification retards it. Mason sees similar influences of gender and family systems with regard to most of the other explanations for fertility transition: mortality reduction through improved child survival is conditional on female status; the economic benefits and costs to women of having children depend on family structure; and opportunity costs are modified by societal accommodation to multiple female roles.

Harriet Presser (this volume) calls attention to the restrictions women in developed countries experience from having children, particularly the restrictions on their leisure time rather than on their employment. Women's sense of entitlement to use their time as they choose, she argues, is a central explanation for low fertility levels.

Given the variety of paths through which family and gender systems might affect fertility, their impact could be large if these influences all operated in the same direction. No evidence is adduced for such a unifying influence, however. In addition, the evidence Mason adduces for individual paths of influence is mixed, comes from a variety of settings, and in at least one case suggests an inverse influence in which greater gender inequality, in the post-transitional setting, produces lower rather than higher fertility.

Since trends in family and gender systems have seldom been successfully predicted, their impact on the future course of fertility is difficult to anticipate (Cherlin 2000). Changes in global fertility might be accounted for in an ad hoc manner, drawing on the variety of pathways of influence incorporated in the gender perspective. But the perspective does not suggest why and when these changes occur.

Even if one assumes that gender equality will increase, this assumption does not help predict the course of future fertility. Fertility might more closely approximate women's preferences, and these preferences are likely to be low when women emphasize their own consumption. But to what extent having children will itself be considered an important source of personal satisfaction, and what level of fertility will result, are indeterminate.

Policy perspective

From a policy perspective, the question is less why fertility declines than whether policy plays a role in decline. Amy Ong Tsui (this volume) affirms the effect of population policy in developing countries in recent decades through family planning programs, which promote access to contraceptives and diffuse attitudes favorable to their use. Tsui provides a brief summary of the debate on this role.

She then speculates about the role of institutions—including ministries, health care providers, and nongovernmental organizations—in shaping behavior in modern societies and the implications of organizational dynamics for modifying the effects of policy on fertility. She directs attention to institutional decisionmaking, institutional evolution, and decentralization—not merely as intervening factors for the effect of policy on fertility but as factors that actually help define policy.

Geoffrey McNicoll (this volume) also considers the contribution of state policies and activities. First he surveys psychosocial and economic explanations for fertility decline—essentially the "demand" explanations already considered—and then argues that these would be enriched by an appreciation of state influences. Government can influence fertility not only through deliberate programs to provide contraception or diffuse supportive ideas but also by altering the institutional context for individual fertility choices. Choices depend on perceived costs and benefits of childbearing, which are modified by publicly enforced intergenerational transfers. The opportunity costs of childbearing are also partly defined by the types of social equalities and inequalities that governments tolerate or enforce.

Both of these perspectives recognize a potential direct effect of policy on fertility transition through improving access to fertility-regulation methods and through diffusion of supportive ideas. Both perspectives also emphasize broader, though indirect, government influences on fertility that originate in organizational or institutional factors. From a policy perspective, then, one should in principle be able to point to government dictates to explain modulations in the pace of fertility decline (e.g., Cleland 1994), though neither Tsui nor McNicoll—their approach being largely speculative—presents evidence of this nature.

What a policy perspective implies about the future course of fertility is also of interest. Both Tsui and McNicoll argue that government may have a continuing interest in modifying fertility levels. Tsui suggests a continuing government interest in family planning programs as well as possible future reorientation to other demographic problems. McNicoll is even more expansive, suggesting that low-fertility societies might validly be concerned about their demographic futures and that some interventions to assure desired outcomes could be consistent with democracy. In particular, he notes proposed designs of incentives for childbearing that could help avert some of the socioeconomic problems attendant on very low fertility (see also Massimo Livi Bacci, this volume). Therefore, while a policy perspective may not suggest any specific future level of fertility, it supports the possibility that levels that may be deemed desirable may be approached through government action.

Theoretical integration and predictions

Each theoretical approach outlined above seeks comprehensiveness, attempting to include in some fashion the range of acceptable explanations for fertility transition. To a great extent, each draws on the same set of eight basic explanations, arranging them in different ways. Different theoretical approaches favor particular arguments, but generally they do not impose any hierarchy on them.

The exceptions are two. The demographic approach gives mortality reduction priority, making it the main driving force that triggers the other explanations. The economic approach typically strives for integration with economic theory generally, paying little attention to factors that are not susceptible to economic analysis. This is not invariably true, however, of economic approaches (e.g., Easterlin 1978).

The basic agreements among the theoretical approaches may be briefly summarized:

—Fertility decline is a largely rational process. It is based on individual calculations that lower fertility makes sense, not solely in economic terms but also for social and psychological reasons.

—As with most rational actions, both the motivation and the means must exist. "Demand" explanations that account for the desire for smaller families and "supply" explanations that account for access to methods of fertility regulation each receive attention from most perspectives.

—As a predominantly rational process, fertility transition involves a multitude of individual decisions. Some theoretical approaches analyze these decisions more closely than others, but none ignores them.

—The framework for individual decisions is set by social-structural and economic factors. These factors are conceived in different ways, with different emphases. They may include the gender rules society enforces, the labor market requirements produced by globalization, and the policy prescriptions that governments adopt.

—Taking such factors into account in their calculations, individuals still must have reference to goals and values that are not themselves readily subject to rational analysis. Lifestyle choices are not entirely rational, nor are preferences for sons or daughters. And the propagation through diffusion of such attitudes, or of contrary attitudes, is only partly a matter of rational argument.

For the most part, these theoretical approaches appear to be evolving toward greater elaboration. Given relative agreement on the main factors motivating fertility decisions, attention has turned increasingly to the micro-level processes that affect these factors: the process of diffusion and the variables that moderate it; the social positions of individuals and the way these shape their preferences and determine the influence they have on fertility decisions; and the psychological processes involved in reaching decisions. An increased focus on process, position, or psychology—or on all of these at once—ties together the historical approach and the sociological approach, affects the gender perspective as well, and is implicit in the policy perspective, which focuses on institutional and organizational processes.

What about the future? The chapters that follow are more concerned with understanding the past than with prediction. Their consensus would be that fertility will continue to fall, although at what pace requires empirical investigation and cannot be determined purely on theoretical grounds. With the attention to path dependence, diffusion effects, and gender and other factors that moderate influences on fertility, the theoretical approaches provide no clear guidance about whether future fertility decline, for countries where fertility is still high, will be faster or slower than declines experienced by low-fertility countries in the past.

At what level fertility will eventually settle, or around what level it may fluctuate in the long run, is even more indeterminate. On the one hand, the demographic approach appears to imply an equilibrium replacement level. On the other hand, the gender perspective implies that personal preferences will become the central factor, and the psychological approach suggests these preferences will favor low fertility. Finally, the economic approach, the gender perspective, and the policy perspective imply that public policy could have an important role in influencing future fertility levels, potentially in an upward direction.

Empirical perspectives

Perhaps the question of long-run fertility levels might be settled by careful empirical analysis, without recourse to theory about how fertility is related to social trends. Empirical analysis is the focus of two of the chapters in this volume. Their answers, however, are at least partly divergent. Assembling detailed data on trends in low-fertility societies, Tomas Frejka and John Ross document the variety of low-fertility societies and the diversity of paths they followed to low fertility. They interpret the patterns as indicating that below-replacement fertility is likely to persist for some indefinite period in every region where it predominates.

John Bongaarts, on the other hand, focuses on reproductive preferences and changes in the tempo of individual childbearing. With the delay in childbearing driving fertility below women's reproductive preferences, he foresees an eventual rise in fertility in societies where childbearing age is now rising rapidly.

Contrasting inferences can therefore be drawn from empirical data, and theory remains critical in projecting future fertility trends.

References

Becker, Gary S. 1960. "An economic analysis of fertility," in *Demographic and Economic Change in Developed Countries*. Universities-National Bureau Committee for Economic Research, Conference Series 11. Princeton: Princeton University Press, pp. 209–231.

Bulatao, Rodolfo A. 1979. *On the Nature of the Transition in the Value of Children*. Papers of the East-West Population Institute, No. 60-A. Honolulu: East-West Center.

———. 1982. "The transition in the value of children and the fertility transition," in Charlotte Höhn and Rainer Mackensen (eds.), *Determinants of Fertility Trends: Theories Re-examined*. Liège: Ordina Editions, pp. 97–122.

Bulatao, Rodolfo A. and Ronald D. Lee (eds.). 1983. *Determinants of Fertility in Developing Countries*. 2 vols. New York: Academic Press.

Caldwell, John C. 1976. "Toward a restatement of demographic transition theory," *Population and Development Review* 2(3/4): 321–366.

Carlsson, Gösta. 1966. "The decline of fertility: Innovation or adjustment process," *Population Studies* 20(2): 149–174.

Cherlin, Andrew J. 2000. "Thoughts on the future of the family," paper presented at the Annual Meeting of the Population Association of America, Los Angeles.

Cleland, John. 1994. "Different pathways to demographic transition," in F. Graham-Smith (ed.), *Population: The Complex Reality*. Golden, CO: North American Press, pp. 229–247.

Cleland, John and Christopher Wilson. 1987. "Demand theories of the fertility transition: An iconoclastic view," *Population Studies* 4(1): 5–30.

Coale, Ansley J. 1973. "The demographic transition," in *International Population Conference, Liège, 1973*, Vol. 1. Liège: International Union for the Scientific Study of Population, pp. 53–72.

Cohen, Barney and Mark R. Montgomery. 1998. "Introduction," in Mark R. Montgomery and Barney Cohen (eds.), *From Death to Birth: Mortality Decline and Reproductive Change*. Washington, DC: National Academy Press, pp. 1–38.

Davis, Kingsley. 1963. "The theory of change and response in modern demographic history," *Population Index* 29(4): 345–366.

Easterlin, Richard A. 1978. "The economics and sociology of fertility: A synthesis," in Charles Tilly (ed.), *Historical Studies of Changing Fertility*. Princeton, NJ: Princeton University Press, pp. 57–133.

Hirschman, Charles. 1994. "Why fertility changes," *Annual Review of Sociology* 20: 203–233.

Lesthaeghe, Ron and Johan Surkyn. 1988. "Cultural dynamics and economic theories of fertility change," *Population and Development Review* 14(1): 1–45.

Lesthaeghe, Ron and C. Vanderhoeft. 1997. "Ready, willing and able: A conceptualization of transitions to new behavioral forms," IPD Working Paper, No. 1997-8. Interface Demography, Vrije Universiteit Brussel.

Mason, Karen Oppenheim. 1997. "Explaining fertility transitions," *Demography* 34(4): 443–454.

Montgomery, Mark R. 1998. "Mortality decline and the fertility transition: Toward a new agenda," paper prepared for the Conference on Global Fertility Transition, Bellagio, Italy, 18–22 May.

National Research Council. 2000. "Appendix B: Accuracy of population projections from the 1970s to the 1990s," in John Bongaarts and Rodolfo A. Bulatao (eds.), *Beyond Six Billion: Forecasting the World's Population*, pp. 254–302. Washington, DC: National Academy Press. Online at «http://www.nap.edu/books/0309069904/html».

Notestein, Frank W. 1953. "Economic problems of population change," in *Proceedings of the Eighth International Conference of Agricultural Economists*. London: Oxford University Press, pp. 13–31.

Palloni, Alberto, and Hantamala Rafalimanana. 1999. "The effects of infant mortality on fertility revisited: New evidence from Latin America," *Demography* 36(1): 41–58.

Potter, Joseph E. 1999. "The persistence of outmoded contraceptive regimes: The cases of Mexico and Brazil," *Population and Development Review* 25(4): 703–739.

Van de Kaa, Dirk J. 1987. "Europe's second demographic transition," *Population Bulletin* 42(1).

Willis, Robert J. 1998. "Economic transformation and fertility," paper prepared for the Conference on Global Fertility Transition, Bellagio, Italy, 18–22 May.

PART ONE

GLOBAL FERTILITY PATTERNS

The Pace of Fertility Transition: National Patterns in the Second Half of the Twentieth Century

JOHN B. CASTERLINE

THE DECLINE IN fertility that began in the late eighteenth century and will in all likelihood come to conclusion sometime in the twenty-first century is a profound demographic transformation. One can argue about its significance in comparison to the other demographic transitions occurring during this same period: the sharp decline in mortality, the aging of populations (a consequence of declines in fertility and mortality), and the urbanization of populations. Most of the key demographic parameters for the world's population in the middle of the twenty-first century will differ substantially from the same parameters at the beginning of the nineteenth. This demographic transformation has not occurred in isolation from other societal changes. Indeed, in their determination to describe and explain the profound demographic changes of the past two centuries, demographers can be faulted for failing to appreciate the scale of the other significant societal transformations that have occurred during this same period, in particular the vast growth in income and wealth in a subset of countries (and the resulting spread of intercountry economic inequalities) and the unprecedented development of science and technology (Ray 1998).

Demographers are also liable to the criticism of being overly focused on the *number* of children as the first and foremost among many fertility parameters. But family size may often be secondary to other family and fertility goals, as Santow and Bracher (1999) suggest in their evocative description of fertility decline among southern Europeans in Australia. Other aspects of family structure and function can show a remarkable capacity to accommodate radical changes in the level of fertility occurring in the space of one generation or less (Hirschman 1994; McDonald 1994). Perhaps it is not so surprising that demographers have been unable to reach consensus on a short list of causes of fertility change: if individuals are less attached to any given family size than our theories implicitly assume, then less powerful and systematic causal forces may suffice to overturn any particular reproductive regime than we have thought necessary.

If demographers are guilty of an exaggerated sense of the significance of fertility levels per se, it remains the case that the quantum of fertility has wide-ranging implications at both the household and societal level, in high- and low-fertility societies alike (Lee and Casterline 1996). Few topics in the social sciences have been pursued with such dedication and resources as the determinants and consequences of fertility. As a result of this investment, we are now in a relatively advantaged position to understand why fertility changes (Hirschman 1994; Mason 1997). A considerable body of pertinent theory has been developed, and there is abundant empirical material that can be exploited for the testing of specific hypotheses. If anything, the empirical materials have been underutilized—if this is possible, considering the enormous number of articles and books on fertility published since 1950.

This chapter examines the *pace* of fertility decline. The pace of transition is a relatively unexplored topic, despite its short- and mid-term demographic consequences and despite the deep impression that the apparent rapidity of transition has left on many scholars (e.g., Watkins 1986; Cleland and Wilson 1987).[1] The classic statements about the determinants of fertility decline are addressed much more to the question of *why* fertility declines than to *how rapidly* it declines (Notestein 1953; Davis 1963; Coale 1973; Freedman 1979; Caldwell 1982), although hypotheses about pace can be readily derived from these statements. As Bongaarts and Watkins (1996) note, at present there is little agreement about why some fertility declines are precipitous while others occur at a leisurely pace. The chapter is motivated by prospective concerns—will fertility decline proceed rapidly or slowly during the next few decades?—hence the empirical analysis is confined to Asia, Africa, and Latin America. I begin with an examination of empirical data on fertility transitions that have commenced since 1950, documenting the variation in pace of decline at the national level. I then shift to a conceptual framework for understanding variation in the pace of fertility transition, followed by an extended discussion of those factors likely to accelerate or hamper fertility decline.

The pace of contemporary fertility declines

What is at stake?

While the transition to low fertility was either completed or well underway in a large number of countries as of the mid-1990s, a substantial fraction of the population of the globe currently resides in countries where fertility transition is far from complete. As a rough indicator that fertility decline is underway but not complete, consider countries with total fertility rates (TFRs) in the range of 2.5 to 5.5 births per woman. According to United Nations estimates for 1990–95, 80 countries fall into this category, and in 1995 they contained 44 percent of the world's population (53 percent of the population of Asia, Africa, and Latin America). Under the UN's assumptions about trends in fertility and mortality, 59 percent of world population growth during the three decades between 1995 and 2025 will occur in these countries.[2] Alternatively, classifying countries in terms of date of onset of fertility decline (see Appendix), 49 percent of the world's population in 1995 resides in countries where sustained fertility transition began after 1965 (but only 9 percent in countries where declines began after 1980), and 61 percent of the projected growth between 1995 and 2025 will occur in these countries. From these figures it is clear that near-term demographic trends in those countries mid-stream in fertility transition will have considerable bearing on the size and structure of the world's population in the twenty-first century (Kandiah and Horiuchi 1995). Fertility decline in these countries could proceed either more gradually or more rapidly than "medium variant" projections assume. As demographers, acutely aware of the uncertainty intrinsic to population projections, we are compelled to consider the range of demographic futures that variations in pace of decline would produce.

To be more concrete, the continuing pace of ongoing fertility declines will affect both the size of future populations and their age structure. Considering first effects on size, the effect of pace of decline on population size was considered by the World Bank (1994) when producing their 1994 round of projections. Projections were produced for three alternative rates of decline: the World Bank "standard," a "slow decline" in which the number of years required to reach replacement-level fertility is twice as long as the standard decline, and a "rapid decline" in which the number of years to replacement level is half as long as the standard decline. The exercise was carried out country-by-country, but the published volume shows only results aggregated across countries within regions. We can briefly consider the global results and the results by region. Comparing the two extremes at the global level, the increase in global population between 2000 and 2050 will be 25 percentage points greater (66 percent versus 41 percent) if fertility decline is "slow" rather than "rapid" (an absolute difference of 1.5 billion persons). The increase over the same period will be 9 percentage points greater (increase of 66 percent versus 57 percent) if the decline follows the World Bank "standard" expectations rather than proceeding "rapidly." Naturally the differences widen by 2100: the increase in global population between 2000 and 2100 will be 47 percentage points greater (100 percent versus 53 percent) if fertility decline is "slow" rather than "rapid" (an absolute difference of 2.8 billion persons). These substantial differences can be attributed almost entirely to the pace of decline over the next two to four decades in those countries where fertility decline is now underway. The effects of pace are greatest, of course, in those regions where fertility was highest in the 1990s, namely, Africa and some subregions of Asia. The alternative scenarios for these regions are shown in Figure 1. In sub-Saharan Africa and Southwest Asia, the increase in population between 2000 and 2050 will be 73–105 percentage points greater if a slow-decline path is followed rather than a fast-decline path. The differences are less pronounced in the more populous South Asia but large nevertheless: under the slow-decline scenario, the growth in population in this region will be 33 percentage points greater over this 50-year period than under the rapid-decline scenario (a difference of almost one-half billion persons).

It follows from this analysis that the future regional distribution of population will be affected by the pace of fertility decline. For example, if fertility declines rapidly in all regions, sub-Saharan Africa will contain 13 percent of the world's population in 2050, compared with 18 percent if fertility declines slowly in all regions. If fertility declines slowly in sub-Saharan Africa but rapidly everywhere else, then sub-Saharan Africa will con-

FIGURE 1 Percentage growth in population size 2000–2050 under alternative rates of fertility decline, by region

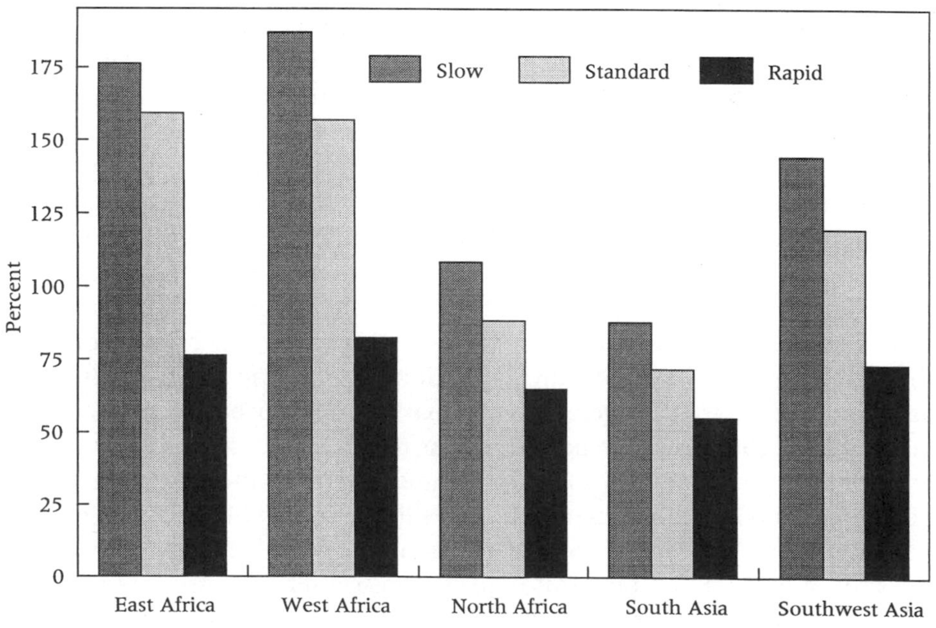

SOURCE: World Bank 1994.

tain almost 20 percent of the world's population in 2050. Naturally all these effects are magnified by 2100. In short, the pace at which fertility declines over the next few decades will have an enormous impact on both the size of the world's population and its regional distribution throughout the twenty-first century.

The overall nature of the effects of the pace of decline on age structure is well known. In general, rapid declines (in fertility and mortality, but especially the former) cause more perturbance in the age structure of a population than slow declines. The most immediate consequence of a decline in fertility is a drop in the fraction of the population at young ages. Since Coale and Hoover (1958), the assumption has been that such age-structure changes are beneficial for the economy and, in addition, encourage higher per capita investment in younger generations (with attendant longer-term economic and social benefits). In the 1990s, interest in Coale and Hoover's argument was revived as several studies appeared to confirm its central conclusions—namely, that fertility decline presents the economy with a "demographic gift" in the form of a surge in the relative size of the working-age population (Higgins and Williamson 1997; Asian Development Bank 1997).

One means of illustrating the plausible effects of the pace of fertility decline on the size of the demographic gift is to use United Nations data to compare age structures for countries that have experienced slow or rapid declines during the past three decades. Figures 2a and 2b show trends in age-dependency ratios until 2050 in two sets of Asian countries selected to contrast slow and rapid fertility declines up to the mid-1990s: South Korea, Thailand, and the Philippines in East and Southeast Asia; and Bangladesh and Pakistan in South Asia. The age-dependency measure selected is the ratio of persons aged 15–64 years to the sum of persons under age 15 and over age 64, multiplied by 100. Higher values indicate a greater concentration of the population in the "working ages," 15–64.[3] The country differences in the dependency ratio are large. In Figure 2a, the age-dependency ratio reaches exceptional heights in Korea, reflecting the country's very rapid fertility decline, with Thailand's age-dependency ratio peaking not far below Korea's (but ten years later). In the Philippines, where the decline continues at a gradual pace, the ratio peaks several decades later and falls well short of the heights achieved in Korea and Thailand. The contrast is not so sharp in the comparison between Bangladesh and Pakistan in Figure 2b but is the same in form: the more rapid fertility decline in Bangladesh delivers a more generous, and earlier, "demographic gift."

From these demographic projections it is clear that a quickening or a slowing of the present rate of fertility decline could have substantial implications for the size and structure of populations in the twenty-first century. Certainly the prospect of smaller population sizes and, in particular,

FIGURE 2 Age-dependency ratios[a] in countries with rapid and slow fertility declines 1970–95 and projected evolution[b] of these ratios 1995–2050

a. Korea, Phillipines, and Thailand

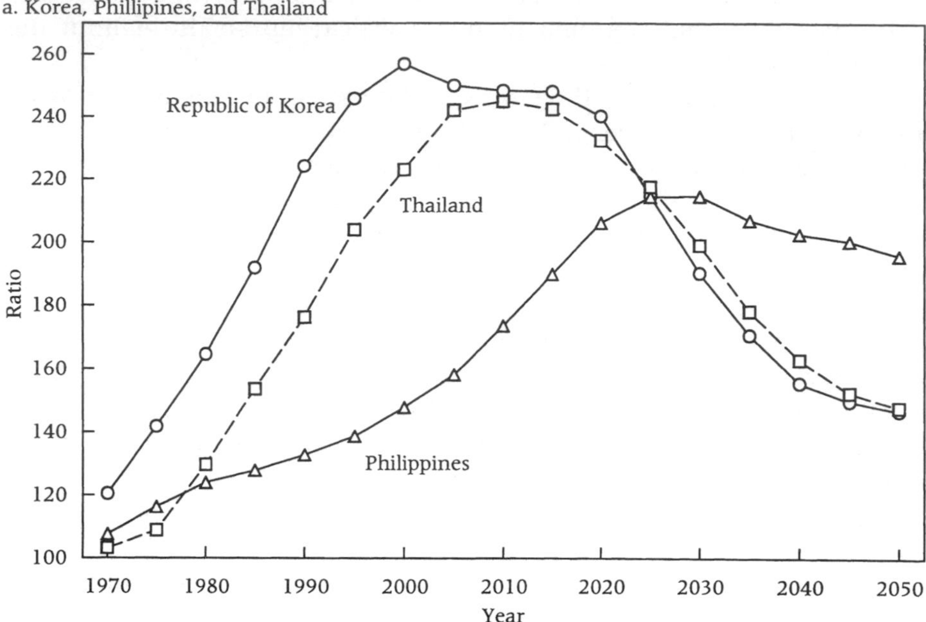

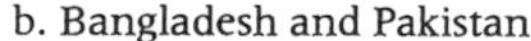

b. Bangladesh and Pakistan

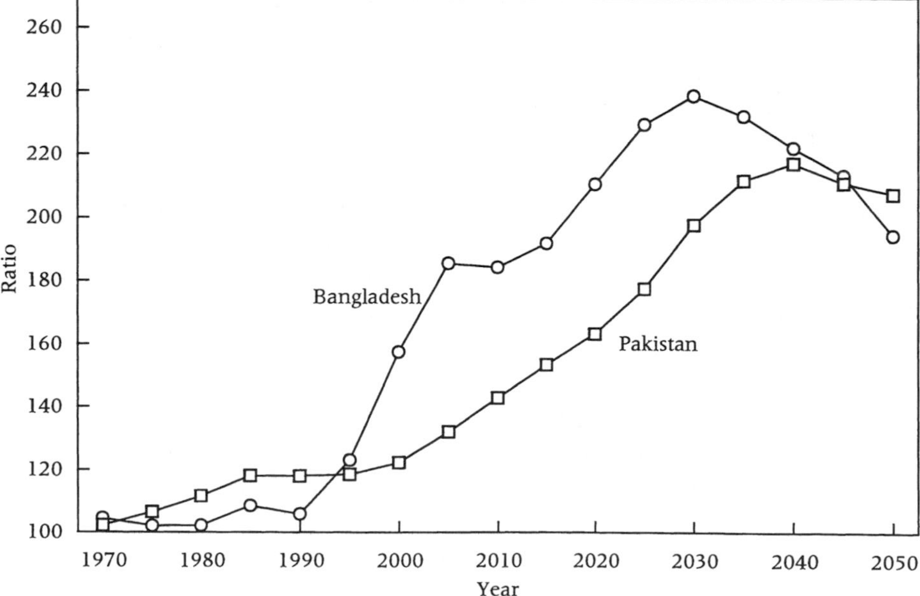

[a]100∗[(15–64)/(<15 + >64)]

[b]United Nations 1996 (medium assumption).

more favorable age structures is appealing on many grounds. But populations whose age structures are concentrated in the working ages eventually grow older. The larger the demographic gift to the economy, the sharper the subsequent aging of the population, as the countries of East Asia have come to realize.

Empirical analysis of contemporary transitions

I proceed to a descriptive analysis of the pace of contemporary fertility declines, using recent United Nations estimates and projections (UN 1996). I examine trends in the total fertility rate (TFR) since 1950 in those countries in Asia, Africa, and Latin America with a population in excess of one million in 1970, omitting countries whose fertility transition was already well advanced as of 1950 and a few other countries on other grounds. For each country, the five-year historical period during which sustained fertility decline begins is determined. I adhere to the Princeton rule that transitions can be safely assumed to be underway if fertility has declined by 10 percent or more from a peak or plateau (Coale and Treadway 1986). However, in contrast to the Princeton studies, I designate the pre-decline peak or plateau as the starting point for the decline, rather than the point at which fertility has declined by 10 percent. As indicated in the Appendix, this has a noticeable effect on the determination of the date of the onset of decline (often a decade or more earlier than under the Princeton approach) and the level of fertility at onset (often 0.5 births or more higher under this approach).[4] The selection of countries and the rules for determining the historical date of the onset of fertility decline are specified in the Appendix.[5]

These data are both left- and right-censored. The left-censoring problem—fertility decline beginning prior to the period of observation—is dealt with by simply discarding those countries judged to have begun fertility transition before 1950. It is certainly possible, however, that left-censoring of fertility decline remains in the data analyzed. The problem is complicated by the fact that the 1940s was a decade of political, economic, social, and demographic turmoil, making it difficult to identify long-term processes in the period 1920–50. Thus there are many advantages to starting the historical clock at 1950. The right-censoring in these data—transitions incomplete at the end of the period of observation—can be compensated for through standard analytical techniques. Large fractions of the fertility declines in these regions are not yet experienced and hence unobservable at this time. I make use of the UN projections to fill in the missing futures, being careful to maintain the distinction between observed and projected experience.

The record to date. Seventy-two countries are judged to have begun fertility transition as of the early 1990s. The pace of decline has been highly variable. Countries with unusually rapid or slow declines are listed in Table 1. The differences in the rate of decline between the fastest and slowest declines are remarkable. During the first ten years of decline, the percentage decline was around 50 percent in several East Asian countries, whereas at the other extreme the decline amounted to less than 5 percent in Papua New Guinea, Guatemala, and the North African Maghreb countries of Morocco and Algeria. The range is even greater for the second through the fourth five-year periods of decline (i.e., years 5–20 of decline), with the largest percentage declines found in East and Southeast Asia (and, interestingly, Cuba) and the smallest percentage declines in Iran (where decline stalled after the Islamic revolution of 1979), Ghana, and Guatemala. Over the first 25 years of decline, fertility fell by more than two-thirds in three countries in East Asia (Hong Kong, North Korea, and China) and in Singapore and by less than one-fifth in Guatemala, Ghana, Iran, and Papua New Guinea.

TABLE 1 Countries experiencing the fastest and slowest declines in fertility by number of years since the beginning of the decline

Fastest	Percent decline	Slowest	Percent decline
First 10 years of decline (n = 72 countries)			
Korea, PDR	53	Papua N.G.	3
Hong Kong	46	Guatemala	3
China	45	Morocco	4
Colombia	31	Algeria	4
Jamaica	31	Botswana	4
Years 5–20 of decline (n = 56 countries)			
Korea, PDR	63	Iran	2
Cuba	57	Ghana	4
Singapore	56	Guatemala	7
Hong Kong	55	Papua N.G.	13
Thailand	52	Iraq	14
First 25 years of decline (n = 51 countries)			
Hong Kong	75	Guatemala	10
Singapore	71	Ghana	16
Korea, PDR	70	Iran	17
China	68	Papua N.G.	18
Cuba	61	Iraq	20
Korea, Rep.	61	Cambodia	20
Thailand	60	Haiti	21
Jamaica	55	Botswana	24

TABLE 2 Variability in the pace of fertility decline, by region

	First quartile	Median	Third quartile	N (countries)
Percent decline during first 10 years				
Sub-Saharan Africa	6	9	14	(16)
Latin America and the Caribbean	11	15	23	(20)
North Africa and West Asia	4	11	19	(11)
East, Southeast, and South Asia	8	14	22	(20)
Central Asia	—	12	—	(5)
Total	9	12	19	(72)
Percent decline during years 5–20				
Sub-Saharan Africa	—	17	—	(4)
Latin America and the Caribbean	21	33	44	(20)
North Africa and West Asia	22	23	29	(9)
East, Southeast, and South Asia	22	39	49	(18)
Central Asia	—	24	—	(5)
Total	20	28	42	(56)
Percent decline during first 25 years				
Sub-Saharan Africa	—	27	—	(4)
Latin America and the Caribbean	34	45	52	(19)
North Africa and West Asia	34	38	42	(9)
East, Southeast, and South Asia	30	40	68	(15)
Central Asia	—	33	—	(4)
Total	31	40	50	(51)

More precise indicators of the variability in the pace of decline are shown in Table 2. The percentage decline is calculated country-by-country for the first ten years, the second through the fourth five-year periods, and the first 25 years of decline, and summary statistics for these percentage declines are calculated for all countries combined and by regional grouping. For all countries, the inter-quartile range (i.e., the difference between the 25th and the 75th percentile) is 10 percentage points for decline over the first ten years, 22 percentage points for decline from the second through the fourth five-year periods, and 19 percentage points for decline over the first 25 years. On average, fertility has declined more rapidly in Latin America and in the countries of East, Southeast, and South Asia grouped together, and more slowly in sub-Saharan Africa. There are large differences among the three Asian subregions that are grouped together; for the 25-year period, the first quartile for this regional grouping is 30 percent decline and the third quartile is 68 percent decline. As is evident from Table 1, some of the declines in East Asia were spectacularly rapid, and these countries are concentrated in the third and fourth quartiles of the Asian regional grouping used in Table 2. The highlight of Table 2 is the considerable inter-country diversity in pace of fertility decline, and on average Asian and Latin American transitions have been more rapid (although in both cases there is considerable intra-regional variability). Again, these conclusions concern the rate of decline once it has begun. There is also, of course, substantial regional variation in the timing of the onset of transition that separately contributes to regional differences in fertility observed during any given period.

A common assertion is that fertility declines have accelerated over time (Kirk 1971 and 1996; Bongaarts and Watkins 1996). Here I examine the proposition that the pace of transition, once transition is underway, is more rapid in later-starting transitions.[6] This proposition appears to be correct if based on a comparison between the historical European transitions and the transitions of the second half of the twentieth century. It is an incorrect description, however, of the experience of developing countries during the past four decades.[7] Figure 3 plots each country's percentage decline against the period when the decline began. The first ten years of decline (Figure 3a) proceeded most rapidly for those declines that began in the 1960s; the rate of decline in this early stage has, if anything, slowed over the past few decades. The percentage decline during the first 20 years (Figure 3b) shows no detectable trend over time; what is most impressive is the inter-country variability in the amount of decline during those two decades.

The patterns in Figure 3 are confounded by regional variations in the pace of decline. It is difficult in these data to separate regional and historical patterns, because of the association between the two and the relatively small number of observations. We can, however, construct graphs of regional distributions that are similar to the graphs in Figure 3. These are presented in Figure 4. The regional differences summarized numerically in Table 2 are readily visible in Figure 4. The pace of Asian and Latin American transitions is more variable, and the transitions in sub-Saharan Africa and the Arab region are slower on average. An unmistakable conclusion from Figure 4b is that, to this point, African transitions are markedly slower than transitions in other regions—this despite the sharp decline of fertility in Kenya that has attracted much attention. From a comparative perspective, even this African transition has not been especially rapid.

That more recent transitions are not proceeding more rapidly—indeed, if anything, are somewhat slower than the transitions that began in the 1960s—runs counter to conventional wisdom, which has assumed that improvements in transportation and communication infrastructure and the increasing reach of modern mass media would be an impetus to rapid fertility decline. On formal grounds, however, this outcome should come as no surprise. As Strang (1991) points out, it is a feature of duration-depen-

FIGURE 3 Pace of fertility decline by period of onset

a. Percent decline during first 10 years

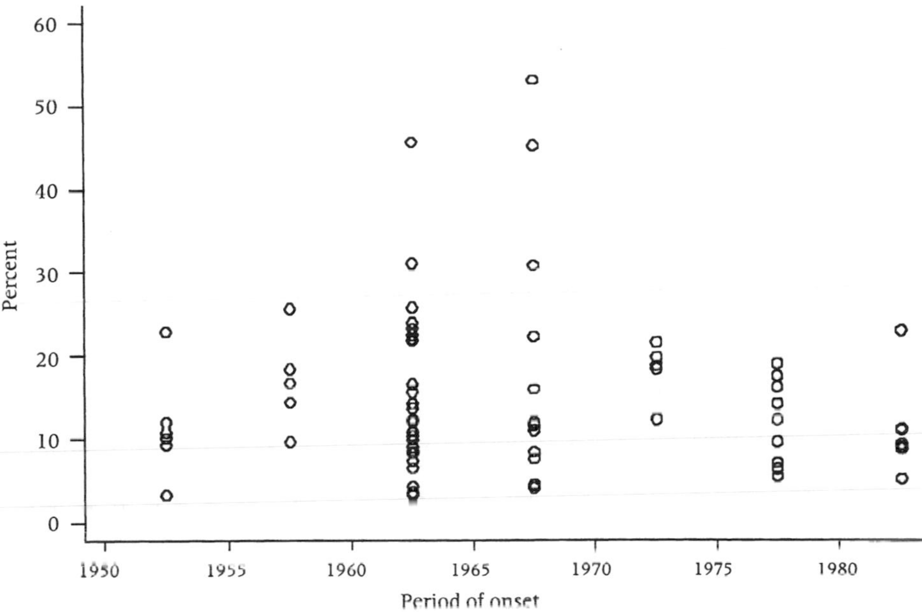

b. Percent decline during first 20 years

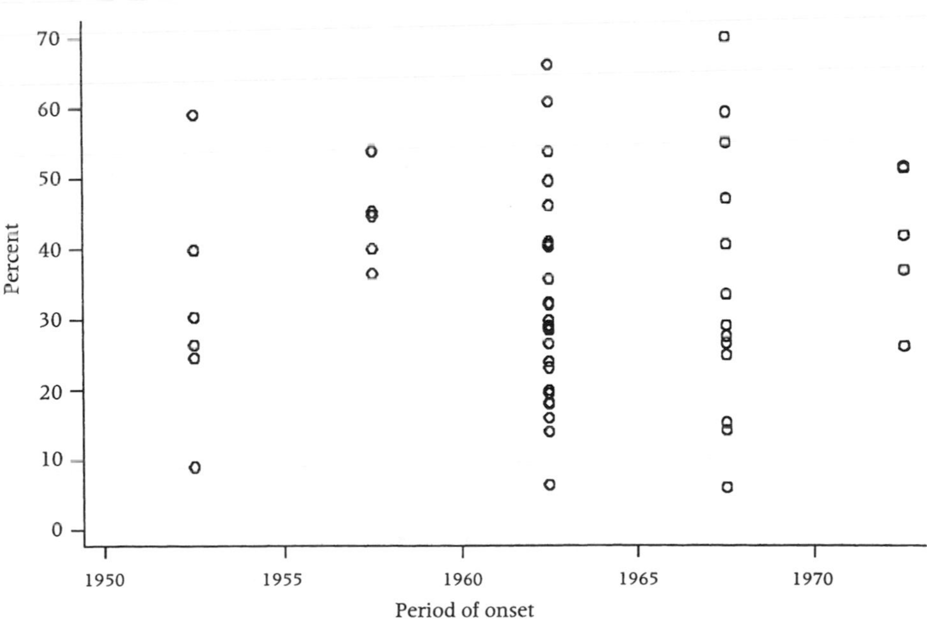

FIGURE 4 Pace of fertility decline by region

a. Percent decline during first 10 years

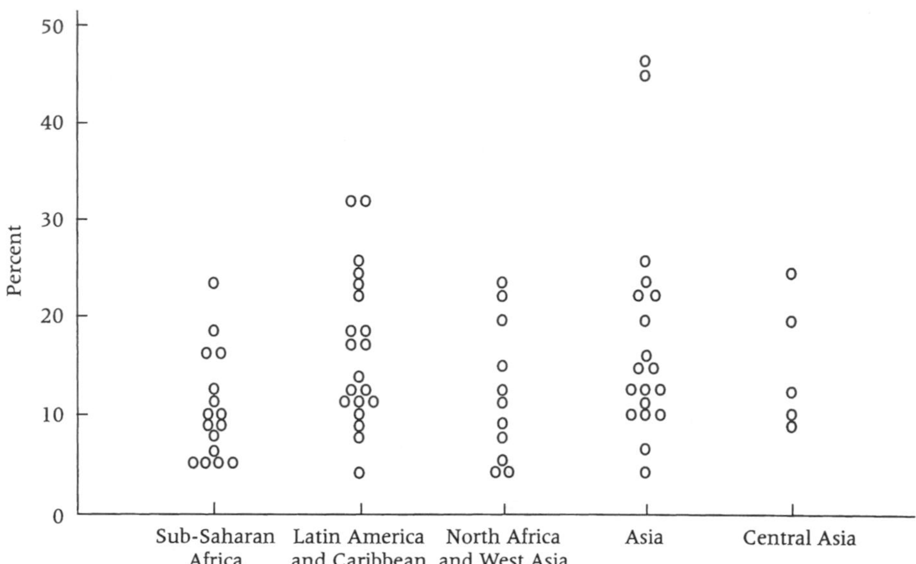

b. Percent decline during first 20 years

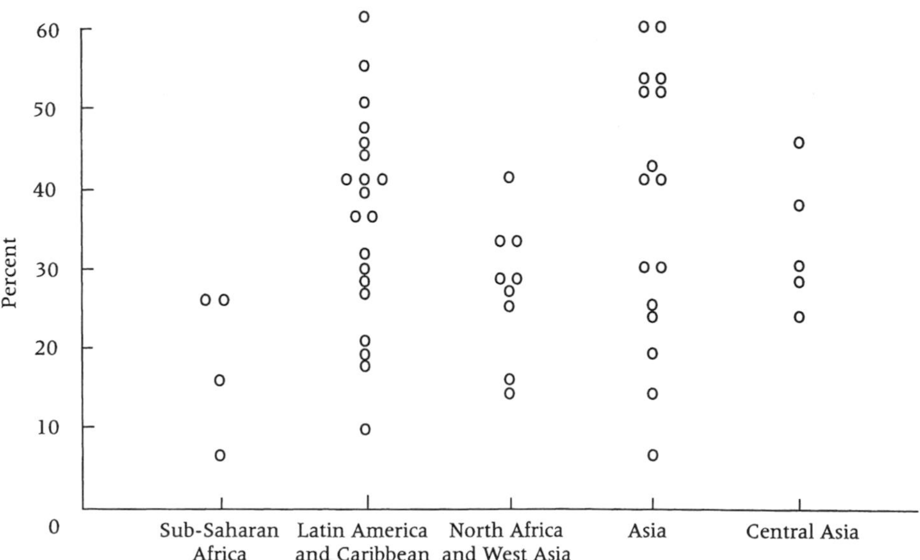

NOTE: Asia refers to East, Southeast, and South Asia.

dent processes (including historical processes) that transition rates decline over time. That is, those societies most receptive to fertility decline begin first, and late declines are therefore selective of societies that are relatively resistent to decline. Reasoning of this sort led Lesthaeghe and Wilson (1986) to posit that onset and pace of decline should be negatively associated (the later the onset, the slower the decline), which, as they indicate in a footnote, proved to be the case in Europe.

These are of course national-level estimates, a circumstance that defines the character of this investigation: this is an analysis of the pace of decline observed in national populations. An analysis at the regional level or at the subnational level would present a different picture and might well yield different conclusions about the nature of contemporary fertility declines. A country may show a slow decline either because reproductive behavior evolves slowly throughout the population or because the decline commences at different dates in various subgroups of the population yet proceeds quickly within these groups (Watkins 1991). These fundamentally different processes can present the same picture at the national level. The more general point is that the "onset of decline" is an elusive concept at the national level because it is affected by the heterogeneity of national populations and the extent to which declines within subgroups of heterogeneous populations are synchronous (Rosero-Bixby, personal communication).

How reasonable are the UN projections? The experience of the recent past provides one basis for assessing the reasonableness of the 1996 set of UN projections. A cursory review of these projections country-by-country suggests that they do not contain the variability of the experience of the past four decades evident in Tables 1 and 2 and Figures 3 and 4. A more specific concern is whether the UN projections allow for the stalls and plateaus that have been a feature of a subset of declines in recent decades in countries such as Costa Rica, Egypt, Iran, and Malaysia (Gendall 1984; Cleland 1995). Most of these and other cases can be explained by the intervention of specific economic or political developments; there is no reason to expect, however, that future declines will be immune to such developments.

Roughly the same conclusion emerges from Figure 5, which plots the pace of decline as observed from the early 1950s through the early 1990s (denoted by "o") and as projected for future time periods by the UN (denoted by "x"). By no means are the rates of decline implicit in the UN projections out of line with the historical experience of the past four decades. Rather, two features of the UN projections stand out: first, the small amount of variability across countries; second, the assumption that African transitions that commence later will proceed more rapidly (this is most evident in the top graph). The first feature is entirely sensible: projections cannot anticipate the many historical contingencies that cause temporary accelerations or slowdowns. The second feature, a trend toward more rapid

FIGURE 5 Pace of fertility decline by region, observed and projected

a. Percent decline during first 10 years

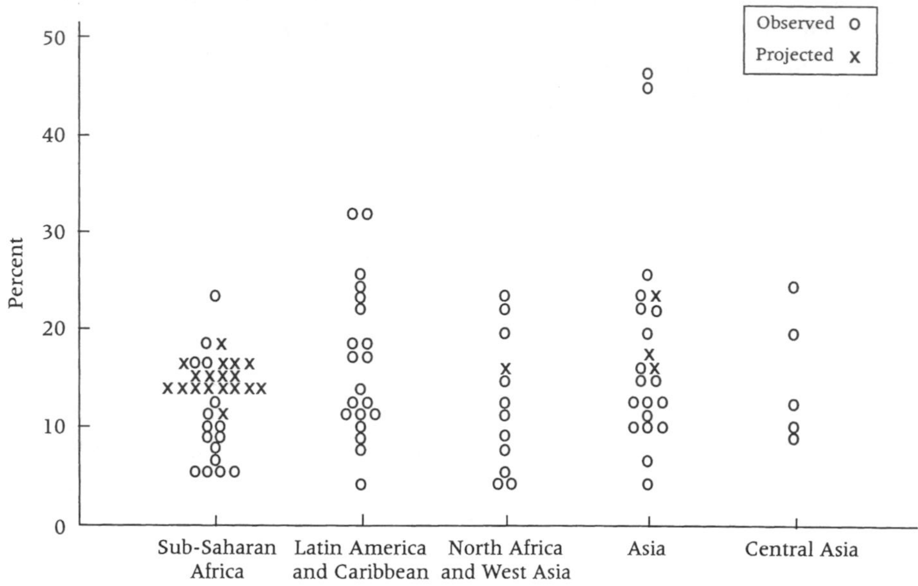

b. Percent decline during first 20 years

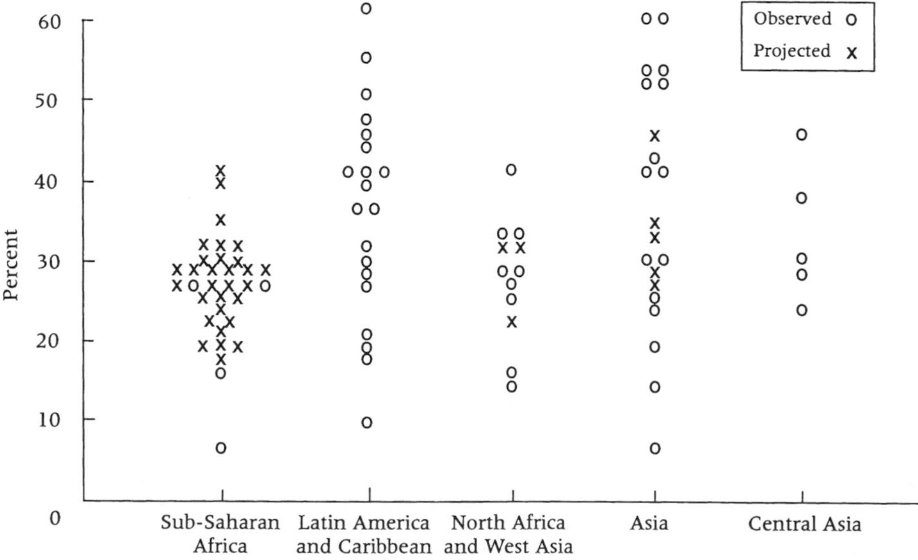

NOTE: Asia refers to East, Southeast, and South Asia.

African transitions, is more debatable. African transitions may well accelerate during the next decade, following a trajectory typical of the majority of countries in other regions. But many aspects of African transitions set them apart from the transitions elsewhere: low levels of income and weak national governments; the AIDS pandemic; and the pattern to date of employing contraception primarily at younger ages and to space rather than limit births. That African transitions will proceed at the pace assumed by the UN projections must be regarded for now as an open question.[8]

Determinants of the pace of fertility decline

The theorizing about fertility decline is as much about the pace of decline as it is about why fertility declines in the first place, although this fact is often not recognized. Hence the research literature hardly leaves us bereft of theory (and empirical evidence) about the determinants of the pace of decline. One can assume that each of the blocks of determinants identified in the literature as determinants of the onset of fertility decline also has some bearing on the pace of decline. For example, a reasonable hypothesis is that where mortality declines more rapidly and where economies change more rapidly, the pace of decline will be more rapid. The aim in this section is to identify a small set of factors that determine whether transitions proceed slowly or rapidly.

The model

For this purpose it is useful to specify a simple model. The model is an algebraic representation of Easterlin's (1975) "synthesis framework," and I have taken it from Bongaarts (1993) and Lee, Galloway, and Hammel (1994) who employ essentially the same equation:

$$f = f_n - [(f_n - (f_d + f_m)) * c]$$

where: f = total fertility
f_n = natural fertility
f_d = desired surviving children
f_m = child deaths (expected)
c = willingness and ability to avert unwanted births (ranges 0–1), a function of birth control costs

In this equation, desired fertility is the sum of desired surviving children (f_d) and expected child deaths (f_m). If natural fertility (f_n) exceeds this sum—that is, $(f_n - (f_d + f_m) > 0)$—then couples run the risk of having unwanted births and will practice birth control, provided they have sufficient willingness and means to do so. Achieved fertility equals either natural fertility or natural fertility minus the fraction of unwanted births that are averted.[9] For our purposes, the most important feature of this equation is the specification of the nature of the effect of *c* (the willingness and ability to avert unwanted births, an inverse function of birth control costs): *c* interacts with the motivation to practice birth control $(f_n - (f_d + f_m))$: that is, the extent to which motivation converts into actual practice of birth control is a function of birth control costs; and, in turn, the impact of birth control costs on fertility is a function of the strength of the motivation to avoid births. This is a theoretical assertion. The argument is that where birth control costs are relatively high, fertility desires will be less consequential, because birth control costs will prevent those who want to limit fertility from doing so. Or, equivalently, where motivation is lacking, birth control costs have little bearing on fertility outcomes, because whatever the costs there is little reason to limit fertility. This interactive relationship between motivation and costs drives many of the results presented below.

What is the effect of social and economic changes on the pace of fertility decline?

The alleged rapidity of fertility declines is a linchpin of the case made by many scholars against conventional demographic transition theory, which attributes fertility decline to falls in mortality and improvements in socioeconomic conditions. Knodel (1977) claims that the pace of development has not matched the pace of fertility decline—either in historical Europe or in twentieth-century Asia—and that this constitutes evidence against Carlsson's (1966) "adjustment" explanation. Cleland and Wilson (1987: 25) argue:

> The fact that falls in marital fertility of one-third or more in a decade are common is a further powerful rebuttal to the more narrowly deterministic microeconomic theories in which fertility change is interpreted largely as the outcome of shifts in the costs and benefits of childbearing. It is implausible to maintain that the social or economic structure of these societies has changed so profoundly within a decade as to account for this demographic response.

In the same vein, Watkins (1987: 659) asserts that

> It is the pace and pervasiveness of the declines in marital fertility that offer the most serious challenges to conventional interpretations of fertility transition.... [C]hange in the economic circumstances of couples has not been as rapid as changes in their reproductive behavior.

This is a familiar argument in support of "diffusionist" interpretations of fertility decline, but it can be shown to be in error on a number of grounds. To begin with, this argument rests on unstated assumptions about what would constitute an appropriate fertility response to social and economic change; without some such standard for comparison, how can fertility be judged implausibly responsive? The implicit assumption is that fertility is highly *insensitive* to changes in social and economic conditions—that substantial changes are required—but it is not at all clear that this needs to be the case in settings where mortality has already declined substantially and there is rapid growth in the size of successive birth cohorts, features that characterized virtually every developing country in the decades following World War II. The argument also assumes that something akin to a linear response of fertility to changes in social and economic conditions is to be expected. The accumulating evidence, however, is that social change is often highly nonlinear and even discontinuous (Hallinan 1997).

There are additional compelling counter-arguments. First, consider how the tradeoff between the quantity and quality of children might manifest itself. In an essay first written two decades ago, Becker (1991) proposed an interaction between production of the quantity and the quality of children. By this he means not that quantity and quality are simple substitutes for each other—although this too probably obtains—but rather that changes in the price of one lead directly to changes in the price of the other. This results in a highly nonlinear dynamic: an increase in the fixed costs of bearing a certain quantity of children induces a shift from quantity to quality, which in turn by raising the costs of children induces a further shift in couples' priorities from quantity to quality. Becker suggests that the response of one to the other may be on the order of two to three times larger than if they were not linked by this peculiar interaction; consequently, the response of fertility levels to social and economic changes will appear to be greatly exaggerated.[10] The dynamic Becker describes is highly plausible, and it is consistent with results from interviews in developing countries in which quality considerations (especially schooling) are repeatedly emphasized as fundamental motivations for lowered fertility. Notice that Becker's explanation for rapid fertility decline rests entirely on socioeconomic effects on the demand for children.

Second, consider how the economic aspirations and expectations that directly impinge on fertility desires (f_d) are linked to changes in social and economic conditions. I argued earlier that aspirations and expectations should not be supposed to move in lockstep with changes in economic conditions. Rather, there will be leads and lags, and these will result in leads and lags in the connection between macro- and micro-level social and economic changes and fertility behavior. These leads and lags, in turn, will be expressed in stalls and accelerations in fertility declines—declines that appear to be too slow or too fast in comparison to structural changes in the society. A common condition will be for aspirations to run ahead of expectations, either because good times nurture aspirations that most households fall short of achieving or because economic reversals leave households struggling to maintain previous gains (let alone advance economically). In either case, it may require only a modest change in aspirations or in expectations (i.e., the evaluation of economic prospects) for individuals to perceive that they are falling short of their goals and—an important further step that is a key to this argument—that curtailment of childbearing will assist them in reducing the gap between economic aspirations and achievements. In my view this perception probably accounts for a large proportion of the apparent misfit between social and economic changes and fertility change. If so, the misfit in no sense refutes the hypothesis that fertility decline is motivated by social and economic changes.

Third, consider how changes in desired fertility might result in changes in observed period fertility. Lee (1980) explores this question for low-fertility societies where trends in desired fertility appear to follow cyclical patterns, but some of his conclusions apply to fertility undergoing transition. His most pertinent conclusion is that levels of period fertility normally decline more sharply than desired fertility when the latter is falling. This is so for reasons that are entirely intuitive: if couples participating in fertility transition adjust their desired fertility downward over the course of their reproductive careers (i.e., they are not wedded to one target family size), then their childbearing will be perpetually "ahead of schedule" as their fertility desires continuously fall. This conclusion is weakened somewhat when Lee allows for unwanted births (e.g., contraceptive failures), but the fundamental conclusion remains: declines in period fertility appear to be steeper than declines in desired fertility.

A fourth, if probably minor point is that social and economic changes can affect both f_d (desired number of surviving children) and f_m (child deaths). This compounds the fertility impact of these changes and, in particular, means that the fertility response can exceed the response that would be appropriate to changes in the costs and benefits of surviving children alone.

Thus far, birth control costs (c) have been left out of the argument. In a moment I will consider what the above equation suggests about the impact on pace of decline of changes in c. For now, I simply note that if birth control costs are large in the pre-decline stage (i.e., c approaches 0), then small changes in c may lead to large changes in fertility by releasing the natural response of desired fertility (f_d) to social and economic change. The result can be a sharp acceleration in fertility decline that is a kind of "catching up" as pent-up desires for limiting fertility are released. This dynamic is described by Retherford (1985), who stresses a further conditioning factor, namely the shape of the fertility preference function. Where this preference function is steep—that is, what couples find acceptable is a narrow range of family sizes—latent receptivity to birth control can be high and a sudden and rapid fertility decline can occur in response to small reductions in birth control costs.[11] Clearly this dynamic results from the interactive effects of the demand for children and birth control costs (see equation). As described here, however, the nonlinear and possibly rapid decline in fertility that results is primarily an expression of those factors that have reduced the demand for children.

What is the effect of changes in birth control costs on the pace of fertility decline?

Having argued that rapid fertility decline can be readily explained simply as a response to social and economic factors operating through fertility desires and child survival, I now consider the expected effect of accompanying declines in birth control costs. An important conclusion emerges immediately. Examining the equation again, it is clear that when c increases (i.e., birth control costs decline) at the same time as f_d and f_m decline (i.e., the desired number of births declines), the decline in fertility will be all the more rapid. That is, the two sets of changes will be mutually reinforcing, as Lee et al. (1994) emphasize. And augmenting the two arguments above about how rapidly fertility desires can change as a result of the quantity–quality tradeoff and of surging economic aspirations and expectations, it can be readily shown that if changes in birth control costs lag behind changes in fertility desires, then once these costs begin to fall the decline in fertility can be precipitous. All this follows directly from the specification of an interaction between motivation and the willingness to employ birth control. Numerical exercises suggest that under plausible circumstances slight reductions in costs can lead to large and rapid declines in fertility. This is Retherford's argument (1985), and, as he demonstrates, it need not require a reductionistic emphasis on birth control costs to the exclusion of fertility desires.

Why are some fertility declines more rapid than others?

With this backdrop, I turn to the question of which factors are the decisive determinants of the pace of fertility decline. As Aminzade (1992) observes, we receive little guidance on this from the mainstream social science literature. On one important point the sociological and anthropological literature is instructive, however. A common assumption in the demographic literature is that ideas/values/culture are intrinsically susceptible to more rapid change than economic and social institutions. Cleland and Wilson (1987: 25) take this view:

> At least part of the explanation [for the rapidity of fertility declines] must lie in social or psychological elements, such as aspirations, knowledge, attitudes or social norms, which are capable of rapid transformation.

It is clear that ideational systems can undergo sudden change, but a general rule that these systems change more easily and rapidly than social and economic institutions runs against a large body of social science thought. Indeed, the more common stance has been that changes in cultural systems lag behind changes in economic and social systems. As a selective sampling, this was the consensus view of social scientists in the first half of the twentieth century (for a representative statement, see Ogburn 1922); it is a common view in sociocultural anthropology (e.g., Geertz 1973); it is confirmed in the classic social psychological experiments of Sherif in the 1940s; it is a prevailing view among development economists (Ray 1998); and it can be found in recent game-theoretic explorations of the formation and maintenance of norms (Bicchieri et al. 1997). In all these literatures, norms are perceived as "sluggish" and slow to change. As we shall see below, "aspirations, knowledge, attitudes or social norms" may indeed be the key to understanding why fertility declines vary in their pace, but the reason is not that these ideational systems are subject to rapid change; in fact, in this instance it is just the opposite feature that gives them such large explanatory power.

Two concepts—*path dependence* and *social effects*—are essential building-blocks of our argument.

Path dependence. At the heart of this concept is the notion that initial conditions and events drive long-term outcomes, often in a manner that is not predictable in advance. Because of self-reinforcement and positive feedback, once a path is chosen—however weak the foundation for that choice—it can be difficult to shift to a different path (i.e., after "lock-in" has occurred). A variety of behavioral mechanisms can explain this phenomenon: for the economist, increasing marginal returns (Arthur 1994); for the sociologist, learning curves, durable commitments, social "sunk costs," and risk aversion (Aminzade 1992). Many of the most salient features of path dependence have little bearing on the pace of change per se, hence I will not dwell on the concept. What path dependence contributes to an understanding of the pace of change is the insight that choices can be self-reinforcing and therefore self-fulfilling. In a sense, means become ends. This permits a more rapid attachment to some behavioral choices and a greater reluctance to relinquish certain choices than circumstances might seem to warrant. That is, path dependence can result in changes that proceed either more quickly or more slowly than would be expected. When choices are bundled, the path-dependence effect can be magnified.[12]

Social effects. Elsewhere we have developed the concept of "social effects" and applied it to fertility (Montgomery and Casterline 1996). The core concept is that actions by some individuals can affect the actions of others. Several powerful behavioral mechanisms can be invoked to explain why this might be so: *social learning*, in which individuals provide information to others regarding new technologies and the consequences of certain decisions (the latter commonly termed "demonstration effects," or what Cialdini (1984) calls the "principle of social proof"—when in doubt about what to do, look to other actors for guidance); *social influence*, in which certain actors impose constraints on the behaviors of other actors by exercising authority derived from power or deference; and *social norms*, which constrain decisions and which themselves are in part a function of the attitudes and behaviors of other members of a social group. A relevant point emphasized in Montgomery and Casterline (1996) is that social effects can operate on all the determinants of fertility: the costs of contraception, fertility desires, perceptions of mortality conditions, evaluations of the costs and benefits of sending children to school, aspirations for consumer durables, and so forth. Social effects can lead to processes that have the appearance of "imitation" ("rational imitation," as Hedstrom (1998) calls it) or "contagion." Like path dependence—and, in fact, social effects can be viewed as a set of mechanisms that account for path dependence—social effects can either retard or accelerate change. Bongaarts and Watkins (1996) argue that social effects ("social interaction," as they call it) explain a good deal that otherwise is puzzling about the timing and pace of contemporary fertility transitions.

What are the key determinants of the pace of fertility decline?

A number of reasonable propositions about which factors determine the pace of decline emerge from the earlier discussion. We specify several of these propositions, with brief commentary. The pace of decline is a positive function of:

a. The pace of social and economic change. At issue are social and economic changes that bear on fertility desires. If birth control costs (c) are stable, then the rate of change in fertility is directly proportional to changes in $(f_d + f_m)$. But as long as c is less than 1, that is, costs discourage birth control practice, then unwanted fertility persists and—very importantly—increases in absolute amount as $(f_d + f_m)$ declines. Hence, fertility decline can closely track social and economic change even as the potential for a more rapid phase of decline is building. A corollary of this point is that the later the onset of transition—late in relation to changes in social and economic conditions—the more rapidly it should proceed, everything else being equal. This follows directly from the model: the larger the fraction of couples having achieved or exceeded their desired fertility, the larger the potential drop in fertility as birth control practices spread. Equivalently, the pace of decline should be a positive function of prior levels of "unmet need for family planning," everything else being equal. This corollary is inconsistent with the empirical evidence presented above. This evidence does not refute the corollary, however, as the ceteris paribus condition may not hold—late-starting countries may differ in their social and economic conditions in ways that impede a rapid pace of decline.

b. The pace of change in economic aspirations and expectations. It is clear that economic aspirations and expectations can evolve somewhat independently of economic conditions. Rapid escalation of economic aspirations, and the perception that reduced fertility should be part of a strategy for achieving them, undoubtedly goes a long way toward explaining the exceptional rapidity of the East Asian declines (Greenhalgh 1988). By accelerating the Asian declines (and probably some of the rapid Latin American declines as well), this factor is, in my view, the most decisive determinant of cross-national variation in the pace of decline in the period since 1950. However, changes in economic aspirations and expectations need not have a similar impact in South Asia and sub-Saharan Africa, especially if individuals see little prospect of achieving their aspirations even if they curtail childbearing. An important characteristic of the late twentieth century is the enormous cross-national disparities in income and wealth, and, more distinctively, widespread awareness of these disparities (Ray 1998). Whether awareness of more affluent lives in distant places constitutes a compelling motive to adopt new reproductive strategies remains unclear.[13] A final point is that rising material aspirations and falling material expectations (e.g., in response to worsening macro-economic conditions) would seem a potent combination.

c. The pace of improvement in the provision of birth control services. A large body of research has accumulated over the past two decades on the impact of improved family planning services on fertility. The weight of the evidence (Bongaarts 1997a) suggests, consistent with the model presented above, that the impact can be substantial and, moreover, that the magnitude of the impact is conditional on the level of social and economic development. While the question often posed is, "Are family planning programs a cause of fertility decline?," in fact most demographers have long recognized that the contribution of these programs would be to *accelerate* decline, that is, to modify the pace of decline.

d. The pace of reduction in the moral and social costs of birth control. For Cleland this is the decisive determinant of the timing and pace of fertility declines (Cleland and Wilson 1987; Cleland forthcoming). The evidence he marshals on this point is persuasive, and in accepting it one does not have to deny the contributions of other factors. In recent research in Pakistan, for example, we have concluded that a sense that family planning is immoral and socially unacceptable has a great deal to do with the lack of significant decline in marital fertility until the 1990s, when these obstacles began to collapse (Sathar and Casterline 1998). While doubts about the morality of limiting family size may constitute a profound obstacle to fertility decline, there are numerous cases where the view that contraceptives per se are immoral disappeared almost overnight.

These four propositions are direct implications of the literature on the determinants of fertility change. Of more interest for this chapter, and the focus of the remainder of the discussion, are structural factors that bear on points b and d above via the mechanism of social effects. Changes in economic aspirations/expectations and reduction in the moral and social costs of contraception are both susceptible to social effects as defined above. That is, social learning, social influence, and social norms can either facilitate or stymie these two sets of changes. Under what conditions will social effects be strong or weak? A common assertion is that the development of intra-national transportation and communication infrastructures increases the power of social effects within countries (see, e.g., Bongaarts and Watkins 1996). A more challenging hypothesis is that social effects are more efficacious under some patterns of social relations than others. This is plausible in an abstract sense. But can we specify certain types of social structure that are more conducive to rapid social change (including fertility change) than others?

Demographers have formulated many notions along these lines. Crook (1977), in a perceptive early contribution to the "diffusionist" literature, speaks of "deviant" and "conformist" communities, the former intrinsically more tolerant of eccentric or innovative behavior. He notes that new fertility behavior is easier to introduce into "deviant" communities but will spread more rapidly in "conformist" communities once it gets a foothold. I return to this argument below. Retherford (1985) and Retherford and Palmore (1983) assert that, everything else being equal, fertility change will occur more rapidly in "socially integrated" societies. By "social integration," they mean shared values, norms, and institutions, and well-developed transportation and communication networks. Bongaarts and Watkins (1996) are more precise in their specification of "social integration," tying it to informal social interaction and arguing that fertility change will be more rapid in societies with a multiplicity of channels of social interaction connecting communities. There is a tendency toward tautological reasoning in this literature: social integration promotes the flow of information and values, but social integration in turn is defined in terms of communication patterns. What is needed is a conceptualization of social structure in terms that are distinct from the social effects (social learning, social influence, social norms) it is meant to explain.

In my research I find the sociological literature unhelpful on this score. Strang (1991) has complained that most diffusion research in sociology assumes random, unstructured patterns of social interaction contrary to all sociological theory and evidence. There are scattered examples of research on the adoption of innovations in which the manner in which social relations are constrained and channeled is taken into account (e.g., Coleman et al. 1966). But the literature that considers the question of whether certain social structures are more conducive to social change remains undeveloped.[14] By far the most influential notion is Granovetter's (1973) "strength of weak ties." Granovetter argues that innovations are most rapidly spread through "weak ties." The phrase "weak ties" refers not so much to the frequency of social interactions and the value placed on those interactions but rather to the number of connections between an individual and a social group. If an individual has interactions with a few members of a group (or just one), then he or she has a weak tie to that group. Granovetter imagines that weak ties serve as a bridge between social groups, thereby expediting the spread of innovations. Indeed, we might imagine that the greater the fraction of social relations in a society that are "weak ties"—in effect, the less that social groups are cleanly circumscribed (i.e., the less that your friends are also my friends)—the greater the opportunity for social effects to operate. This conclusion, however, runs counter to an equally plausible hypothesis, which enjoys some empirical support, that innovations spread more rapidly within tightly knit social networks (i.e., where the degree of inter-connectedness among members of the group is greater) (Valente 1995). Empirical research suggests a further positive effect on the spread of innovations of "network centrality"—the extent to which one or several persons are linked to everyone else and therefore are in a position to serve as communication nodes. We are left with a mixed bag of hypotheses, some of which appear to be contradictory: change occurs more rapidly in tightly knit—or is it loosely knit?—communities.

The apparent contradictions can be resolved through a more careful specification of the differing contribution of "weak ties" and "close-knittedness" (Valente 1995). Social effects are maximally effective if both types of relations are present, that is, if the society is composed of tightly knit groups that also contain a discrete number of functioning bridges crossing between groups. Weak ties are instrumental in introducing innovations (knowledge, attitudes, behaviors) into a social group (where *social learning* may dominate, among the mechanisms for social effects identified above), whereas dense and centralized networks lead to more rapid within-group change (where *social influence* and *social norms* may be the potent mechanisms). This is plausible in an abstract sense, but it will take further effort to apply this type of reasoning to fertility declines. Speculating about the pace of fertility decline, one might describe the Chinese and Indonesian cases as conforming to the optimal design: close-knit local groups linked through a limited set of "weak ties" (in both instances provided most explicitly by government officials). The cross-national variations also suggest that, as Granovetter would predict, the existence of weak ties is more critical. Fertility has been slow to change in the northern portions of the Indian sub-continent and throughout the Arab world where women move about in limited tightly knit social spheres.[15] In contrast, fertility declined unusually rapidly in Thailand with its distinctive "loosely structured" kinship system (Potter 1976)[16] and in Colombia following the decade-long "La Violencia" that was highly disruptive of local and primary social relations. And West African societies, with their dense overlapping networks of local groups and organizations, appear to be less receptive to fertility change than East African societies, with their more individualistic and nucleated social structure. Tight-knittedness is a two-edged sword, an efficient mechanism for the diffusion of information (e.g., through "gossip"; Merry 1984) but also an instrument through which social conformity is enforced. Innovations in reproductive behavior, by threatening highly salient social norms, may bring the conservative impulse of tightly knit social structures to the fore. All this is untested speculation on my part.

This discussion has taken a static view of social structure, as an exogenous and relatively unchanging characteristic of any setting. But of course social relations themselves undergo change, possibly radical and rapid change in contemporary developing countries. The enlargement of circles of social interaction, and in particular the proliferation of "indirect" social relationships, is one of the distinguishing features of modern society (Calhoun 1992). The magnitude and rate of change in patterns of social relations may substantially affect the pace of fertility decline. Rosero-Bixby and Casterline (1993) conclude that a pure diffusionist explanation for rapid fertility decline in Costa Rica is only defensible if social relations were expanding and intensifying during the period of decline, that is, evolving historically in a direction that facilitated social effects on fertility. Otherwise, the existence of low fertility in certain subgroups of the population for many decades prior to the national fertility decline must be taken as evidence against the diffusionist argument.

An altogether different effect of social structure on the pace of fertility change should be noted before closing. Merton (1968) develops the notion of social comparison, in which individuals' evaluations of their own circumstances are constructed through observation of the circumstances of others. I argued above that the evolving relationship between economic aspirations and expectations is a critical factor in determining the pace of fertility change. It is plausible that these economic aspirations and expectations in turn are developed through social comparison: the observed material circumstances of others define in part what is both desirable and attainable. It follows that by setting boundaries on who can be observed and how fully they can be observed, social structure affects the pace of change. This is not a matter of *social effects* as defined above, although it is closely related. Whether this contribution of social structure continues to carry much weight when the mass media penetrate all segments of the society is an open question. Certainly in the latter half of the twentieth century the capacity for individuals to compare their personal material circumstances with the circumstances of relatively remote social groups increased multifold, in the process sharply reducing the salience of all conventional social divisions.

Concluding remarks

The size and structure of the populations of Asia, Africa, and Latin America in the twenty-first century will be determined by the pace of fertility decline during the next two or three decades and by the level of post-decline fertility. The timing of onset is now of little consequence, as only a few countries that in the aggregate make up a small fraction of the population of these regions have not yet begun fertility decline. As time goes by, the level of post-decline fertility will be the critical determinant. Although I have not addressed this here, it merits extensive thought and research (Demeny 1997). The UN "medium variant" projections assume that the post-transition TFR will settle at replacement level (although projections assuming that fertility is one-half child lower or higher than replacement are also presented). Judging from the experience of the West and of East Asia, an assumption of replacement-level fertility errs on the high side. But other regions may find other equilibria; Argentina's TFR, after dropping rapidly in the first half of the twentieth century, has remained near 3.0 for decades, only recently showing signs of further decline. There is no obvious reason why low-mortality regimes and advanced economies cannot readily accommodate TFRs ranging from 1.5 to 2.5 (and perhaps outside those bounds). Suppose that post-decline TFRs in populous South Asia settle around 2.5; this would result in continued population growth in that region and significant and continued increments to the world's population. With only the experience of the West and East Asia to go on, we are relatively uninformed about the character of low-fertility regimes.

For the near term—the next several decades—the decisive variable is the pace of fertility decline in the large number of countries where fertility decline is mid-stream. The experience of the past four decades indicates the tremendous range that is possible, from the spectacularly rapid declines of East Asia to the more drawn-out declines in countries such as Guatemala, Haiti, Iran, Iraq, and Cambodia. In several of these latter cases, one can point to political upheavals that threw the transition off track. But of course there is no reason to assume that political upheavals will subside during the next several decades, and thus unanticipated interruptions in fertility declines can be expected to occur again, even if these cannot be incorporated in UN projections. In this respect the UN projections can be criticized for being too optimistic about the likely pace of fertility decline, even though the country-by-country projected rates of decline are of the same order of magnitude as declines in the period since 1950. Contrary to a common assumption, the evidence reviewed in this chapter suggests that more recent declines are proceeding more slowly than earlier declines. This conclusion applies to the very early stages of decline; the slow start could easily be offset by rapid acceleration in the next stages. The declines just getting underway—chiefly in sub-Saharan Africa—could follow rather different trajectories from earlier transitions in Asia and Latin America.

I have reviewed the reasons why fertility decline might be rapid or slow. Rapid decline is often cited as evidence against theories of fertility transition that revolve around reduction in the demand for children, itself a response to changing social and economic circumstances. This argument does not hold up. In fact, nonlinear and possibly rapid decline should be the usual response of fertility to structural change, for several reasons: because of the interaction between quantity and quality of children, because of lags and leads in economic aspirations and expectations, and because period fertility does not perfectly track trends in desired fertility. My own interpretation of the period since 1950 is that variation in the pace of change in economic aspirations and expectations constitutes the primary explanation for inter-country variation in the pace of fertility decline. The key historical development is the spread through a population of the conviction that achievable economic aspirations are undermined by continued childbearing. This conviction might occur in the presence of rapidly escalating aspirations that outstrip the growth in economic opportunities, or conversely in the presence of economic contraction that threatens the achievement of existing aspirations. Either circumstance can set in motion a calculus that quickly shifts against childbearing. Nevertheless, the multi-dimensional costs of birth control—their levels and trends—also stand as a powerful and parsimonious alternative explanation for variation in the pace of decline. It is highly plausible that in many settings fertility decline proceeds slowly because of the obstacles presented by high birth control costs, costs that fall precipitously once these obstacles collapse. Clearly, improvements in access to birth control services lead to significant reductions of birth control costs in many settings, with the potential therefore of accelerating fertility decline.

Motivated by concerns about population size, the international population community has been dedicated to nurturing rapid fertility decline. Against these widely held preferences for rapid demographic change, it is interesting to observe that other social scientists have stressed the destabilizing and harmful effects on social and political life of rapid change. Several decades ago Mancur Olson (1963) spoke of "rapid growth as a destabilizing force," and in several essays on social change written during the 1960s Neil Smelser stressed that rapid change leads to social disorganization and many concomitant threats to social well-being (e.g., Smelser 1968). In his study of African decolonization, Wallerstein (1961) argued that a slower pace of decolonization was associated with a more successful start in independent African states. Demographers have naturally been more attuned to the demographic consequences of the pace of decline (in mortality and in fertility) than to the social and economic consequences. In research in the 1990s, much more attention was given to the economic benefits of rapid demographic change (e.g., through age structure) than to the social consequences—for example, for kinship systems and for local community institutions. But there may have been some wisdom in demographers' lack of sensitivity to the possibility that rapid fertility decline can cause social damage. Wilson and Airey (1999) argue that for most of human history social institutions must have been designed to accommodate relatively small numbers of surviving children. If this is correct, then rapid transition from large to small family sizes need not be socially disruptive and, indeed, should be less threatening to social institutions than a persistence of high fertility.

Appendix: Selection and transformation of UN data

The analysis in this chapter relies entirely on the 1996 Revision of the United Nations' *World Population Prospects* (UN 1996). The "medium variant" projections are used for dates beyond 1995.

Selection of countries

The aim is to examine fertility transitions that commenced after World War II. The analysis therefore is confined to Asia (including the central Asian republics of the former Soviet Union), Africa, Latin America, and the Caribbean. In addition, the analysis is limited to those countries with a population in excess of one million in 1970; this eliminates 33 small countries that collectively contain a very small fraction of the aggregate population of these regions. An exception to the population size criterion is made for Botswana (estimated population of 637,000 in 1970) because of its confirmed status in the vanguard of transitions in sub-Saharan Africa. Further exceptions among countries otherwise meeting the regional and population size criteria are as follows:

—Japan, because its fertility transition was largely completed by 1950.

—Saudi Arabia, Libya, and Israel, because of the wealth of their economies and, in the case of Israel, the large fraction of the population native to Europe and North America. (Note that the other wealthy oil-producing countries of West Asia fail to meet the population size criterion.)

—Armenia, Georgia, and Kazakhstan, because substantial fertility decline occurred prior to 1950, undoubtedly in part a reflection of their membership in the Soviet Union.

—Argentina and Uruguay, two South American countries with substantial fertility decline prior to 1950.

Ninety-four countries comprise the sample for analysis.

Ascertaining that fertility decline is underway

The usual solution to the problem of determining when fertility transition has commenced is the 10 percent rule popularized by the Princeton European Fertility project: fertility transition is confirmed when fertility has fallen by 10 percent or greater in a secular decline that persists until a relatively low level of fertility is attained (Coale and Treadway 1986). I apply this rule to the UN estimates of total fertility rates for five-year periods from 1950–55 onward: a peak TFR is identified (note that the UN estimates show some countries' fertility increasing before it declines—see discussion below), and transition is confirmed if the TFR at some later point is 90 percent or less of that peak. I experimented with alternative rules, but these proved to have little bearing on which countries were classified as having begun their transition prior to 1995.[17] The exceptions to this generalization are some countries in sub-Saharan Africa—among them Cameroon, Senegal, and Tanzania—where alternative rules lead to different conclusions about whether transition is underway as of the 1990s. Because of the manner in which I define the starting point of the decline (see next section), the rule for ascertaining that a decline is underway has no bearing on the parameters of the decline itself (e.g. the pace of decline by time since onset), in contrast to the Princeton approach (as adopted, for example, by Bongaarts and Watkins 1996).

The data are right-censored: countries that have not yet experienced a 10 percent reduction in fertility as of 1990–95 presumably will do so after 1995. In the case of a few countries, there is evidence as of 1990–95 that, despite their fertility not yet having declined by 10 percent, transition was underway, as indicated by their relatively rapid rate of decline from the early 1980s to the early 1990s (using the rate of early decline of those countries that have already attained a 10 percent decline as a standard for comparison). On this basis I classify four African countries as having begun fertility decline despite their not meeting the 10 percent criterion: Burkina Faso (decline in the TFR from 7.80 in 1980–85 to 7.10 in 1990–95); Lesotho (decline from 5.74 in 1980–85 to 5.20 in 1990–95); Malawi (decline from 7.60 in 1980–85 to 7.20 in 1990–95); and Niger (decline from 8.12 in 1980–85 to 7.40 in 1990–95). In each of the four countries the decline is projected to exceed 10 percent in 1995–2000.

This results in 72 out of the 94 countries being classified as having begun fertility transition prior to 1990–95. Undoubtedly many countries among those remaining have also begun a sustained fertility decline, but their declines had not progressed far enough as of the early 1990s to render a judgment with confidence.

Defining the starting point of the fertility decline

In the Princeton project and analyses modeled after it, the point at which a 10 percent decline is attained is regarded as the onset of transition. Contemporary societies typically begin transition with a TFR around 7.0 births per woman. If the Princeton practice is followed, the decline is not said to begin until fertility has dropped by 0.7 births, which, assuming that post-decline fertility settles around 2.0 births per woman, amounts to about 15 percent of the total decline. A more defensible approach is to regard the peak from which fertility declines as the starting point for the decline. Applying this approach rather than the Princeton approach yields a different level of fertility at onset and, more importantly, a different historical date. A question that is frequently posed is what conditions (of mortality, urbanization, income, literacy) obtain at the onset of fertility decline. In those transitions that proceed slowly, the answer will differ markedly depending on whether the point of onset is regarded as peak fertility or 10 percent below peak fertility. To take the most extreme case in the data under analysis here, Guatemala required 30 years to attain a 10 percent reduction: the TFR is estimated as 7.09 in 1950–55 and it declines steadily (albeit very slowly) thereafter, exceeding the 10 percent threshold of 6.38 in 1980–85 when the TFR is estimated as 6.12. Admittedly, this is the most extreme case. But Ghana required 25 years to achieve a 10 percent TFR decline, five countries (including Guatemala and Ghana) required 20 or more years, and 25 out of 72 countries that are classified as having begun decline prior to 1995 (i.e., about one-third of these countries) required 15 years or more.[18] Social and economic conditions can change substantially over a 15-year period.

The problem of identifying the origins of the decline is exacerbated by the fact that the departure from traditional reproductive regimes often begins with a rise in fertility rates; indeed, judging from the evidence assembled by Dyson and Murphy (1985), this may well be the norm. (See also Kirk 1996 for comments on the historical European experience.) It seems pointless for descriptive purposes to back-date the onset of fertility *decline* to a period during which fertility *rises*. But if the aim is to explore the underlying social, economic, and cultural causes of fertility *transition*, one can argue persuasively that much might be learned by focusing on conditions and developments during a period of rising fertility that is followed by sustained decline. In the data analyzed here, 45 of 72 countries that are classified as having begun their decline prior to 1995 (i.e., almost two-thirds) show some rise in fertility prior to sustained decline. Among the more substantial increases, listed by major region:

	Pre-decline low		Starting point of decline	
Country	**TFR**	**Period**	**TFR**	**Period**
Angola	6.39	1950–55	7.20	1990–95
Burkina Faso	6.33	1950–55	7.80	1980–85
Cameroon	5.68	1950–55	6.45	1975–80
Kenya	7.51	1950–55	8.12	1975–80
Malawi	6.78	1950–55	7.60	1980–85
Niger	7.10	1950–55	8.12	1980–85
Rwanda	7.08	1950–55	8.49	1975–80
Costa Rica	6.72	1950–55	7.11	1955–60
Egypt	6.56	1950–55	7.07	1960–65
Syria	7.09	1950–55	7.79	1965–70
Bangladesh	6.62	1950–55	7.02	1970–75
Pakistan	6.50	1950–55	7.00	1975–80

Mechanical application of the rules specified above—fertility decline confirmed when the TFR declines by 10 percent from a peak that is taken as the starting point for the decline—yields an unambiguous identification of the date of onset for each country. A closer look at the historical trajectories in the UN data, however, suggests that in many instances the result is not sensible by other criteria. In particular, some countries show a very slow decline for a decade or more before accelerating into substantial and sustained transition. These gradual declines may reflect slight changes in reproductive behavior dispersed throughout the population or marked changes concentrated in a small subgroup. While it is important to allow for slow declines, in my judgment some of the five-year declines in the UN data are too small to be viewed as the initial stage of a sustained fertility decline. I make these judgments through country-by-country examination of the TFR trends. In the following countries, the starting point of the decline is reset to one or more periods later than the absolute peak in fertility:

	Starting point according to rules		Adjusted starting point	
Country	**TFR**	**Period**	**TFR**	**Period**
Central African Rep.	5.89	1975–80	5.69	1985–90
Chad	6.05	1965–70	5.89	1990–95
Eritrea	6.62	1955–60	6.00	1985–90
Ethiopia	7.15	1950–55	7.00	1995–00*
Ghana	6.90	1960–65	6.80	1965–70
Lesotho	5.86	1955–60	5.74	1980–85
Bolivia	6.75	1955–60	6.50	1970–75
Honduras	7.50	1955–60	7.42	1965–70
Mexico	6.96	1955–60	6.82	1965–70
Morocco	7.17	1955–60	7.15	1960–65
Yemen	7.61	1975–80	7.60	1995–00*
Afghanistan	7.21	1975–80	6.90	1995–00*
Bhutan	6.05	1950–55	5.89	1995–00*
China	6.22	1950–55	6.06	1965–70
India	5.97	1950–55	5.81	1960–65
Indonesia	5.67	1950–55	5.57	1965–70
Nepal	6.30	1970–75	6.10	1980–85
Thailand	6.59	1950–55	6.39	1960–65
Vietnam	6.05	1960–65	5.85	1970–75

*Denotes projected starting point

Included among those countries with adjusted starting points are the three most populous countries in the regions represented here: China, India, and Indonesia.

Historical time in the UN data

The UN presents fertility estimates in terms of five-year periods: 1950–55 through 1990–95, and projections for 1995–2000 through 2045–50. Hence, in this analysis, all dating is in terms of five-year historical periods: starting points for declines are assigned to five-year periods, not precise years, and historical change is calculated in terms of five-year intervals (e.g., the first five years of decline, the second five years of decline, the first ten years of decline, etc.).

Notes

1 The pace of change has also been neglected in the sociological literature (on this see Aminzade 1992). This stands in contrast to the literature on political and economic development, where pace of change is a primary concern. See, for example, the economic development textbooks by Todaro (1994) and Ray (1998) and the review of development literature by Gereffi and Fonda (1992).

2 A further 23 percent of future growth will occur in those countries with TFRs in excess of 5.5 as of 1995.

3 Because the UN projections typically assume an acceleration in the pace of fertility decline in those countries where the decline has proceeded slowly to date, such as the Philippines and Pakistan, these comparisons by no means reveal the full potential consequence of the pace of fertility decline on age structure. Further, the discussion here assumes that the differences in age structure between the two groups of countries are due entirely to fertility trends. Trends in mortality and international migration can also contribute to age-structure variation, but in the five populations shown here their contributions are almost certainly minor over most of the period examined.

4 Even so, in many instances the starting point may be placed later than it should be. As observed by Dyson and Murphy (1985), Kirk (1996), and van de Kaa (1996), upheaval in reproductive regimes often precedes the steep decline in fertility by several decades.

5 This is an analysis of trends in the TFR, and as such reflects the joint effects of trends in marital fertility and nuptiality. Nuptiality is neglected in the major international demographic data bases, making it very difficult to construct, even through indirect techniques, a comprehensive portrait of *marital* fertility change in the developing world in the postwar period. In most settings the motivations for reducing marital fertility and for delaying marriage are probably quite distinct (McDonald 1981). However, as Coale (1992) has demonstrated, transitions in nuptiality and marital fertility are strongly associated empirically, so that trends in total fertility present an exaggerated impression of the extent of change in marital fertility.

6 A more general assertion is that the rate of fertility decline (for specific countries or agglomerations of countries) has increased over time. This empirical pattern could be the result of a more rapid pace of decline once underway or of the onset of decline occurring earlier, as judged by one or more criteria (in the case of Bongaarts and Watkins (1996), a country's score on the UN Human Development Index).

7 Nor does this generalization correctly characterize the European experience, where, as Watkins (1991) notes, the relatively late Mediterranean declines proceeded more slowly than the earlier declines in northern Europe and Scandinavia.

8 Since this analysis was completed, the UN has released a revised set of estimates and projections that shows slower fertility decline in the 1990s than the earlier set. Demographic surveys in the late 1990s have revealed that fertility is declining less rapidly than the UN assumed in some populations in South Asia and Africa (UN 2000).

9 $(f_n - (f_d + f_m))$ is constrained to be ≥ 0: fertility cannot exceed natural fertility.

10 Mark Montgomery has pointed out to me that Becker assumes no differentials among siblings in parental investment. Unequal investment undoubtedly complicates the model, but it is unclear whether it threatens the basic conclusion that the shift from quantity to quality can be expected to occur very rapidly. Most patterns of unequal investment probably on

balance work against the dynamic Becker describes, especially if the pattern results in an inverse association between birth order and the amount of investment per child.

11 Bongaarts (1997b) describes a similar scenario. If over the course of fertility transition the extent of implementation of fertility preferences rises (i.e., birth control costs fall), then the relationship between changes in actual and wanted fertility will be nonlinear: early in the transition, actual fertility will fall more slowly than wanted fertility, while later in the transition actual fertility will fall more rapidly than wanted fertility as couples strive to close the gap between their fertility preferences and fertility outcomes.

12 Hechter (1993) and White (1993) argue that values come in "packages," making them highly resistant to change but, once resistance is lowered, susceptible to rapid change.

13 Although this is a frequent assertion about the effects of globalization, this line of reasoning rarely appears in the qualitative interviews from South Asia and sub-Saharan Africa that I have read. Couples' fears and ambitions concern developments and opportunities much closer to home.

14 Interesting research appears to be underway, for example the theoretical piece by Gould (1993) on network structures and collective action. His results are discouraging, however, for he concludes that the effects of social structure are highly contingent (e.g., on individual characteristics and positions in networks) and not readily reduced to a small set of primary determinants.

15 Fertility has declined relatively rapidly in Bangladesh, but only with determined programmatic efforts to transcend the social structural obstacles.

16 Carter (forthcoming) also credits social structural factors for the rapid spread of modern contraception in rural Thailand, but his hypothesis is more concrete and richer than the loosely structured explanation proposed here. Carter notes that postnuptial living arrangements in Thai society result in women living near their sisters and female cousins to an extent that is unusual from a cross-societal perspective, and he speculates that this facilitated local conversations about modern contraception and fertility limitation.

17 Kandiah and Horiuchi (1995) employ a more demanding criterion: the TFR must fall by 0.5 births within a five year period for a fertility transition to be considered underway. Many countries will satisfy the Princeton 10 percent rule before they meet this eligibility requirement.

18 These calculations are based on the adjusted starting points described in the Appendix. Without these adjustments, even more declines would appear to proceed very gradually over the first one or two decades.

References

Aminzade, Ron. 1992. "Historical sociology and time," *Sociological Methods and Research* 20(4): 456–480.

Arthur, W. Brian. 1994. *Increasing Returns and Path Dependence in the Economy*. Ann Arbor: University of Michigan Press.

Asian Development Bank. 1997. *Emerging Asia: Changes and Challenges*. Manila: ADB.

Becker, Gary S. 1991. *A Treatise on the Family*. Enlarged Edition. Cambridge: Harvard University Press.

Bicchieri, Cristina, Richard Jeffrey, and Brian Skyrms. 1997. *The Dynamics of Norms*. Cambridge: Cambridge University Press.

Bongaarts, John. 1993. "The supply-demand framework for the determinants of fertility: An alternative implementation," *Population Studies* 47(3): 437–456.

———. 1997a. "The role of family planning programmes in contemporary fertility transitions," in *The Continuing Demographic Transition*, G. W. Jones, R. M. Douglas, J. C. Caldwell, and R. M. D'Souza (eds.), pp. 422–443. Oxford: Clarendon.

———. 1997b. "Trends in unwanted childbearing in the developing world," *Studies in Family Planning* 28(4): 267–277.

Bongaarts, John and Susan Cotts Watkins. 1996. "Social interactions and contemporary fertility transitions," *Population and Development Review* 22(4): 639–682.

Caldwell, John C. 1982. *Theory of Fertility Decline*. London: Academic Press.

Calhoun, Craig. 1992. "The infrastructure of modernity: Indirect social relationships, information technology, and social integration," in H. Haferkamp and N. Smelser (eds.), *Social Change and Modernity*, pp. 205–236. Berkeley: University of California Press.

Carlsson, Gösta. 1966. "The decline of fertility: Innovation or adjustment process," *Population Studies* 20(2): 149–174.

Carter, Anthony. Forthcoming. "Anthropological perspectives on diffusion and social processes," in J. Casterline (ed.), *Diffusion Processes and Fertility Transition: Selected Perspectives*. Washington, DC: National Academy Press.

Cialdini, Robert B. 1984. *The Psychology of Persuasion*. New York: Quill.

Cleland, John. 1995. "Different pathways to demographic transition," in F. Graham-Smith (ed.), *Population—The Complex Reality*, pp. 229–247. Golden, CO: North American Press.

———. Forthcoming. "Potatoes and pills: An overview of innovation-diffusion contributions to explanations of fertility decline," in J. Casterline (ed.), *Diffusion Processes and Fertility Transition: Selected Perspectives*. Washington, DC: National Academy Press.

Cleland, John and Christopher Wilson. 1987. "Demand theories of the fertility transition: An iconoclastic view," *Population Studies* 41(1): 5–30.

Coale, Ansley J. 1973. "The demographic transition reconsidered," in *International Population Conference, Liège, 1973*, Volume I, pp. 53–72. Liège: International Union for the Scientific Study of Population.

———. 1992. "Age of entry into marriage and the date of the initiation of voluntary birth control," *Demography* 29(3): 333–341.

Coale, Ansley J. and Edgar M. Hoover. 1958. *Population Growth and Economic Development in Low-Income Countries*. Princeton: Princeton University Press.

Coale, Ansley J. and Roy Treadway. 1986. "A summary of the changing distribution of overall fertility, marital fertility, and the proportion married in the provinces of Europe," in A. J. Coale and S. C. Watkins (eds.), *The Decline of Fertility in Europe*, pp. 31–181. Princeton: Princeton University Press.

Coleman, James, Elihu Katz, and Herbert Menzel. 1966. *Medical Innovation: A Diffusion Study*. Indianapolis: Bobbs-Merrill.

Crook, Nigel. 1977. "On social norms and fertility decline," *Journal of Development Studies* 14(4): 198–210.

Davis, Kingsley. 1963. "The theory of change and response in modern demographic history," *Population Index* 29(4): 345–366.

Demeny, Paul. 1997. "Replacement-level fertility: The implausible endpoint of the demographic transition," in G. W. Jones, R. M. Douglas, J. C. Caldwell, and R. M. D'Souza (eds.), *The Continuing Demographic Transition*, pp. 94–110. Oxford: Clarendon.

Dyson, Tim and Mike Murphy. 1985. "The onset of fertility transition," *Population and Development Review* 11(3): 399–440.

Easterlin, Richard. 1975. "An economic framework for fertility analysis," *Studies in Family Planning* 6(1): 54–63.

Freedman, Ronald. 1979. "Theories of fertility decline: A reappraisal," *Social Forces* 58(1): 1–17.

Geertz, Clifford. 1973. *An Interpretation of Culture*. New York: Basic Books.

Gendall, Murray. 1984. "Stalls in fertility decline in Costa Rica, Korea, and Sri Lanka," World Bank Staff Working Paper No. 693. Washington, DC: World Bank.

Gereffi, Gary and Stephanie Fonda. 1992. "Regional paths of development," *Annual Review of Sociology* 18: 419–448.

Gould, Roger V. 1993. "Collective action and network structure," *American Sociological Review* 58(2): 182–196.

Granovetter, Mark. 1973. "The strength of weak ties," *American Journal of Sociology* 78(6): 1360–1380.

Greenhalgh, Susan. 1988. "Fertility as mobility: Sinic transitions," *Population and Development Review* 14(4): 629–674.

Hallinan, Maureen T. 1997. "The sociological study of social change," *American Sociological Review* 62(1): 1–11.

Hechter, Michael. 1993. "Values research in the social and behavioral sciences," in M. Hechter, L. Nadel, and R. E. Michod (eds.), *The Origin of Values*, pp. 1–30. New York: Aldine de Gruyter.

Hedstrom, Peter. 1998. "Rational imitation," in P. Hedstrom and R. Swedburg (eds.), *Social Mechanisms: An Analytical Approach to Social Theory*, pp. 306–327. Cambridge: Cambridge University Press.

Higgins, Matthew and Jeffrey G. Williamson. 1997. "Age structure dynamics in Asia and dependence on foreign capital," *Population and Development Review* 23(2): 261–293.

Hirschman, Charles. 1994. "Why fertility changes," *Annual Review of Sociology* 20: 203–233.

Kandiah, Vasantha and Shiro Horiuchi. 1995. "Recent trends and prospects in world population growth," *Population Bulletin of the United Nations* no 39. New York: United Nations.

Kirk, Dudley. 1971. "A new demographic transition?" in *Rapid Population Growth: Consequences and Policy Implications*, pp. 123–147. Baltimore: Johns Hopkins Press.

———. 1996. "Demographic transition theory," *Population Studies* 50(3): 361–387.

Knodel, John. 1977. "Family limitation and the fertility transition: Evidence from the age patterns of fertility in Europe and Asia," *Population Studies* 31(2): 219–249.

Lee, R. D. 1980. "Aiming at a moving target: Period fertility and changing reproductive goals," *Population Studies* 34(2): 205–226.

Lee, Ronald D. and John B. Casterline. 1996. "Introduction," in J. B. Casterline, R. D. Lee, and K. A. Foote (eds.), *Fertility in the United States: New Patterns, New Theories*, pp. 1–15. Supplement to *Population and Development Review* 22. New York: Population Council.

Lee, Ronald D., Patrick R. Galloway, and Eugene A. Hammel 1994. "Fertility decline in Prussia: Estimating influences on supply, demand, and degree of control," *Demography* 31(2): 347–373.

Lesthaeghe, Ron and Chris Wilson. 1986. "Modes of production, secularization, and the pace of fertility decline in Western Europe, 1870–1930," in A. J. Coale and S. C. Watkins (eds.), *The Decline of Fertility in Europe*, pp. 261–292. Princeton: Princeton University Press.

Mason, Karen Oppenheim. 1997. "Explaining fertility transitions," *Demography* 34(4): 443–454.

McDonald, Peter. 1981. "Social change and age at marriage," in *International Population Conference, Manila, 1981*, Volume I, pp. 413–432. Liège: International Union for the Scientific Study of Population.

———. 1994. "Fertility transition hypotheses," in R. Leete and I. Alam (eds.), *The Revolution in Asian Fertility: Dimensions, Causes, and Implications*, pp. 3–14. Oxford: Clarendon Press.

Merry, S. E. 1984. "Rethinking gossip and scandal," in D. Black (ed.), *Toward a General Theory of Social Control*, pp. 271–302. New York: Academic Press.

Merton, Robert K. 1968. *Social Theory and Social Structure*. New York: Free Press.

Montgomery, Mark R. and John B. Casterline. 1996. "Social learning, social influence, and new models of fertility," in J. B. Casterline, R. D. Lee, and K. A. Foote (eds.), *Fertility in the United States: New Patterns, New Theories*, pp. 151–175. Supplement to *Population and Development Review* 22. New York: Population Council.

Notestein, Frank W. 1953. "Economic problems of population change," in *Proceedings of the Eighth International Conference of Agricultural Economics*, pp. 13–31. London: Oxford University Press.

Ogburn, William F. 1922. *Social Change*. New York: B.W. Huebsch, Inc.

Olson, Mancur. 1963. "Rapid growth as a destabilizing force," *Journal of Economic History* 23(December): 529–552.

Potter, Jack M. 1976. *Thai Peasant Social Structure*. Chicago: University of Chicago Press.

Ray, Debraj. 1998. *Development Economics*. Princeton: Princeton University Press.

Retherford, R. D. 1985. "A theory of marital fertility transition," *Population Studies* 39(2): 249–268.

Retherford, Robert and James Palmore. 1983. "Diffusion processes affecting fertility regulation," in R. A. Bulatao and R. D. Lee (eds.), *Determinants of Fertility in Developing Countries*, Volume 2, pp. 295–339. New York: Academic Press.

Rosero-Bixby, Luis and John B. Casterline. 1993. "Modelling diffusion effects in fertility transition," *Population Studies* 47(1): 147–167.

Sathar, Zeba A. and John B. Casterline. 1998. "The onset of fertility transition in Pakistan," *Population and Development Review* 24(4): 773–796.

Santow, Gigi and Michael D. Bracher. 1999. "Traditional families and fertility decline: Lessons from Australia's southern Europeans," in R. Leete (ed.), *Dynamics of Values in Fertility Change*, pp. 51–77. Oxford: Oxford University Press.

Smelser, Neil. 1968. *Essays in Sociological Explanation*. Englewood Cliffs, NJ: Prentice-Hall.

Strang, David. 1991. "Adding social structure to diffusion models: An event history framework," *Sociological Methods and Research* 19(3): 324–353.

Todaro, Michael P. 1994. *Economic Development*. New York: Longman.

United Nations. 1996. *World Population Prospects: 1996 Revision*. New York.

———. 2000. *World Population Prospects: 2000 Revision*. New York.

Valente, Thomas W. 1995. *Network Models of the Diffusion of Innovations*. Cresskill, NJ: Hampton Press.

Van de Kaa, Dirk. 1996. "Anchored narratives: The story and findings of a half century of research into the determinants of fertility," *Population Studies* 50(3): 389–432.

Wallerstein, Immanuel. 1961. *Africa: The Politics of Independence*. New York: Vintage.

Watkins, Susan Cotts. 1986. "Conclusions," in A. J. Coale and S. C. Watkins (eds.), *The Decline of Fertility in Europe*, pp. 420–449. Princeton: Princeton University Press.

———. 1987. "The fertility transition: Europe and the third world compared," *Sociological Forum* 2(4): 645–673.

———. 1991. *From Provinces into Nations: Demographic Integration in Western Europe, 1870–1960*. Princeton: Princeton University Press.

White, Harrison C. 1993. "Values come in styles, which mate to change," in M. Hechter, L. Nadel, and R. E. Michod (eds.), *The Origin of Values*, pp. 63–93. New York: Aldine de Gruyter.

Wilson, Chris and Pauline Airey. 1999. "How can a homeostatic perspective enhance demographic transition theory?" *Population Studies* 53(2): 117–128.

World Bank. 1994. *World Population Projections*. Washington, DC: World Bank.

Comment: The Pace of Fertility Decline and the Utility of Evolutionary Approaches

John G. Haaga

John Casterline's chapter makes two important contributions: (1) his data analysis shows that some widely held perceptions about the pace of fertility decline are wrong (notably, that the transitions have speeded up in recent decades in developing countries); and (2) his interpretation re-opens the question whether the pace of fertility decline disproves neoclassical economic theories of its causes. I would like to extend his argument by claiming that the rapidity of fertility decline is also consistent with evolutionary approaches to human behavior.

Slow processes can cause sudden changes. Karen Mason (1997: 449) recalls the image of plate tectonics—a slow grinding of sections of the earth's crust that can cause a terrifying, albeit brief earthquake. I find helpful the image of a brushfire. Creosote and mesquite bushes cover thousands of acres of mountainside in southern California, growing slowly for decades, drying out nearly completely each summer. Once a fire starts somewhere in this expanse, it spreads "like wildfire," whipped by the seasonal dry winds. Once the fire is going strong, it generates stormwinds that in turn spread it all the faster. If we were to discuss the onset and pace of brushfires, we could legitimately include multiple levels of analysis. Some might focus on proximate causes of the onset (e.g., lightning or arsonists). "Diffusionists" would point out that every scorched bush caught fire only after one or more of its neighbors were ablaze, and that the whole process had an element of self-reinforcement (path dependence) about it. Yet a more basic line of inquiry would seek to understand why all this land ends up covered by scrubby aromatic plants, and why they were all so dry at the same time, as if waiting to catch fire. We would seek theory and evidence about the evolution of an ecosystem subject to—in fact, adapted to—such fires.

The social sciences are currently being shaken by a search for evolutionary explanations of the workings of the human mind/brain (for excellent summaries, see Pinker 1997; Tooby and Cosmides 1990). Can this line of inquiry help us solve the problems of determining why fertility preferences start to change, why they can change so fast (within a generation or two), and why they always fall and almost never, and never for very long, rise? Both the ideational change explanations of fertility decline and the economic aspirations theories that Casterline seeks to revive are unsatisfying in this regard. Preferences are the primum mobile: they are set or changed outside the models, and fertility behavior responds. If evolutionary approaches are to add anything, it would be by explaining where preferences come from.

Before we can even begin borrowing insights from the evolutionary study of human psychology and behavior, though, we have to deal with misconceptions. First is the notion that the pace of fertility decline shows that evolution tells us nothing because the genetic composition of a population does not change within a decade, while fertility rates do. This argument would only make sense if we were seeking in effect a "gene for fertility rates," which is not the expected relationship between the genome and any complex behavior, particularly one touching on such a fundamental part of life history strategy as the number of offspring. Another common misperception concerns the general strategy by which primates maximize inclusive fitness. ("Evolution must want us to have more children, not fewer.") Natural selection cannot operate directly on something so abstract as a fertility rate, or even family size. Instead it produces incremental changes in frequencies of genes governing behavior or structures at the level of the organism, resulting in greater or lesser representation of those genes in future generations.

Natural selection does not guarantee instant success when the environment changes. The workings of an organ system or a behavioral response would not need to explain reproductive success in the contemporary United States, if it plausibly could explain, instead, reproductive success in the environment of a mobile band of about 100 individuals, most of whom are related to each other. Our bodies, brains, and minds evolved in the latter kind of social environment. Finally, many social scientists believe that evolutionary explanations of human behavior are concerned with differences among human populations, that they lead toward Social Darwinism and racism. On the contrary, they are mostly about uncovering human, and even primate or mammalian, universals.

The quest for uniformity provides a clue that evolutionary approaches might help to explain fertility declines. The transitions that Casterline analyzes are all sustained fertility declines, never sustained rises. He proposes greater use of path-dependence models, but these by themselves could not explain why we are on a one-way street. In a slight majority of the countries in his sample, there were rises in fertility rates before declines began, but somehow these never turned into self-reinforcing contagions. We could remember the cliché that mutual-fund salesmen used to employ on potential customers reluctant to trust their savings to the stock market: "I can't tell you what direction the next 10-percent change in the Dow will be, but I can tell you what direction the next 100-percent change will be," meaning, they want us to infer, up. For demographers the analogous line could be: "I can't tell you the direction of the next 0.3 child-per-woman change in the TFR of China, but I can tell you the direction of the next 3.0 children-per-woman change in any country where TFR is currently 5.0," namely, down. This is an important ability, not to be taken for granted.

The importance of cognitive dimensions

Why should aspirations and thus, in Casterline's persuasive view, fertility preferences change among large groups fairly suddenly (within one or two generations), all leading to the same behavioral response? Casterline is right to find the variability in the pace of decline worth renewed attention, since even continued declines at different rates within the range of recent experience can lead to vastly different eventual population sizes, as the result of population momentum. But in a comparative and historical perspective, the variation is not so impressive, especially since the units of analysis are somewhat arbitrary political creations.

One possibility is widespread sensitivity to particular cues from the social environment; when people get these cues, they can modify behavior relatively quickly. One cannot afford to be left behind. As Casterline points out, a great deal of the literature suggests that aspirations—anxieties might be a better term—for the education of one's children are connected to fertility decisions. An excellent source is the rich body of interviews in Thailand conducted by John Knodel and his colleagues (1987):

> "If there are many children you cannot send them to school, but if you have only one or two children, you can manage. Nowadays education must come first."
>
> "I don't want my children to do this type of work. I want my children to have knowledge, to do work sitting in a chair, like other people." (pp. 129–131)

"Like other people...." These are familiar voices of anxious parents who know that the rules are changing—opportunities will be open to their children, at least some of them, but social mobility is not a foregone conclusion. All depends on schooling. Susan Watkins's observations (2000) about the Luo of Kenya between the 1930s and the 1990s show similarities to the circumstances of the Thai villagers. Once education is established as the principal determinant of status, of economic and social mobility, the rules of the game have changed.

It is unfortunate how little direct evidence demographers usually have, or even seek, on what Casterline terms the "mediating cognitive factors," factors that might connect aspirations and fertility behaviors. Knodel and his colleagues reported survey results of two items that lie at the heart of hypotheses about the influence of mass education on fertility, mediated through aspirations: In rural areas in 1975, over a third of adult respondents felt that the minimum education required for a boy to get by these days was upper secondary or beyond; and over 40 percent anticipated a "heavy burden" providing their own sons with that much schooling (Knodel et al. 1987: table 7.3). These villagers spoke about their inability to afford as many children as their parents had, even though the researchers could see in their homes radios, motorbikes, and other goods that previous generations never had. "Afford" seemed to mean enabling their sons and daughters to succeed in the world that is coming, rather than simply to avoid starving. I suspect that the questionnaire items from the 1975 Thailand survey would have been powerful predictors of subsequent fertility decline for other countries, as powerful as the more commonly asked items about intentions to use contraceptives.

Anxieties about social status, and why they might be important for fertility

The central paradox for economic demography in both the Becker and the Easterlin traditions, what drove modeling in its heyday, was this finding that people who appear to be able to afford more children than their parents nevertheless want, have—and even say they can afford —fewer children.

John Kenneth Galbraith, over 40 years ago, argued that Americans had achieved an Affluent Society, in which the chief economic problem had become figuring out what to do with all that they earned, and how to dispose profitably of leisure time (Galbraith 1958). The chief problem for manufacturers would be getting people to want things they clearly did not need. Since then, real disposable income per person in the United States has more than doubled, in part as a result of increased, not decreased, labor supply per household, and few Americans are troubled by an inability to think of what to do with their greater incomes. They could have taken their improved standard of living in the form of radically shorter working hours, or greater numbers of dependents per working adult, or in any number of ways. Instead they work almost as hard as ever for incomes that would allow them to raise dozens of children—children that Americans, like the Thai villagers, believe they cannot afford. Robert Frank and Philip Cook (1995) may resolve the paradox by pointing out that we are motivated by the need for "positional goods." We can never have enough if what we really need is more status than the next person has. And the besetting problem of modern life is that we know about more and more other people and what they have.

If we have evolved to respond to cues about social position in relation to the people we know about, then the widening of our social worlds makes life more stressful. We will behave as though we inhabit a low, or at least precarious, position, not like the extraordinarily successful animals we actually are.

On an even more basic level: "[L]ow dominance status does indeed seem to be associated routinely with lower reproductive success in mammals" (Bronson 1989: 142). Primates, in particular, enjoy a relatively low rate of adult mortality, "hence they can afford a relatively low reproductive potential" (ibid.: 217). Human reproductive potential is the lowest among primates. Females invest a great deal in each liveborn child and hence have to get the timing and mate selection just right. Robert Foley (1995: 209) dates our ancestors' transition to the "expensive offspring life-history strategy" to *Homo erectus* (beginning 1.6 to 2 million years ago). In this longer perspective, human evolution has been a progression from maximizing fitness through having large numbers of children, toward having well-timed, well-reared children, secure enough in a local dominance hierarchy to reproduce themselves eventually. From an evolutionary perspective, the value of children is that they are the means to having grandchildren. Most mammals do not react directly to information from the environment about available space and resources (Freedman 1980: 189–190), but to information about their own and their potential mates' position in social hierarchies. John Christian (1970) has elaborated an influential theory for the evolution of social hierarchies among mammals, including reasons for subordinates to adapt fertility-related behavior to current information about their place in the hierarchy: if it is high, take advantage of that fact and mate; if it is low, be ready to move somewhere else.

Returning to humans, we are made very anxious by threats to our social position, and respond quickly to opportunities to advance our, or our children's, social position. We are not much reassured by the direct evidence of our ability to take care of physical needs; that is not what we, or our closest animal relatives, respond to. These biological regularities would lead us to look at social hierarchies, and at cues about social status and how it might change, for explanations of widely shared fertility behavior—not to changes in resource availability in any absolute sense.

The paradoxes besetting both economic and cultural models of fertility might be resolved (or moved to a higher level of abstraction) by a search for stable, widely shared "if…then" rules linking social status to preferences and behavior. The very rapidity (within one or two generations) of fertility declines in the modern era, and their unidirectionality, suggest that the engine is something that most people in most countries have in common. People do not need to collect much information about possible outcomes or observe long-term consequences of alternate fertility decisions. They respond a certain way when a cue about the social environment changes. To return to the metaphor with which I began, the brush is already dry.

Social structure would matter, in this view, not so much by determining whether people received specific birth planning information through a particular network, and when, but by determining the boundaries of status competition: Whom might my children surpass? What do I see my potential rivals providing for their children?

It is probably fruitless to look for any psychosocial mechanism that responds directly to crowding, somehow keeping the net reproduction rate equal to one. For one thing, we can infer from patterns of human movement in the past that some human populations have gone for long periods of time with a net reproduction rate above one (see, for example, the evidence from analyses of blood proteins explained by Cavalli-Sforza and Cavalli-Sforza 1995). Human populations also can go for decades with a net reproduction rate below one, as Paul Demeny (1997) has pointed out. The capacity to migrate complicates the picture. Humans do not in fact know much about the dynamics of the populations to which they are assigned by our statistical systems (as anyone who teaches undergraduate courses on population studies knows). We have not evolved any so-called epideictic behaviors like those of birds. Evolutionary biologists explain this behavior, in which birds flock together every morning and squawk loudly, as a way for birds to keep track of local population numbers for their species. Birds of these species take censuses by instinct; for humans the matter is not so straightforward.

These thoughts lead to two implications for the data-collection and research agenda. One is that we need much more direct evidence on the "psychological proximate determinants" of fertility preferences, including aspirations for one's children, perceptions of status, and the avenues of status change. What are the cues that convince large numbers of people that the rules of their society are changing? A second implication is that we need better direct information on the size and composition of reference groups: Who are the Joneses with whom we, or our children, must keep up?

References

Bronson, F. H. 1989. *Mammalian Reproductive Biology*. Chicago: University of Chicago Press.

Cavalli-Sforza, Luigi and Francesco Cavalli-Sforza. 1995. *The Great Human Diasporas: The History of Diversity and Evolution*. Reading, MA: Addison-Wesley.

Christian, John J. 1970. "Social subordination, population density, and mammalian evolution," *Science* 168: 84–90.

Cleland, John and Christopher Wilson. 1987. "Demand theories of the fertility transition: An iconoclastic view," *Population Studies* 41: 5–30.

Demeny, Paul. 1997. "Replacement-level fertility: The implausible endpoint of the demographic transition," in G. W. Jones, R. M. Douglas, J. C. Caldwell, and R. M. D'Souza (eds.), *The Continuing Demographic Transition*, pp. 94–110. Oxford: Clarendon.

Foley, Robert. 1995. *Humans Before Humanity: An Evolutionary Perspective*. Oxford: Blackwell.

Frank, Robert H. and Philip J. Cook. 1995. *The Winner-Take-All Society: How More and More Americans Compete for Ever Fewer and Bigger Prizes, Encouraging Economic Waste, Income Inequality, and an Impoverished Cultural Life*. New York: Free Press.

Freedman, Jonathan. 1980. "Human reactions to population density," in Mark Nathan Cohen, Roy S. Malpass, and Harold G. Klein (eds.), *Biosocial Mechanisms of Population Regulation*. New Haven: Yale University Press, pp. 189–224.

Galbraith, John Kenneth. 1958. *The Affluent Society*. Boston: Houghton Mifflin.

Knodel, John, Aphichat Chamratrithirong, and Nibhon Debavalya. 1987. *Thailand's Reproductive Revolution: Rapid Fertility Decline in a Third-World Setting*. Madison: University of Wisconsin Press.

Mason, Karen Oppenheim. 1997. "Explaining fertility transitions," *Demography* 34(4): 443–451.

Pinker, Steven. 1997. *How the Mind Works*. New York: W.W. Norton.

Tooby, John and Leda Cosmides. 1990. "The past explains the present: Emotional adaptations and the structure of ancestral environments," *Ethology and Sociobiology* 11: 375–424.

Watkins, Susan Cotts. 2000. "Local and foreign models of reproduction in Nyanza Province, Kenya," *Population and Development Review* 26(4): 725–759.

The Effects of Improved Survival on Fertility: A Reassessment

JOHN CLELAND

NEARLY ALL CLASSICAL representations of demographic transition depict the following chronological sequence: a fall in death rates, an ensuing period of rapid natural increase, a lagged decline of birth rates, and an eventual return to population equilibrium. The characterization of the link between mortality and fertility varies, however. For Notestein (1953), improved survival was perhaps a necessary but not a sufficient cause of a fertility response. While "falling death rates at once increased the size of the family to be supported and lowered the inducement to have many births" (p. 16), other factors (including changing costs and benefits of children, new economic roles for women, and the erosion of the family as a productive unit) were seen as critically important precursors of the trend toward low fertility. Within this framework, the structural modernization of societies acts as the common cause of both mortality and fertility decline.

Kingsley Davis (1963), in his theory of the multi-phasic response, assigns a more emphatic causal role to improved survival than Notestein. In his view large mortality declines constitute both a necessary and a sufficient stimulus for fertility decline. For the family, improved survival brings an inevitable "train of disadvantages" (p. 352). More children have to be reared and educated and their inheritance of resources is both fragmented, because of an increased number of siblings, and delayed because of longer parental survival. Under most circumstances improved survival imposes a severe strain on the maintenance of the economic and social status of families across the generations. A response is inevitable. The possible solutions are out-migration, marriage postponement and celibacy, and fertility regulation within marriage. Economic modernization is largely irrelevant because the "train of disadvantages" impinges just as strongly on subsistence agrarian families as on urban wage earners.

Since these two early contributions to fertility transition theory, there have been no notable theoretical advances in the interpretation of macrolevel mortality–fertility links. Chesnais (1992) reasserts the temporal precedence of mortality transition but offers no new insights into the nature of its effects on reproduction. A number of writers have proposed explanatory frameworks that include improved survival as one of several determinants (e.g., Easterlin and Crimmins 1985; Retherford 1985). Others have acknowledged its importance as an underlying determinant (e.g., Cleland 1993; Mason 1997). But, in general, interest in the mortality–fertility link has faded. The reason for this relative neglect can be traced to the disappointing results of research in the 1960s and 1970s.

The nature of mortality–fertility links was once a research priority. The dominant line of inquiry focused on reproductive physiology and behavioral responses to child loss (replacement) or the anticipation of future losses (insurance or hoarding). As evidence about the effect of lactation on ovulation accumulated, it was realized that one pathway of influence was purely physiological. An early child death truncates breastfeeding and thus permits an early return to ovulation and a shortened interval to the next birth. A recent multi-country analysis by Grummer-Strawn, Stupp, and Mei (1998) estimates that the median birth interval is 60 percent longer if a child lives than if it dies in early infancy. Most of the relationship is explained by curtailment of lactation. While this is an appreciably larger effect than many previous estimates, it is nevertheless a relatively minor pathway of influence, even under extreme assumptions. Assume for instance that a birth interval will be 30 months in length if a child survives but only 18 months if the child dies early in infancy. With a reproductive span of, say, 20 years, the effect of a reduction of early infant deaths from 500 per thousand live births (an extreme pretransitional situation) to zero would be to decrease fertility from ten to eight births.

Behavioral responses to child death (i.e., the replacement effect) have also proved to be modest in magnitude. Preston (1978) concluded that parents who had lost a child were only 20–30 percent more likely to proceed to the next birth than parents who had not lost a child.

Investigation of the insurance, or hoarding, effect has proved more difficult. One approach, championed by Heer, used simulation models. Heer and Smith (1968, 1969) examined how many births a couple would need under varying mortality conditions to be 95 percent certain of having a living son when the husband reached his sixty-fifth birthday. At an expectation of life at birth of 20 years, more than nine births would be needed and this number approaches two births as expectation of life at birth rises to 74 years. These simulations, though interesting, are not very convincing partly because the choice of the confidence level is arbitrary and yet crucial to the numerical results. Moreover, there is no evidence that Heer and Smith's model corresponds to real-life decisions. The second main attempt to capture an insurance effect has been to measure perceived mortality and to use answers on this and related topics as predictors of behavior. Here again results have been disappointing: effects of such perceptions on reproductive behavior have been weak or nonexistent (e.g., Rutstein 1974; Pebley, Delgado, and Brinemann 1979). Montgomery (1998) raised further doubts about the insurance hypothesis. After reviewing relevant evidence from cognitive and social psychology, he finds ample reason to believe that the relationship between actual mortality change and perceived change may be weak. Individuals appear to be inherently poor at probabilistic reasoning. Furthermore, improved survival of children is rarely proffered by individuals as a reason for wanting fewer births or for using contraception. On balance, therefore, one finds little evidence that the insurance motive is a powerful direct link between mortality and fertility at the individual level.

Empirical investigation at the individual level has been paralleled by aggregate-level investigation, in which the unit of analysis is a population, typically a nation-state. Life expectancy, under-five mortality, or infant mortality is assessed as a predictor of some fertility measure, usually with a lag. In most such analyses, mortality, along with adult education or literacy, emerged as the strongest predictors of fertility (e.g., Cutright 1983; Bongaarts and Watkins 1996). The causal implication of such statistical associations is far from obvious, however, particularly because there is no straightforward mechanical relationship between mortality decline and a fertility response. For instance, in the last 40 years the onset of fertility transition has occurred in settings where infant mortality is 150 per thousand live births and survival at older ages is correspondingly low. In other settings, birth rates have remained unchanged until infant mortality dropped to 50 per thousand.

In the search for simple dose–response relationships, the net reproduction rate (NRR) is in some ways preferable to a mortality measure, because it better represents the extent of departure from the long-run historical equilibrium between mortality and fertility on one hand and low population growth on the other. But even the use of this measure as a predictor of the onset or speed of fertility decline serves merely to illustrate the absence of any mechanical relationship. Figure 1 shows the value of the NRR at the onset of fertility decline, as indicated by a 10 percent fall in total fertility, for 41 developing countries using data from the United Nations Population Division. It is immediately obvious that NRRs vary considerably at time of fertility transition onset. In some countries, the NRR was over 2.7 (Syria, Kenya, Mexico, and Paraguay). In others, fertility started its decline when the NRR was below 2.0 (Myanmar, Chile, India, and Indonesia). Similarly, the NRR value at onset of transition was unrelated to the pace of decline in the subsequent ten years (results not shown). In short, no simple relationship between net reproduction and the timing or speed of fertility decline is evident.

FIGURE 1 Net reproduction rate at time of fertility transition in 41 developing countries

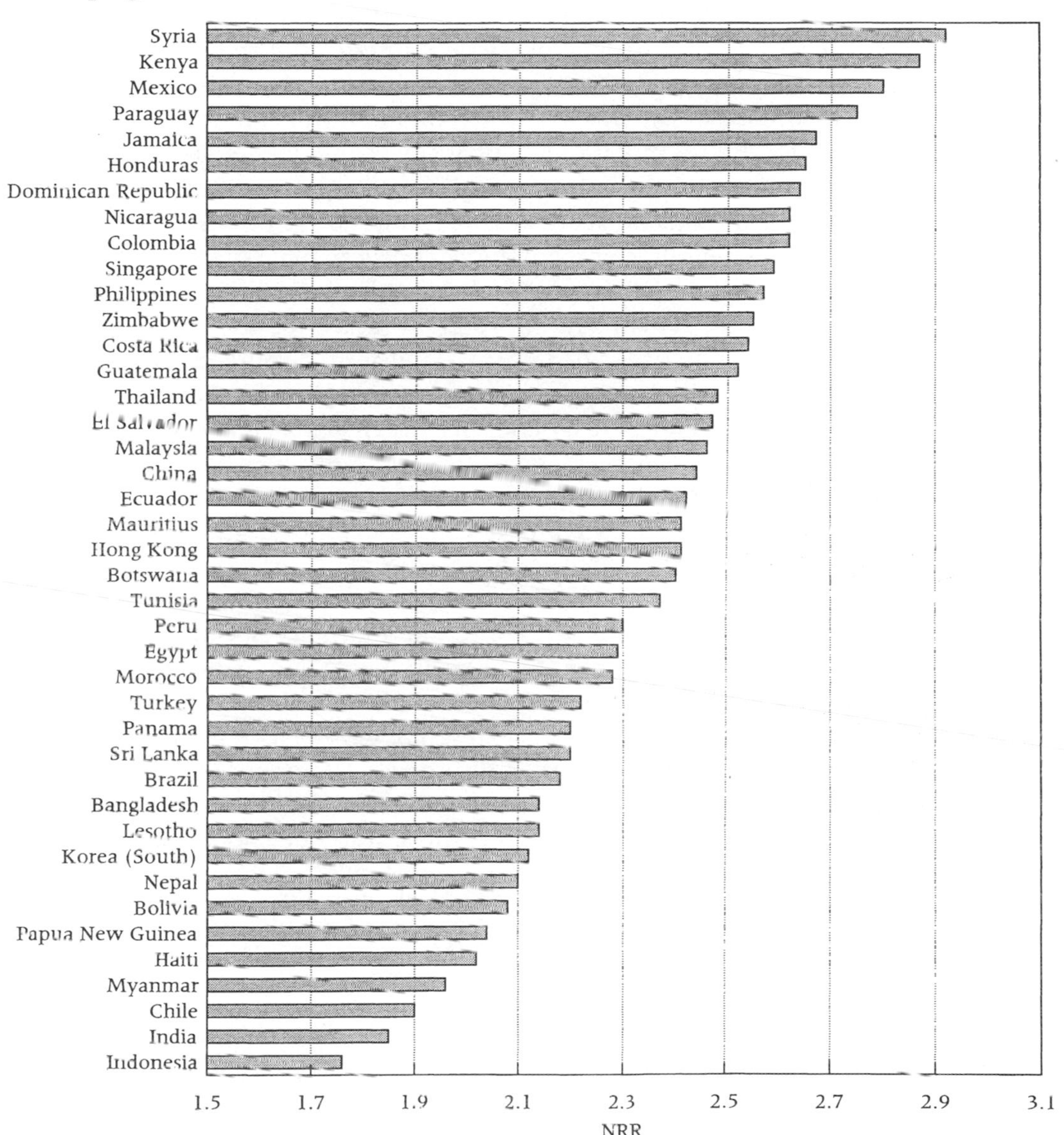

SOURCE: UN *World Population Prospects*.

To summarize, empirical research on mortality–fertility relationships in developing countries has succeeded in demonstrating and quantifying rather weak links at the individual level, derived from biological and behavioral responses to child death. Little support has been found for the highly plausible thesis that mortality exerts a direct, albeit lagged, influence on fertility through the conscious realization by parents that they no longer need to have so many children as an insurance against possible future child losses. At the aggregate level, mortality decline in the developing world has always preceded falls in natality but no further empirical regularities, or generalizations, about their interrelationship have been identified. When combined with major challenges to the causal role of prior mortality decline arising from research on the European transition (van de Walle 1986), this disappointingly inconclusive body of evidence has led to an impasse. The basic instinct of many demographers remains that mortality and fertility decline must be causally connected. For instance Kirk (1996) writes, "Whilst definitive proof of this connection may not be possible, there exist cogent reasons for supposing that it exists" (p. 368). And Galloway, Lee, and Hammel (1998) say "it is difficult to escape the conclusion that, in some vague and unspecified way, ... long-term decline in fertility is ultimately due to a very long-term decline in mortality, or the two are interlinked" (p. 184). Yet, in the absence of convincing evidence to support this central proposition of classical transition theory, the attention of most population scientists has drifted elsewhere.

The purpose of this chapter is to reassess mortality–fertility links in the context of less developed countries. In the first section, I examine the nature of pretransitional reproductive regimes. I then describe the massive disruption to these regimes caused by the mortality declines in the early half of the twentieth century and follow this account by distilling explanatory lessons from the evidence about fertility transitions in the second half of that century. I then assemble these building blocks in support of the conclusion that Davis was essentially correct. Mortality decline is indeed the common underlying cause—both necessary and sufficient—of the fertility declines that have swept across most of the developing world in the past 40 years.

Pretransitional reproductive regimes

Any theory of profound social change must start with a detailed analysis of the relevant system prior to the change. With demographic, or fertility transition, theory a careful appraisal of the nature of pretransitional reproductive systems is indispensable, because the identification of the forces or conditions responsible for the pretransitional state of affairs is likely to lead to the specification of the factor or factors responsible for its destabilization. Misspecification of the system prior to the point of departure inevitably results in misspecification of the forces of change.

The familiar characterization of pretransitional fertility is that the levels of childbearing and of demand, or need, for surviving children were both high. Elevated mortality necessitated an offsetting level of at least moderate fertility, but, more importantly, surviving offspring constituted an advantage to parents, extended families, and clans or lineages because the economic and social returns from children outweighed the costs. From this characterization it is but a modest leap to the position held by many social biologists (e.g., Cronk 1991) and some demographers (e.g., Caldwell 1982) that human reproductive strategies were designed to maximize the number of surviving offspring in the next generation.

If this pervasive view of maximal or high demand for children in pretransitional societies stemming from strongly positive net returns from childbearing is broadly correct, it logically follows that the central explanation for fertility decline must focus on factors that erode the utility of children and/or raise the costs of their nurture. Accordingly, from the earliest theories to current writing, much of the literature has been dominated by the search for the determinants of an assumed fall in the demand for children. Despite subsequent attacks from proponents of alternative ideational and diffusionist explanations, demand theories of fertility transition will remain dominant for as long as the view prevails that traditional societies were characterized by high demand for children.

The purpose of this section is to reconsider the nature of pretransitional reproductive regimes and to question common assumptions about them. What follows has been heavily influenced by an article by Wilson and Airey (1999), who like Davis (1963) argue that a return to a more holistic approach to the study of demographic change is needed, an approach in which fertility, mortality, and migration are analyzed together rather than in isolation.

It is beyond dispute that, until the recent past, growth of the planet's human population has been little above zero. At this very high level of temporal and spatial abstraction, births and deaths have been in balance; net reproduction rates have been close to unity, implying that the average couple saw only two offspring survive to maturity. Such near-stability in terms of size at the global level over thousands of years is in part a consequence of offsetting temporal and spatial disequilibria. Some populations have grown, only to suffer severe reversals because of disease, famine, or warfare (e.g., the bubonic plague in fourteenth-century Europe). Other populations have sustained rapid growth over centuries. Livi-Bacci (1992) cites, as a striking demographic success story, the example of the French Canadians whose population rose in size from about 5,000 to over 2 million in 300 years, largely by natural increase. Conversely, the collapse between 1500 and 1800 of the indigenous populations of the Americas following European contact is a vivid example of demographic decline. Even within a country, stability of numbers may be a result of the cancellation of natural growth in some areas by decline in others.

The synthesis of historical evidence for Europe, China, Japan, and India by Wilson and Airey (1999) suggests, however, that long-term stability was achieved in these larger, enduring populations not by violent swings from rapid expansion to sharp decline but by moderate vital rates that yielded very modest rates of population growth. Total fertility was typically between 4 and 6 births, balanced by life expectancy at birth of 25 to 40 years.[1]

Can these moderate levels of childbearing be reconciled with the thesis of maximal or high demand for surviving children because benefits outweighed costs? Reconciliation could be achieved if, for instance, reproduction was constrained by disease or undernutrition, or if the poor and the powerless were denied reproductive opportunities by the rich and the powerful. No doubt such biological and coercive factors have played and continue to play a role in the regulation of childbearing but they do not appear to have been dominant forces. Unlike that of other higher primates (Dunbar 1990), the human reproductive system is relatively impervious to undernutrition and adversity, and, at least in Asian societies, mating and marriage opportunities appear to have been nearly universal. More consistent with the historical evidence is that most pretransitional societies evolved noncoercive social institutions to ensure that aggregate childbearing was restricted to modest levels. The evolution and persistence of these institutions would have been difficult, if not impossible, in the context of a conscious demand for many surviving offspring. It is much more likely that attitudes to childbearing among our ancestors were less positive, and more ambivalent, than is usually taken to be the case. It is surely of great significance that most microeconomic studies in less advanced economies have found that children represent a net economic loss to parents until the teenage years are reached (Mueller 1976; Lindert 1983). Even in West Africa, the one remaining high-fertility subregion of the world, the flow of resources appears to be from the parental generation to the younger generation and is reversed only at very late ages (Stecklov 1997). No doubt in most premodern societies, offspring also cost more than they produced for the first 10 to 15 years. This factor alone provides ample grounds for skepticism about the maximal or high demand stereotype.

Quite apart from narrow economic considerations, the rearing of offspring is demanding of time and energy. The human species has always valued other goals (recreation, leisure, luxury) that compete with childbearing (Douglas 1972), and the direct threat of pregnancy and childbirth to the life of the mother is no small consideration. Assuming a maternal mortality ratio of 1,500 per 100,000 live births and total fertility rate of 6 births, the lifetime risk of dying from maternal causes is nearly one in ten. It would thus hardly be surprising if, in most societies throughout most of history, reproduction has been regarded not as something to maximize but rather as a mixed blessing.

No portrayal of the reproductive values of traditional societies can be stated dogmatically because the evidence is fragmentary and oblique. However, the considerations enumerated above imply that the reproductive systems of societies where the historical evidence is most abundant (Asia and Europe) were not designed to maximize numbers of surviving children. They also suggest that such maximization was not an active goal of couples. With life expectancies of only some 30 years, and subject to short-run fluctuations, mating, marriage, and procreation must have been central concerns; but this does not necessarily imply that couples consciously wanted numerous surviving children. With the clear exception of Africa,[2] the earliest surveys in the late 1950s and the 1960s of reproductive attitudes in low-income countries portray moderately rather than highly pronatalist sentiments, with desired family sizes typically in the range of 3 to 5 children (Mauldin 1965). On balance, it is reasonable to conclude that demand for surviving children in pretransitional societies was similarly moderate.

What do moderate gross reproduction rates and net rates close to 1.0 at the aggregate level imply for individual reproductive patterns? These aggregate averages are deceptive when applied to individual families because pretransitional regimes were characterized by wide variability in outcomes at the family level. Wrigley (1978) has demonstrated that in a stationary population with universal marriage, 20 percent of men would have no surviving offspring at the time of their death, and a further 20 percent would have one or more surviving daughters but no living male heir. Conversely, a substantial minority of men could expect to see several surviving sons at their deathbed. These proportions hold regardless of the combinations of fertility and mortality that underlie equilibrium. This analysis leads to a rarely employed definition of demographic transition in terms of surviving children. According to that definition, the net reproduction rate starts at a value close to unity, rises, and then returns to its original value. The only fundamental changes are a contraction of the variance and the widespread use of new methods of family limitation. By the end of transition, completed family sizes are concentrated in the range of 1 to 3 surviving children, with a severe curtailment of the upper tail of the distribution.

If gross reproduction rates were moderate and net reproduction rates close to 1.0 in the large historical populations for which evidence is available, the next question concerns the mechanisms of fertility control. A great deal has been established about the biosocial constraints on conception and their institutional underpinning in different societies (e.g., checks on sexual access via marriage systems; lactational amenorrhea; postnatal abstinence). However, there is little agreement concerning the extent to which individuals in pretransitional societies were able to consciously plan or adjust the numbers, spacing, and sex of their children. Despite the fact that withdrawal and prolonged abstinence from vaginal intercourse were available, at least theoretically, as means of regulating conception, the evidence suggests that they were used only by minorities or in exceptional circumstances.

Methods of induced abortion were widely known in historical populations but again were probably used only in extreme circumstances, because of their danger or extreme discomfort.[3] Despite numerous attacks on the concept of natural fertility and on the methods of its measurement, the broad generalization remains valid that the reproductive behavior of pretransitional couples was insensitive to the number and sex of children already born and surviving. This verdict is entirely consistent with survey and ethnographic evidence from high-fertility societies in the 1960s and 1970s that the idea of deliberate birth regulation within marriage was unthinkable and/or the means to achieve it unknown (Cleland 1998). As Mason (1997) points out, postnatal adjustments of family size and composition were more common than prenatal control. Examples of the former include infanticide, child abandonment, adoption, and fostering. Mason sees in these examples of control a continuity between past and present in the exercise of conscious rationality vis-à-vis reproduction. In terms of behavior there is a big difference, however, between the use of modern contraception and, for instance, fostering of a child.

For the individual family, it is clear that pretransitional reproduction resembled a lottery, because of the vagaries of both natural fertility and mortality. Parents were equally likely to have no children surviving to maturity as they were to see many surviving. For the latter group, Wrigley suggests, the economic penalty of having to rear many children was offset, at least partially, by the existence of "ecological niches," or opportunities, stemming from families with no or few children—niches that the children from highly fertile families could exploit. As Davis put it, "land and goods flow from the dead to the living in several ways" (1963: 353). Similarly for childless couples, there was a ready supply of "surplus" offspring from other families who could be taken as apprentices, adopted, fostered, or "loaned" in other ways. What these complex redistribution mechanisms imply for reproductive attitudes is unclear, though it is likely that had our ancestors been given the theoretical choice of numerous surviving children versus one or none, they would have opted for the former. In any case their attitudes must have included a large quotient of resignation, if not fatalism, because of the overriding uncertainty of successful reproduction.

The main conclusions from this brief discussion of the nature of pretransitional demographic regimes are as follows:

1. Most historical societies were adapted to moderate levels of childbearing, low net fertility, and very low rates of population growth. This adaptation to low net fertility encompasses marriage systems, inheritance, land tenure, and other social institutions. It is thus incorrect to argue that certain types of traditional social or family structure depend for their maintenance on large numbers of surviving children. Exactly the opposite is true. Asian and African social systems are just as adapted to small families as European systems.

2. Major imbalances between births and deaths, giving rise to high rates of natural increase, have been the exception rather than the norm and have usually occurred in response to the acquisition of new land, resources, or technology.

3. A fundamental understanding of fertility transition cannot be achieved in isolation from consideration of mortality and population growth. Wilson and Airey (1999) assert that "the transition must be understood as an episode of growth, rather than as a decline in fertility" (p. 125). The central theoretical question at an aggregate level then becomes: For what reasons and for how long can societies accommodate high rates of increase before equilibrium is restored? In a similar vein, Cleland (1993) maintains that the central question of fertility transition is not to ask what factors undermine the need of communities, lineages, or families for large numbers of children but to ask instead "for how long, and by what means, can [they] accommodate and tolerate such an unprecedented abundance of children?" (p. 351).

4. While direct evidence regarding parental aspirations for surviving children is fragmentary, the aggregate evidence does not support the view that demand for surviving children was unlimited and casts doubt on whether it could aptly be described as high. Thus the central proposition of many theories of fertility transition, namely that the root cause is falling demand or need for surviving children, is questionable.

5. The use of birth control within marriage was not the major means of fertility restraint. Checks on marriage (particularly in Western Europe) and postnatal adjustments, or control, were more common means of regulation in pretransitional societies. Fertility transition is achieved by an important behavioral innovation: the deployment of contraception (and abortion) within marriage.

Mortality decline and population growth in developing-country transitions

Although the evidence is fragmentary, the demographic situation of developing countries at the start of the twentieth century was probably similar to the situation that characterized Europe, China, and Japan over many centuries. Population growth was modest, with births and deaths approximately in balance. Perhaps vital rates were somewhat higher than in historical Europe and China, with life expectancy typically in the range of 20 to 30 years, balanced by total fertility of 5.0 to 6.5 births.

By 1950, a fundamental change had occurred. In many countries net reproduction rates had doubled from historical levels of close to unity. For the three major developing regions, Latin America (and the Caribbean), Asia, and Africa, these net rates ranged between 1.8 and 2.2 (see Figure 2). A further illustration of the scale of change is given by a compilation of

FIGURE 2 Trends in net reproduction rates for major developing regions, 1950–2000

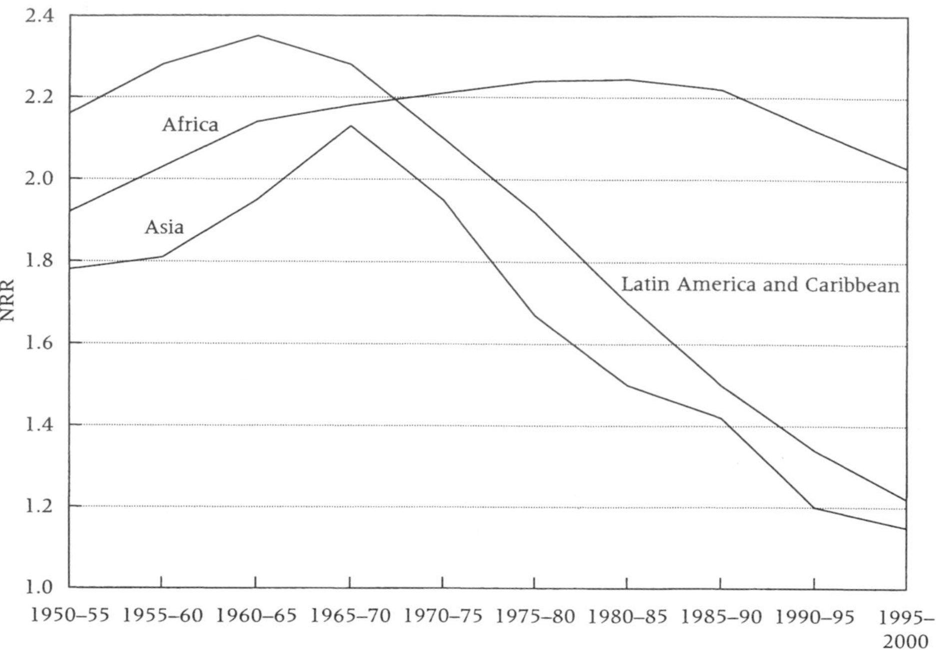

SOURCE: Calculated from UN *World Population Prospects.*

data from the World Fertility Survey (Hodgson and Gibbs 1980). The surveys shown in Table 1 were conducted between 1974 and 1979. Women in the age group 40–44 years at that time experienced their peak childbearing in the 1950s. As Table 1 shows, the mean number of surviving children for this cohort ranges between 3.9 and 7.2. Most of these children had already passed the hazardous years of infancy and early childhood and thus all but a few were destined to survive to maturity. In 16 out of 19 surveys, over 40 percent of ever-married women aged 40–44 years record 6 or more living children. The proportion childless ranges from 2 to 5 percent in most surveys, though higher levels are apparent for the three Caribbean surveys.

In some countries, one reason for this transformation of demographic regimes was an increase in fertility. Dyson and Murphy (1985) find convincing evidence that marriage ages in Latin America fell and thereby exerted an upward pressure on birth rates. They also suggest that similar trends in nuptiality may have occurred in parts of Africa and Asia, though the evidence is less clearcut than for Latin America. In Africa, erosion of traditional birth spacing mechanisms and falls in pathological sterility both exerted an upward influence on natality. The most compelling evidence that

TABLE 1 Percent distribution of ever-married women aged 40–44 according to number of surviving children in surveys conducted between 1974 and 1979

	Children surviving				
Country	0	1–2	3–5	6+	Mean
Asia and Pacific					
Bangladesh	4.4	12.0	40.4	43.2	5.1
Fiji	4.6	11.9	31.3	52.2	5.6
Indonesia	6.7	21.1	43.6	28.7	4.1
Jordan	2.7	4.9	16.4	76.0	7.2
Korea	1.8	11.9	59.2	27.1	4.5
Malaysia	3.2	12.8	35.1	48.8	5.4
Nepal	6.3	21.8	49.5	22.5	3.9
Pakistan	5.5	10.7	40.4	43.4	5.0
Philippines	2.7	9.4	31.0	57.0	6.0
Sri Lanka	5.0	16.7	37.8	40.6	4.9
Thailand	3.2	14.0	38.0	44.7	5.1
Latin America and Caribbean					
Colombia	3.9	13.8	31.8	50.6	5.7
Costa Rica	2.3	13.3	33.9	50.9	6.0
Dominican Republic	7.3	11.1	32.1	49.6	5.5
Guyana	8.3	11.2	27.1	53.2	5.7
Jamaica	8.1	20.7	27.6	43.8	4.9
Mexico	3.9	12.7	26.1	57.3	6.0
Panama	3.8	13.5	39.0	43.6	5.3
Peru	2.8	11.2	41.9	44.1	5.2

SOURCE: Hodgson and Gibbs (1980).

fertility rose in many developing countries is the simple fact that total fertility rates in excess of 7 births were commonly recorded in the decades following World War II. Many demographers have pointed out that such high levels of childbearing were almost certainly a departure from historically lower levels because they imply the existence of an offsetting mortality regime of such severity that these populations would have been at a serious disadvantage compared to others with more moderate vital rates.

Falls in mortality, of course, were much more important causes of the transformation of developing-country demographic regimes than rises in fertility. A few figures will illustrate the magnitude of the change between the 1930s and 1960s. In India, life expectancy at birth improved from about 27 years to 46 years; in Indonesia the corresponding figures are 32 to 46 years (Preston 1975). Throughout most of Latin America, gains in life expectancy over this period were typically larger: 20 years in Mexico, 24 years in Colombia, and 23 years in Chile, for instance. Preston's analysis suggests that improvements in standards of living or formal schooling can account for only a small proportion of these mortality declines.[4] The spread of new medical knowledge and public health measures appear to have been more decisive influences. The curtailment by colonial regimes of localized warfare and famine may also have played a role. Whatever the causes, economic development and rising prosperity clearly were not the major underlying determinants.

Mortality decline continued to be the dominant influence on natural increase throughout the 1950s in all developing regions with the partial exception of West and Central Africa.[5] In Latin America, the NRR peaked in the early 1960s at about 2.3 before starting to decline as childbearing patterns changed. In Asia, the change came in the 1970s and in Africa in the 1980s.

An inevitable consequence of steep declines in mortality, which started in some low-income countries early in the twentieth century but gathered pace after 1930, coupled with constant or rising fertility, was population growth. Rates of increase in the range of 2 to 4 percent per annum, implying doubling times of 35 to 17 years, became commonplace. To underscore the point that the transition must be understood as an era of growth, Chesnais's concept (1992) of a transitional population multiplier (i.e., the ratio of population size at the end of transition to size at the start) can be adapted to developing countries to illustrate the approximate increase in sizes that they are likely to experience over the course of transition. Population size in the first decade of the twentieth century is used as a crude indicator of pretransitional size, and World Bank long-term projections are chosen to indicate projected population size. After excluding small countries of less than one million, reasonably reliable estimates of population size at the start of the century were found for only 20 developing countries.[6]

The results of this exercise are shown in Table 2. Two World Bank projections are used: projected population size at time of reaching replacement-level fertility and projected size at time of achieving a stationary population. The difference between the two reflects population momentum. The figures suggest that the population sizes of these 20 countries will grow by 5- to 14-fold between 1900 and the point at which replacement fertility is reached. After taking population momentum into account, the corresponding figures for reaching a stationary population indicate a range of 8- to 24-fold growth.

In terms of rates of growth and long-term potential increases in size, the demographic transition in developing countries stands apart from the earlier European transition. During the European transition, annual rates of natural increase were typically below one percent and net reproduction rates below 1.5. Between 1800 and 1950, the population of Europe and its overseas offshoots of European extraction increased from about 200 mil-

TABLE 2 Projected population transition multipliers for 20 developing countries

	Population size (millions)			Ratios	
	c. 1900	Replacement	Stationary	Replacement (col. 2 ÷ col. 1)	Stationary (col. 3 ÷ col. 1)
Algeria	4.7	41.4	67	8.8	14.3
Egypt	11.2	77.3	121	6.9	10.8
Madagascar	2.2	30.0	49	13.6	22.3
Sierra Leone	1.0	11.5	23	11.5	23.0
South Africa	5.2	65.2	103	12.5	19.8
Tunisia	1.9	12.6	20	6.6	10.5
Brazil	17.4	174.2	285	9.9	16.4
Chile	2.9	15.1	23	5.2	7.9
Colombia	4.3	37.5	62	8.7	14.4
Cuba	1.6	10.6	13	6.6	8.1
Guatemala	1.4	20.4	33	14.6	23.6
Mexico	13.6	114.0	182	8.4	13.4
Venezuela	2.3	26.3	45	11.4	19.6
India	235.5	1170.0	1888	5.0	8.0
Indonesia	37.7	218.9	355	5.8	9.4
Myanmar	10.8	69.1	172	6.4	15.9
Pakistan	45.5	259.0	400	5.7	8.8
Philippines	7.6	108.2	172	14.2	22.6
Sri Lanka	3.6	19.0	29	5.3	8.1
Thailand	8.3	56.3	104	6.8	12.5

NOTE: See note 6 for sources of 1900 population estimates.

lion to about 750 million, giving a ratio, or transition multiplier, that is far below the ratios in Table 2.

The reasons for these differences between Europe and the developing countries of Asia, Latin America, and Africa lie beyond the scope of this chapter. The key point is that, by the middle of the twentieth century, the population equilibrium of the developing world had been disrupted on an unprecedented scale by huge declines in mortality, amplified in some instances by rises in fertility. The net result—population sizes that were doubling every 25 years or so—is clearly unsustainable in the long term. Sooner or later, balance has to be restored by a resurgence in mortality or by a reduction in fertility. But does this long-term inevitability of a return to equilibrium imply that mortality decline giving rise to rapid growth can be taken as the underlying cause of what has emerged as the major means of restoring equilibrium, namely fertility declines? To answer the question, we now examine the conditions under which fertility in low-income countries has fallen in recent decades.

The globalization of fertility decline and its theoretical implications

Recent trends in childbearing—in both industrialized and developing countries—are forcing fundamental reappraisals of fertility theories. The emergence of below-replacement fertility in parts of Europe and East Asia has raised questions that were never foreseen in theories of demographic transition. In the developing world, the apparently inexorable spread of fertility decline carries implications for an understanding of the underlying forces of change.

Regional examples

By the late 1980s, fertility transition was well established throughout East and Southeast Asia, Latin America, and the Caribbean. Elsewhere the situation was very different and future trends uncertain. In South Asia, representing about 20 percent of the world's population, sustained decline was confined to Sri Lanka and some of the southcentral states of India. In the populous north Indian states of Uttar Pradesh, Bihar, Rajasthan, and Madhya Pradesh, fertility remained high and there were concerns that the modest earlier falls had leveled off (Khan et al. 1988; Satia and Jejeebhoy 1991). In the neighboring countries of Bangladesh, Nepal, and Pakistan, birth rates remained resolutely high.

Plausible reasons were advanced for this persistence of high fertility throughout much of South Asia. These populations are among the poorest in the world with low levels of adult literacy and low rates of women's participation in the paid labor force. Gender inequality is severe and there is a clearcut preference for sons over daughters. One common interpretation was that this cluster of interrelated factors represented an insurmountable barrier to the achievement of lower fertility and eventual population stabilization. It was argued that national family planning programs would achieve little in the absence of structural reform.

A mere decade later, demographic realities have changed radically. The most surprising development is the steep fertility decline in Bangladesh, one of the poorest countries in the world. Between 1980 and 1995, total fertility in that country fell by approximately 50 percent. This trend is all the more remarkable because it coincides with a switch from reliance on surgical contraception to reversible methods. Neither coercion nor financial incentives to promote sterilization played a significant role during the years of steepest decline. Moreover, changes in reproductive behavior have been registered in all socioeconomic strata, thereby undermining the view that Bangladesh's fertility transition was a response to deepening poverty and desperation (see also Cleland et al. 1994).

In Nepal and Pakistan the pace of change has been slower, but in both countries there is now unmistakable evidence that levels of childbearing have started to drop. In Nepal the 1996 Family Health Survey estimated contraceptive prevalence to be 28.5 percent and total fertility to be 4.6 births (Retherford and Thapa 1998). In Pakistan the 1996/97 National Fertility and Family Planning Survey registered a continued upward movement in contraceptive use, from 12 percent in 1991 to 24 percent in 1996/97 (Hakim et al. 1998). Confident fertility estimation is precluded by the poor quality of birth history data, but the total fertility rate has almost certainly fallen from a historical level of about 7.0 births per woman to below 5.5. In the high-fertility north Indian states, evidence from both the 1992/93 National Family Health Survey and the Sample Registration System indicates that earlier concerns that fertility had stabilized at high levels were unwarranted. In the latter half of the 1980s and early 1990s fertility fell, although levels remain much higher than in other states (Narasimhan et al. 1996).

This selective and brief review of fertility trends in South Asia over the last decade demonstrates that fertility decline is now ubiquitous in this region; Afghanistan and Bhutan are possibly the only exceptions. Moreover, it is implausible to argue that these recent demographic trends have been the result of massive structural improvements. Contrary to entrenched earlier beliefs, fertility declines are not incompatible with considerable material poverty, low adult literacy and school enrollments, and gender inequality. With 1993 incomes of about US$200 per head, Nepal and Bangladesh remain among the poorest of countries (UNDP 1997). In north India, Pakistan, and Bangladesh, adult literacy is in the range of 30 to 40 percent and in Nepal it is much lower. Combined first- and second-level gross enrollment ratios are below 50 percent in Bangladesh and Pakistan, although an implausibly high figure of 75 percent is given for Nepal (UNDP 1997). In the face of this evidence, it is no longer tenable to argue that development (at least as defined conventionally) is a necessary precondition for fertility transition.

We now consider recent trends in the Arab states. These comprise a linguistic and cultural grouping rather than a geographic entity and include an exceptionally wide range of economic circumstances, from high-income oil-rich states of the Persian Gulf to some of the poorest countries in the world: Sudan, Mauritania, and Yemen. Until the 1990s, demographic information was patchy but nevertheless sufficient to constitute a severe challenge to conventional explanations of fertility transition. Contrary to expectations, fertility appeared to remain extremely high among the rich, urbanized, and increasingly well-educated Arab countries, particularly so if attention was restricted to the indigenous populations. Conversely, declining trends were most clearly documented among the poorer countries, such as Morocco, Egypt, and Tunisia.

The advent in the 1990s of new data sets allows a reappraisal of this characterization. The compilation by Farid (1996) of results from 27 surveys for the indigenous populations of 18 Arab states shows that, just as in

South Asia, national fertility transitions are now close to universal. Farid's analysis suggests that most countries in the group experienced steep declines in total fertility in the 1980s. These falls equalled or exceeded 3 births in Libya, Qatar, Syria, the United Arab Emirates, and Oman and were in the range of 2.0–2.9 births in Bahrain, Morocco, Algeria, Sudan, and Saudi Arabia. Only Yemen registered no decline, but a more recent DHS survey, not included in Farid's compilation, suggests that fertility has started to fall in this country also (Yemen, Central Statistical Organization 1998). Farid also presents data on nuptiality and contraceptive use, and it is apparent that the declines in total fertility are attributable both to rising ages at first marriage and to increases in contraceptive use.

The Arab states still present a demographic enigma, with many countries exhibiting much higher fertility rates than might be expected from their ranking on the UNDP Human Development Index. Within the group, the lack of the expected association between income and natality also remains: among the four states with recent total fertility of 6 or more births are three—Kuwait, Saudi Arabia, and Oman—whose indigenous populations are wealthy. Nevertheless the main point for the purpose of this chapter is that patterns of family formation are changing rapidly and the Arab states have undeniably entered an era of fertility transition.

Sub-Saharan Africa is the last region to be considered here. Until recently most commentators were pessimistic about the prospects for fertility decline, citing cultural and economic barriers that appeared insurmountable in the short term and that distinguished this region from most others. Among these perceived barriers were the pronatalist influence of traditional African religious beliefs, the separation of men's and women's economic domains, the weakness of the nuclear family relative to the lineage, the custom of child fosterage, and communal land ownership (e.g., Frank and McNicoll 1987; Caldwell and Caldwell 1987). Interpretations drawing on these factors were buttressed by more conventional considerations. In many African countries, child mortality remained high by international standards, educational levels were low, and government attitudes toward control of population growth and promotion of family planning were neutral or hostile. Moreover, family-size desires as reported in surveys were much higher than those ever recorded in Asia or Latin America.

The change in reality and perceptions is well documented. Because of doubts about data quality, the first signs of fertility decline in East and Southern Africa in the 1980s were regarded with considerable skepticism or were thought to reflect a temporary response to economic recessions. However, as the evidence accumulated, largely from DHS inquiries, it became increasingly clear that fertility decline was being established in many countries in East and Southern Africa and was starting elsewhere in the region. Recent reviews have reached broadly similar conclusions. Cohen (1998) adduces evidence of decline in 21 out of 41 countries for which sufficient data are available. In most cases, the falls are modest, but in ten countries they amount to 1.5 births or more. Similarly Kirk and Pillet (1998) conclude that childbearing levels have fallen in about two-thirds of countries that conducted a DHS inquiry prior to 1995. Appreciable rises in age at first marriage and less-marked increases in age at first birth are widespread and contribute to observed declines in total fertility (Westoff 1992). However, the major proximate determinant of change is increased use of contraception, buttressed no doubt by more frequent resort to induced abortion.

Is it justified to claim that sub-Saharan Africa has started a fertility transition that will unfold over the next few decades with a speed and magnitude similar to transitions in other regions? The fertility decline in Europe and its overseas colonies or ex-colonies was clearly distinct in its timing from trends elsewhere, and the pattern holds broadly true for Latin America and East Asia. Why should the same syncronicity not apply to Africa? Opposed to this historical argument are the facts that sub-Saharan Africa contains a wide diversity of cultures and that East and Southern Africa differ from West and Central Africa in many characteristics (Gould and Brown 1996). The idea that fertility transition will spread rapidly across East and Southern Africa appears justified both by historical precedent and by careful consideration of trends in contraceptive use and fertility preferences. Of particular significance, the use of birth control for family limitation is becoming established (Westoff and Bankole 1995). The most serious complicating factor in this part of the subcontinent is likely to be civil unrest or civil war.

In West and Central Africa, the verdict has to be more cautious. There is increasing evidence that fertility has started to decline in parts of Ivory Coast, Senegal, Nigeria, and Ghana. Yet the example of Ghana serves as a warning that the pace of change may be slow and the onset of decline delayed for another decade or so in the more isolated and least developed countries. In Ghana childbearing levels, until recently, remained unchanged despite historically high levels of urbanization and education. Furthermore, as Bledsoe et al. (1994) deduce from their research in the Gambia, rising levels of contraceptive use may simply reflect the use of new means to achieve the traditional goal of birth spacing, and thus do not necessarily herald falls in the quantum of childbearing

Despite this caution concerning West Africa, the broad conclusion from this review of demographic trends of the last decade is that fertility decline in developing countries is rapidly becoming ubiquitous. In 1960, birth rates outside the industrialized countries were either constant or rising. The few exceptions were clearly idiosyncratic, such as the city-states of East Asia or island territories with unusually high exposure to Western influences. By the year 2010 or so, there will be few, if any, countries where childbearing has not started to fall. Thus, just as in the earlier European transition, it will have taken approximately two generations for fertility decline to spread, starting in East Asia and Latin America, then moving to South Asia and the Arab states, more recently to East and Southern Africa, and lastly to the rest of Africa.

The explanatory possibilities

Of course, the mechanisms of change have not been identical everywhere. In much of Asia and the Arab states, delayed childbearing because of increased ages at marriage made a major contribution to declines in overall fertility. Africa may follow this pathway (United Nations 1990). In Latin America, on the other hand, marriage ages have been relatively stable and therefore nuptiality has made little contribution to the fall in total fertility (Rosero-Bixby 1996). Similarly, the role of induced abortion has varied greatly between countries, reflecting in part differences in its legal status. Nevertheless the dominant instrument of change has been the use of modern methods of contraception, as evidenced by the strong linear association at the country level between contraceptive prevalence and total fertility (Ross and Frankenberg 1993). With few exceptions, such as the Philippines and perhaps Pakistan, so-called traditional methods of regulating births within marriage have been largely overshadowed by resort to modern methods.

Changes in family formation during the fertility transition also exhibit a surprising uniformity in the developing world. Typically, the marital fertility decline has been spearheaded by couples with three or more surviving children who adopted contraception to limit family size.[7] Changes in the spacing of births have been relatively modest. As a net result, the childbearing span is progressively reduced from pretransitional durations of 15 to 20 years to a mere 6 to 10 years. Maternal age at last birth drops from values of 35 to 40 years to around 30 years.

The most striking feature of the fertility transition of the past 40 years is that an essentially similar behavioral change (i.e., limitation of births by newly developed techniques of contraception and abortion) has taken root in diverse economic, social, and cultural conditions over a relatively short time. This diversity encompasses material standards of living, degrees of income inequality, dominant modes of production, levels of school enrollment and adult literacy, the position of women in public life, family systems, religious beliefs, systems of government, and government population policies. A few examples will illustrate this diversity. In Taiwan, South Korea, and Singapore, the decline in fertility was paralleled by a massive expansion of formal schooling, rapid restructuring of the economies, and steep rises in standards of living and, no doubt, aspirations. In East and Southern Africa, by contrast, family sizes are starting to drop in a time of falling living standards and school enrollments, rising unemployment, and disillusionment about the future. In some countries, the decline in fertility started only after the achievement of comparatively high living standards, educational levels, and urbanization (e.g., Philippines, many of the Arab states). By contrast, fertility transition in Egypt, Java, Nepal, and Bangladesh started when material and educational standards were very low, populations were still predominantly rural, and the economies were dominated by agriculture. In countries isolated from global capitalism and consumerism (e.g., North Korea, Vietnam, Myanmar), as well as in those with greater contacts with the outside world, family sizes have started to fall. The policy setting has been equally varied. Fertility has declined in contexts of government indifference or hostility to promotion of family planning (e.g., Saudi Arabia, Mongolia), permissive neutrality (much of Latin America), and strong support (e.g., China, India, Indonesia, and Bangladesh).

One possible reaction to this bewildering diversity of circumstances in which fertility has declined is to abandon simple monocausal explanations and to argue instead that different factors, or combinations of factors, have propelled different populations along the pathway to low fertility (e.g., Freedman 1979; Mason 1997). For instance, it is possible to maintain that in some settings rising aspirations concerning "quality" of children were crucial to parental decisions to reduce the "quantity" of offspring. In other settings, severe threats to living standards or strong government action may have prompted changes in reproductive behavior. Thus each country, or at least each subregion, has to be examined in depth in order to identify a unique constellation of key determinants.

This stance is the correct one for analyses of the precise timing of change, its speed, and its mechanisms. These features of demographic change in a given population cannot be understood without invoking its specific circumstances: economic, social, cultural, political. All persuasive attempts to explain fertility transition in a particular country have involved such nuanced and context-specific accounts (e.g., Knodel, Chamratrithirong, and Debavalya 1987 for Thailand; Caldwell, Reddy, and Caldwell 1982 for south India; Cleland et al. 1994 for Bangladesh).

This approach, however, is inadequate to address the larger question of why, between 1960 and 1995, fertility started to decline in nearly all developing countries. It is implausible to argue that the same outcome was achieved coincidentally by different determinants. On the contrary, it is inherently more convincing to assume some underlying common cause of change (or a logically interrelated cluster of causes). The explanatory search should surely be directed toward a factor, or related factors, that developing countries have in common.

This perspective severely limits the range of explanatory possibilities. Clearly, the structural transformation of economies through industrialization and urbanization, or rapidly rising real incomes, cannot be preconditions, nor can the displacement of familial modes of production by larger units. Increases in the value of women's time, with its implications for the opportunity costs of childbearing—the centerpiece of much economic theorizing—cannot be the common underlying cause, because fertility has dropped in settings where women's roles in public life and paid employment were negligible (e.g., Japan in the 1950s; South Korea in the 1960s). Similarly, the advent of alternatives to the value of children as forms of security in old age, sickness, and adversity must be discarded, because alternative security mechanisms have evolved in only a minority of poorer countries.

One is left with only a handful of competing, or perhaps complementary, explanations. These include the spread of formal education and rise in adult literacy, monetization of economies, the impact of new ideas and aspirations, the international family planning movement, and improved survival. In the next section I argue that the last factor, mortality decline, is the simplest and most convincing candidate. Indeed its centrality in any explanation of developing-country fertility transitions seems to me so compelling that its neglect in much recent writing is remarkable.

Toward a reinstatement of mortality decline at the center of fertility transition theory

Here I attempt to reinstate mortality decline in explanations of fertility transition in developing countries. My underlying assumption is that explanations, or theories, of profound social change are not empirically testable in the strict sense of the natural sciences. For instance, explanations of the rise of capitalism in Western Europe in the eighteenth century or the demise of communism in the late twentieth century are not amenable to straightforward criteria of refutation or verification. Rather the merits, or demerits, of explanations rest on whether they provide a compelling coherence to an otherwise disparate record of historical sequences as well as empirically measurable relationships.

Demographers rarely venture beyond the numerical data at their disposal. We suffer from a "tyranny of the quantifiable" because we allow data availability to dominate the process of conceptualization (Ryder 1984: 300). Of course, many mid-level propositions about demographic transition can be tested: the influence of state-sponsored family planning or the link between population density and fertility decline, for instance. To borrow van de Kaa's words, any explanatory narrative should be firmly anchored in the available empirical evidence (van de Kaa 1996); yet, to reach convincing explanations one has to travel beyond the empirically testable.

Some of the key steps toward a reinstatement of mortality decline in explanations of fertility transition have already been taken in the previous three sections. The analysis of historical societies showed that the human species must be adapted to small rather than large numbers of surviving children and cast doubt on the stereotype that couples wanted to maximize their number of surviving children. The next section served mainly to underscore the obvious point that, by the middle of the last century, steep improvements in survival had more than doubled the average number of surviving children per family over historic levels and the era of rapid population growth had begun. The last section argued that some single underlying factor, or logically related cluster of factors, must be responsible for the near universality of third world fertility transitions over the past 40 years.

With these steps in place, the centrality of mortality decline in explanations of developing-country fertility transitions is compelling, but the task remains of specifying the pathways of influence. These may operate at societal or individual levels.

Neither of the two obvious societal pathways—homeostatic forces and government policies to reduce population growth—can muster much support. The existence of homeostatic forces of a Malthusian nature—negative feedback from population growth that reduces living standards and thereby raises mortality or depresses fertility—has been a major theme in historical demography (e.g., Lee 1987). With regard to developing countries over the past 50 years, this feedback mechanism does not appear to have operated. No clearcut relationship between population growth and resources or real incomes is apparent. In many countries, rises in production of food and other goods have exceeded the growth in human numbers. Fertility has declined both in buoyant economies and in countries where living standards are falling.

The evidence regarding population control policies is somewhat more positive. The international family planning movement has undoubtedly exerted a demonstrable influence on fertility transitions of the past 40 years. Its role in legitimating the idea of a small family and new mechanisms of reproductive control has probably been as powerful a force for change as its role in enhancing access to contraception, though the former effect is difficult to quantify. Nevertheless it cannot constitute either a necessary or sufficient pathway of influence. Fertility has also declined in countries that have been sheltered from the powerful and persistent birth control messages emanating from Washington and New York and in settings where the attitudes of elites have not been conducive to reproductive change (North Korea, Myanmar, Mongolia).

Micro-level linkages are now considered. As shown earlier, the physiological and behavioral responses to child deaths constitute rather trivial effects. Nor is there much evidence to support the insurance or hoarding linkage. However, as also discussed earlier, steep mortality declines impinge on families in profound ways that do not require an accurate perception of demographic change. The parental generation lives longer, hence inheritance of land or other resources by the younger generation is delayed. The number of surviving children per family increases, with concomitant rises in direct costs of upbringing and greater difficulties for parents in meeting obligations to adult children, such as endowing marriages. Whatever advantages and opportunities that may have accrued to families with numerous children in pretransitional settings are eroded by mortality decline. In short, large mortality decline places a strain or pressure on families that sooner or later forces an innovative behavioral response—the limitation of births by contraception and abortion.

Several features of this proposed link between greater survival and reproduction need to be stressed. First, it does not depend on conscious awareness of changing survival probabilities. The misperception that, in the "past," typical family sizes were large is widespread, even among demographers. Hence failure to realize the magnitude of demographic change is understandable, though it does nothing to defray the real costs of raising more children. And, of course, the pressure on families is not increased abruptly but builds up slowly over decades. When life expectancy improves by one year in each calendar year (a common trend between 1930 and 1960), the rise in the average number of children surviving to age 20 is about 0.8 per decade (Bongaarts and Menken 1983). Lastly, improved survival forces adaptations other than birth control, such as migration of adult children and, in some societies, postponement of marriage.

The value of this classical explanation, as mentioned earlier, depends on the extent to which it provides coherence to the mass of empirical evidence that has accumulated in the last few decades. First and foremost, life expectancy is one of several factors that have changed radically in all developing countries, and longer life expectancy is thus a plausible candidate as a common underlying cause. It is consistent with the observation that, outside sub-Saharan Africa, family-size aspirations, as recorded in surveys, have been modest. Even the earliest surveys in Asia and Latin America showed that most women wanted no more than 3 to 5 children (Mauldin 1965). Improved survival provides a natural explanation for the emergence of unwelcome childbearing and "unmet need" for fertility regulation in the 1950s and 1960s. It accords with the subjective rationale that individuals offer for wishing to curtail childbearing. As noted by Casterline in this volume, there is a broad uniformity across countries in these reasons. Parents wish to limit their family size because of the costs of rearing children.

The survival thesis is also consistent with evidence concerning the influence of education. As discussed above, literacy and life expectancy are the two strongest predictors of fertility at the national level. The ways in which the spread of formal schooling may accelerate the fertility response to an improving mortality regime are simple to discern. The costs of childrearing are raised by educational expenses, and literate populations are likely to respond more quickly to external changes because they are better informed and more widely exposed to new ideas. So powerful is the potential impact of education not only on direct costs but on parental aspirations for children that it constitutes a possible alternative underlying cause of developing-country fertility transitions. In terms of the strength and regularity of their temporal and spatial relationships to fertility, there is little to distinguish between education and survival. Just as there is no clearcut survival threshold beyond which a fall in childbearing becomes automatic, so there is no educational threshold. The difficulty of disentangling the two factors is exacerbated by the strong link that has emerged since the 1960s between the levels of schooling in a population and its mortality. Thus it is difficult to imagine a well-educated society with high mortality, or vice versa. However, if the characterization of pretransitional fertility proposed in this chapter is valid, then vastly improved survival is likely to be a sufficiently powerful stimulus to engender a fertility response, regardless of schooling opportunities and costs, and is thus the more convincing underlying determinant.

Can survey data on family-size preferences help to assess the validity of the improved survival explanation versus the more common explanation of reduced demand for children as the root cause of fertility decline? Demand theories lead to the expectation that societal modernization, including the spread of formal schooling, will lead to a downward reappraisal of desired numbers of children and that this change in values will be followed, perhaps with a lag, by appropriate modification of reproductive behavior.

Simple cross-sectional analysis (e.g., Pritchett 1994) appears to support the demand thesis. Couples in countries with low fertility want small family sizes and vice versa. However, examination of longitudinal data for the small number of countries where comparable information on preferences has been gathered in successive surveys casts doubt on the usual causal interpretation. In most such countries, behavioral change preceded attitudinal change. For instance in the Republic of Korea (Cho, Arnold, and Kwon 1982), Taiwan (Freedman, Chang, and Sun 1994), Thailand (Knodel, Chamratrithirong, and Debavalya 1987), and Costa Rica (Rosero-Bixby and Casterline 1994), fertility fell for 10 to 15 years prior to declines in desired family size. In the middle phase of transition, behavior and attitudes changed in parallel, but preferences typically stabilized earlier and at a higher level than behavior (see Figure 3). In most post-transitional societies, desired family size remains slightly above two children whereas period or even cohort fertility is appreciably below replacement level.

There are several possible interpretations of this sequence but the almost identical one reached for Taiwan by Freedman et al. (1994) and for Thailand by Knodel et al. (1987) is the most plausible. Fertility decline is,

FIGURE 3 Stylized representation of trends in net fertility and desired family size during the course of fertility transition

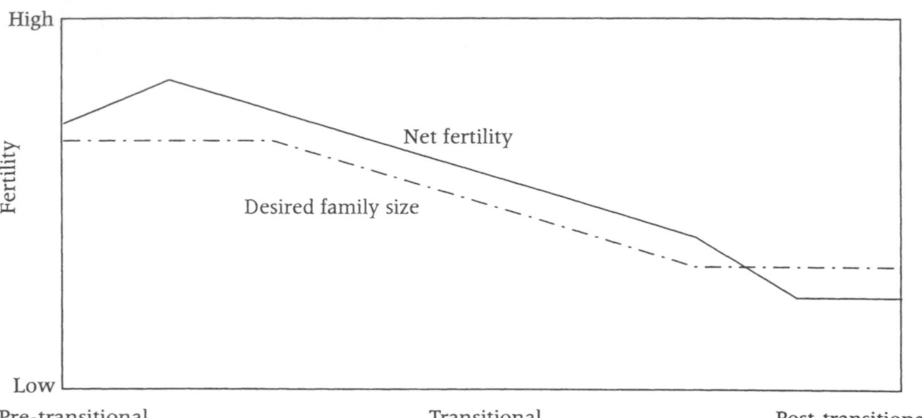

at least initially, a response to prior declines in mortality rather than to any downward reassessment of demand or need for surviving children because of changing socioeconomic circumstances. What then accounts for the lagged drop in preferences? Changing costs and benefits of childbearing are the conventional and obvious explanation, but it is equally likely that the advent and legitimation of new effective methods of fertility regulation destabilize family-size norms. In other words, as in many other spheres of life, new means or technologies allow new motives to emerge and encourage a realignment of preexisting motives.

This interpretation provides a good fit to the evidence for Asia and Latin America. For instance in Pakistan, where fertility decline has started only recently, mean desired family size has shown no change between 1975 and 1997/98. National surveys at these two points document mean desired sizes of about 4 children. Such stability over a generation experiencing considerable socioeconomic change is difficult to reconcile with the demand thesis. No doubt Pakistan will follow the pathway of Thailand: birth control will gain widespread acceptance and this change will permit a reappraisal of family-size norms.

Once again sub-Saharan Africa stands apart from other regions. Family-size aspirations are much higher than elsewhere, and evidence from successive surveys in some countries indicates that demand for children is falling modestly prior to large changes in reproductive behavior (see Table 3). Kenya, however, provides an interesting counter-example. Just a few years before the onset of fertility transition, the 1977/78 Kenya Fertility Survey documented a highly pronatalist society. The mean desired family size was 7.2 children, only 16 percent of married women wanted to stop childbearing, and only 7 percent were practicing any method of contra-

TABLE 3 Trends in mean desired family size among married women aged 15–44 in sub-Saharan Africa, mid-1970s to mid-1990s

	1975–79	1980–84	1985–89	1990–95
East and Southern				
Kenya	7.2		4.7	3.9
Malawi		6.0		5.3
Rwanda		6.3		4.4
Uganda			6.5	5.6
Zimbabwe			4.9	4.7
West and Central				
Cameroon	8.1			7.3
Ghana	6.0		5.5	4.7
Ivory Coast	8.4			6.0
Nigeria		8.3		6.2
Senegal	8.3		7.1	6.3

SOURCE: WFS and DHS inquiries.

ception. Ten years later, both attitudes and behavior had changed sharply. Contraceptive use had risen to 27 percent, and the percentage wishing to limit family size had grown to 49 percent. Clearly something happened in Kenya in the early 1980s to upset an entire reproductive system, and behavior and attitudes changed simultaneously. While this sequence is open to varied interpretations, it appears likely that the reinvigoration of Kenya's family planning program by President Moi and the subsequent legitimation of modern birth control precipitated the rapid transformation of family-size preferences

To sum up, the evidence from the analysis of self-declared desire for children offers more support to the survival thesis than to the demand thesis. During the course of transition, the number of children desired by couples falls, but it does not appear that this change in demand either precedes or precipitates the onset of fertility decline except in sub-Saharan Africa. A steady increase in the number of surviving children against a backdrop of moderate and stable family-size preferences offers a more convincing explanation of the onset of fertility decline.

I do not attempt here a classification of all possible factors that mediate the fertility response to vastly improved mortality. Instead, I restrict my attention to the mediating role of the innovation that provides the main behavioral mechanism for fertility reduction, namely the routine deployment of contraception within marriage. I single out this factor for discussion because it provides a bridge between the classical thesis that has been proposed and innovation–diffusion styles of explanation.

It is sometimes argued that the means of pregnancy regulation can be seamlessly incorporated into reproductive habits, once the motive or need has arisen. This view runs counter to a large body of evidence. Marriage, family, sex, and procreation are key ingredients of any society, and the systems of beliefs and values that surround them are often imbued with moral and religious significance. The concept of deliberate regulation of births within marriage may pose a considerable threat to these values and arouse fierce hostility. It is all too easy to forget the moral uproar that the advent of birth control caused in parts of nineteenth-century Europe. It was condemned by politicians, the medical profession, and the church as a drain on national vitality, a threat to health, and an invitation to promiscuity.

While, in Europe, birth control was essentially a moral innovation, in developing countries it arrived as a technological innovation also. The main mechanism of fertility decline in Asia and elsewhere has been the products of medical and technological progress: contraceptive sterilization, mass-produced latex condoms, intrauterine devices, and hormonal pills, injections, and implants. In some developing countries both the idea of birth control and its material manifestations were greeted enthusiastically. In the 1960s, for instance, women in Taiwan and Thailand flocked from afar to have IUDs fitted. But in many other settings, birth control and its methods have been received initially with suspicion, fear, and sometimes outrage (Bogue 1983; Simmons at al. 1988; Watkins, Rutenberg, and Green 1995; Casterline and Sathar 1997).

There is also abundant evidence from developing countries that the decisions of individuals to limit family size by contraception are subject to social influence and pressures. The idea of birth control, the properties of particular methods, and issues of family size are topics of frequent conversations (e.g., Palmore 1967; Watkins and Danzi 1995; Freedman and Takeshita 1969; Rosenfield, Asavasena, and Mikhanorn 1973; Rogers and Kincaid 1981; Marshall 1971; Blaikie 1975; Lin and Burt 1975). In closely knit communities, the observability of contraceptive adoption is high and decisions of individuals are typically public knowledge (Mita and Simmons 1995; Entwistle et al. 1996). Information exchange within social networks goes hand-in-hand with assessment and evaluation, with particular importance attached to the experience of close friends, neighbors, and relatives (Watkins, Rutenberg, and Green 1995). Thus, while fertility transition involves a change in the mechanism of control, reproductive behavior remains to a large extent socially determined. Indeed it can be argued that the impact of social influences increases during transition because the role of chance or fate in determining reproductive outcomes is steadily reduced.

This brief summary of the key considerations of the innovation–diffusion framework helps to explain otherwise perplexing features of fertility transition. For instance, it offers an explanation for the rapid spread of birth limitation from urban, educated elites to rural, less privileged sectors in many countries (Rodríguez 1996); the fact that fertility transition often follows linguistic or religious contours (Cleland 1985); evidence that actions by governments and other elites to legitimize, or oppose, modern birth control affect the timing and speed of decline (Cleland 1994); and the common finding of a wide gap between stated desires to stop childbearing and adoption of contraception (e.g., Westoff and Ochoa 1991). While improved survival is the engine of fertility change, diffusion processes provide the lubricant.

Conclusion

The view that large mortality declines will stimulate, sooner or later, corresponding adjustments in fertility was a linchpin of classical transition theory, stated most emphatically by Kingsley Davis in 1963. This chapter is essentially a restatement of Davis's position, though with more supporting evidence, both from historical studies and from developing-country research. As emphasized earlier, a causal link cannot be empirically tested. Too many mediating factors obscure any mechanical dose–response relationship between probabilities of survival and fertility trends. The validity of the proposition argued here—namely that mortality decline is the common underlying cause of developing-world fertility transition, chronologically remote but nevertheless fundamental—thus depends on whether or not it provides coherence to an otherwise baffling array of evidence. The explanatory framework provides common ground for both economic determinists and those who emphasize the role of cultural factors and the diffusion of new information, ideas, and attitudes. The main pathway through which mortality decline impinges on reproduction is explicitly economic: the pressure on families of having to rear "abnormally" large numbers of surviving children. Some factors, such as the advent of schooling, may accentuate these costs; others may mitigate them. At the same time, a convincing body of evidence supports the view that the timing and speed of fertility adjustment is also strongly influenced by reactions to the behavioral innovation—namely, contraception—that makes possible this adjustment, and these reactions stem largely from social, cultural, and political factors.

Notes

The author thanks Zelee Hill for the analysis of net reproduction rates and population multipliers, Huyette Shillingford for secretarial assistance, and Ian Timaeus for valuable comments.

1 This is not to suggest that vital rates in these historical populations were entirely stable. On the contrary, population growth, fertility, and mortality exhibited long-term swings, but rates of growth above one percent per annum were rare.

2 There can be no doubt about the strength of pronatalist attitudes in sub-Saharan Africa, compared with other regions. This fea-

ture may have been a longstanding characteristic of African reproductive regimes, reflecting perhaps an adaptation to unusually high mortality stemming from localized warfare or a severe disease environment. It is equally likely that African pronatalism is a recent phenomenon. Although the historical evidence is meager, fertility levels may have risen throughout much of Africa following European colonization. In some parts of Africa, control of sexually transmitted diseases was a major cause (e.g., Romaniuk 1980). In other parts, the collapse of traditional restraints on reproduction are implicated. Certainly in Kenya there is firm evidence of rises in fertility that started before 1950 (Kenya, Central Bureau of Statistics 1996). Total fertility in Kenya rose from 6.2 for the cohort of women born between 1900 and 1904 to 7.7 for those born between 1945 and 1949. In Swaziland there is similar evidence of increased fertility in cohorts born before 1935 (Blacker 1990).

3 Induced abortions performed by traditional means or by untrained persons are associated with a high probability of serious complications (Singh and Wulf 1993).

4 Between the 1960s and 1970s, however, income and literacy probably exercised a far greater influence on mortality than previously (Preston 1986).

5 In parts of West and Central Africa, mortality was still high in the 1950s, but large gains in life expectancy were recorded in subsequent decades (Brass et al. 1968).

6 The main sources of population estimates consulted were: UK Board of Trade 1897–1931; League of Nations 1911–48; Kuczynski 1937, 1948; Durand 1977; McEvedy and Jones 1978; and Mitchell 1993.

7 As predicted by Caldwell, Orubuloye, and Caldwell (1992), sub-Saharan Africa is a partial exception. Contraceptive use for spacing purposes is more common than in other regions and is less strongly related to family size and woman's age. However, as noted earlier, limitation of births is now emerging in East and Southern Africa.

References

Blacker, J. G. C. 1990. "Fertility, mortality and population growth in Swaziland," Mbabane, Central Statistical Office, unpublished report.

Blaikie, P. M. 1975. *Family Planning in India: Diffusion and Policy*. London: Edward Arnold.

Bledsoe, C. H., A. G. Hill, U. D'Alessandro, and P. Langerock. 1994. "Constructing natural fertility: The use of Western contraceptive technologies in rural Gambia," *Population and Development Review* 20: 81–113.

Bogue, D. J. 1983. "Normative and psychic costs of contraception," in R. A. Bulatao and R. D. Lee (eds.), *Determinants of Fertility in Developing Countries*, Vol. 2. New York: Academic Press, pp. 151–192.

Bongaarts, J. and J. Menken. 1983. "The supply of children: A critical essay," in R. A. Bulatao and R. D. Lee (eds.), *Determinants of Fertility in Developing Countries*, Vol. 1. New York: Academic Press, pp. 27–60.

Bongaarts, J. and S. C. Watkins. 1996. "Social interactions and contemporary fertility transitions," *Population and Development Review* 22(4): 639–682.

Brass, W. et al. 1968. *The Demography of Tropical Africa*. Princeton: Princeton University Press.

Caldwell, J. C. 1982. *Theory of Fertility Decline*. London: Academic Press.

Caldwell, J. C. and P. Caldwell. 1987. "The cultural context of high fertility in sub-Saharan Africa," *Population and Development Review* 13: 409–437.

Caldwell, J. C., I. O. Oruboloye, and P. Caldwell. 1992. "Fertility decline in Africa: A new type of transition?" *Population and Development Review* 18: 211–242.

Caldwell, J. C., P. H. Reddy, and P. Caldwell 1982. "The causes of demographic change in rural South India: A micro approach," *Population and Development Review* 8(4): 689–727.

Casterline, J. B. and Z. Sathar. 1997. *The Gap Between Reproductive Intention and Behavior*. Islamabad: Population Council.

Chesnais, J-C. 1992. *The Demographic Transition*. Oxford: Oxford University Press.

Cho, L-J., F. Arnold, and T. H. Kwon 1982. *The Determinants of Fertility in the Republic of Korea*, Committee on Population and Demography Report No. 14. Washington, DC: National Academy Press.

Cleland, J. 1985. "Marital fertility decline: Theories and the evidence," in J. Cleland and J. Hobcraft (eds.), *Reproductive Change in Developing Countries: Insights from the World Fertility Survey*. Oxford University Press, pp. 223–254.

———. 1993. "Equality, security and fertility: A reaction to Thomas," *Population Studies* 47(2): 345–352.

———. 1994. "Different pathways to demographic transition," in F. Graham-Smith (ed.), *Population—The Complex Reality*. Golden, CO: North American Press and London: The Royal Society.

———. 1998. "Potatoes & pills: An overview of innovation—Diffusion contributions to explanations of fertility decline," paper presented at a National Academy of Sciences Workshop, January, Washington, DC.

Cleland, J. et al. 1994. *The Determinants of Reproductive Change in Bangladesh: Success in a Challenging Environment*. Washington, DC: World Bank.

Cohen, B. 1998. "The emerging fertility transition in sub-Saharan Africa," *World Development* 26: 1431–1461.

Cronk, L. 1991. "Human behavioral ecology," *Annual Review of Anthropology* 20: 25–53.

Cutright, P. 1983. "The ingredients of recent fertility decline in developing countries," *International Family Planning Perspectives* 9: 101–109.

Davis, K. 1963. "The theory of change and response in modern demographic history," *Population Index* 29: 345–366.

Douglas, M. 1972. "Population control in primitive groups," in S. T. Reid and D. L. Lyon (eds.), *Population Crisis: An Interdisciplinary Perspective*. Glenview, IL: Scott, Foresman, pp. 49–55.

Dunbar, R. I. M. 1990. "Environmental and social determinants of fecundity in primates," in J. Landers and V. Reynolds (eds.), *Fertility and Resources*. Cambridge: Cambridge University Press, pp. 5–17.

Durand, J. D. 1977. "Historical estimates of world population: An evaluation," *Population and Development Review* 3: 253–296.

Dyson, T. and M. Murphy. 1985. "The onset of fertility transition," *Population and Development Review* 11: 399–440.

Easterlin, R. A. and E. M. Crimmins. 1985. *The Fertility Revolution: A Supply–Demand Analysis*. Chicago: University of Chicago Press.

Entwisle, B. et al. 1996. "Community and contraceptive choice in rural Thailand: A case study of Nang Rong," *Demography* 33(1):1–11.

Farid, S. 1996. "Transitions in demographic and health patterns in the Arab region," in *IUSSP Arab Regional Population Conference, Cairo*, Vol. 1, pp. 435–468.

Frank, O. and G. McNicoll. 1987. "An interpretation of fertility and population policy in Kenya," *Population and Development Review* 13: 209–243.

Freedman, R. 1979. "Theories of fertility decline: A reappraisal," *Social Forces* 58(1): 1–17.

Freedman, R., M-C. Chang, and T-H. Sun. 1994. "Taiwan's transition from high fertility to below-replacement levels," *Studies in Family Planning* 25(6): 317–331.

Freedman, R. and Y. Takeshita. 1969. *Family Planning in Taiwan: An Experiment in Social Change*. Princeton: Princeton University Press.

Galloway, P. R., R. D. Lee, and E. A. Hammel. 1998. "Infant mortality and the fertility transition: Macro evidence from Europe and new findings from Prussia," in M. R. Montgomery and B. Cohen (eds.), *From Death to Birth: Mortality Decline and Reproductive Change*. Washington, DC: National Academy Press, pp. 182–226.

Gould, W. T. S. and M. S. Brown. 1996. "A fertility transition in sub-Saharan Africa?" *International Journal of Population Geography* 2: 1–22.

Grummer-Strawn, L. M., P. W. Stupp, and Z. Mei. 1998. "Effect of a child's death on birth spacing: A cross-national analysis," in M. R. Montgomery and B. Cohen (eds.), *From Death to Birth: Mortality Decline and Reproductive Change*. Washington, DC: National Academy Press, pp. 39–73.

Hakim, A., J. Cleland, and M. H. Bhatti. 1998. *Pakistan Fertility and Family Planning Survey 1996/97: Main Report*. Islamabad: National Institute of Population Studies.

Heer, D. M. and D. O. Smith. 1968. "Mortality level, desired family size, and population increase," *Demography* 5: 104–121.

———. 1969. "Mortality level, desired family size and population increase: Further variations on a basic model," *Demography* 6: 141–149.

Hodgson, M. and J. Gibbs. 1980. "Children ever born," International Statistical Institute, *WFS Comparative Study* No. 12.

Kenya, Central Bureau of Statistics. 1996. "Kenya Population Census 1989," *Analytical Report* No. III. Nairobi.

Khan, M. E. et al. (eds.). 1988. *Performance of Health and Family Welfare Programme in India*. Bombay: Himalaya Publishing House.

Kirk, D. 1996. "Demographic transition theory," *Population Studies* 50(3): 361–387.

Kirk, D. and B. Pillet. 1998. "Fertility levels, trends and differentials in sub-Saharan Africa in the 1980s and 1990s," *Studies in Family Planning* 29(1): 1–22.

Knodel, J., A. Chamratrithirong, and N. Debavalya. 1987. *Thailand's Reproductive Revolution: Rapid Decline in a Third-World Setting*. Madison: University of Wisconsin Press.

Kuczynski, R. R. 1937. *Colonial Population*. Oxford: Oxford University Press.

———. 1948. *Demographic Survey of the British Colonial Empire*. Oxford: Oxford University Press.

Ladier-Fouladi, M. 1996. "La transition de la fécondité en Iran," *Population* 51: 1101–1128.

League of Nations. 1911–1948. *Statistical Yearbook of the League of Nations*. Geneva.

Lee, K., G. Walt, L. Lush, and J. Cleland. 1998. "Family planning policies and programmes in eight low-income countries: A comparative policy analysis," *Social Science and Medicine* 47(7): 949–959.

Lee, K. et al. 1995. *Population Policies and Programmes: Determinants and Consequences in Eight Developing Countries*. London School of Hygiene and Tropical Medicine and United Nations Population Fund.

Lee, R. D. 1987. "Population dynamics of humans and other animals," *Demography* 24(4): 443–465.

Lin, N. and R. S. Burt. 1975. "Differential effect of information channels in the process of innovation diffusion," *Social Forces* 54: 256–274.

Lindert, P. H. 1983. "Changing economic costs and benefits of having children," in R. A. Bulatao and R. D. Lee (eds.), *Determinants of Fertility in Developing Countries*, Vol. 1. New York: Academic Press, pp. 494–516.

Livi-Bacci, M. 1992. *A Concise History of World Population*. Oxford: Blackwell.

Marshall, J. F. 1971. "Topics and networks in intra-village communication," in. S. Polgar (ed.), *Culture and Population: A Collection of Current Studies*. Carolina Population Center, University of North Carolina, pp. 160–166.

Mason, K. O. 1997. "Explaining fertility transitions," *Demography* 34(4): 443–454.

Mauldin, W. P. 1965. "Fertility studies: Knowledge, attitude, and practice," *Studies in Family Planning* 1(7): 1–10

McEvedy, C. and R. Jones. 1978. *Atlas of World Population History*. Harmondsworth: Penguin Books.

Mita, R. and R. Simmons. 1995. "Diffusion of the culture of contraception: Program effects on young women in rural Bangladesh," *Studies in Family Planning* 26(1): 1–13.

Mitchell, B. R. 1993. *International Historical Statistics: Europe, 1750–1988*. New York: Stockton Press.

Montgomery, M. R. 1998. "Learning and lags in mortality perceptions," in M. R. Montgomery and B. Cohen (eds.), *From Death to Birth: Mortality Decline and Reproductive Change.* Washington, DC: National Academy Press, pp. 112–137.

Mueller, E. 1976. "The economic value of children in peasant agriculture," in R. Ridker (ed.), *Population and Development: The Search for Selective Interventions.* Baltimore: Johns Hopkins Press.

Narasimhan, R. L. et al. 1996. "Comparison of fertility estimates from India's National Family Health Survey and Sample Registration System," paper prepared for the IUSSP Seminar on Comparative Perspectives on Fertility Transition in South Asia, Islamabad, Pakistan, 17–20 December.

Notestein, F. W. 1953. "Economic problems of population change," in *Proceedings of the Eighth International Conference of Agricultural Economists*: London: Oxford University Press, pp. 13–31.

Palmore, J. A. 1967. "The Chicago snowball: A study of the flow and diffusion of family planning information," in D. J. Bogue (ed.), *Sociological Contributions to Family Planning Research.* Chicago: University of Chicago Press, pp. 272–363.

Pebley, A. R., H. Delgado, and E. Brinemann. 1979. "Fertility desires and child mortality experience among Guatemalan women," *Studies in Family Planning* 10: 129–136.

Preston, S. H. 1975. "The changing relation between mortality and level of economic development," *Population Studies* 29(2): 231–248.

——— (ed.). 1978. *The Effects of Infant and Child Mortality on Fertility.* New York: Academic Press.

———. 1986. "Mortality and development revisited," *Population Bulletin of the United Nations* 18: 34–40.

Pritchett, L. H. 1994. "Desired fertility and the impact of population policies," *Population and Development Review* 20(1): 1–55.

Retherford, R. D. 1985. "A theory of marital fertility transition," *Population Studies* 39(2): 249–268.

Retherford, R. D. and S. Thapa. 1998. "Fertility trends in Nepal, 1977–1995," *Journal of Centre for Nepal and Asian Studies* 25: 9–58.

Rodríguez, G. 1996. "The spacing and limiting components of the fertility transition in Latin America," in J. M. Guzmán et al. (eds.), *The Fertility Transition in Latin America.* Oxford: Oxford University Press, pp. 27–47.

Rogers, E. M. and D. L. Kincaid. 1981. *Communication Networks: Toward a New Paradigm for Research.* New York: Free Press.

Romaniuk, A. 1980. "Increase in natural fertility during the early stages of modernization: Evidence from an African case study, Zaire," *Population Studies* 34(2): 293–310.

Rosenfield, A. G., W. Asavasena, and J. Mikhanorn. 1973. "Person-to-person communication in Thailand," *Studies in Family Planning* 4(6): 145–149.

Rosero-Bixby, L. 1996. "Nuptiality trends and fertility transition in Latin America," in J. M. Guzmán et al. (eds.), *The Fertility Transition in Latin America.* Oxford: Oxford University Press, pp. 135–150.

Rosero-Bixby, L. and J. B. Casterline 1994. "Interaction diffusion and fertility transition in Costa Rica," *Social Forces* 73(2): 435–462.

Ross, J. A. and E. Frankenberg 1993. *Findings from Two Decades of Family Planning Research.* New York: Population Council

Rutstein, S. O. 1974. "The influence of child mortality on fertility in Taiwan," *Studies in Family Planning* 5(6):182–188.

Ryder, N. 1984. "Fertility and family structure," in *Fertility and Family: Proceedings of the Expert Group on Fertility and Family.* New Delhi, 5–11 January 1983. New York: United Nations ST/ESA/SER.A/88., pp. 279–320.

Satia, J. K. and S. J. Jejeebhoy (eds.). 1991. *The Demographic Challenge: A Study of Four Large Indian States.* Bombay: Oxford University Press.

Simmons, R. et al. 1988. "Beyond supply: The importance of female family planning workers in rural Bangladesh," *Studies in Family Planning* 19(1): 29–38.

Singh, S. and D. Wulf. 1993. "The likelihood of induced abortion among women hospitalized for abortion complications in four Latin American countries," *International Family Planning Perspectives* 19: 134–141.

Stecklov, G. 1997. "Intergenerational resource flows in Côte d'Ivoire: Empirical analysis of aggregate flows," *Population and Development Review* 23: 525–553.

UK Board of Trade. 1897–1931. *Statistical Abstracts for the British Empire.* London.

United Nations. 1990. *Patterns of First Marriage.* New York. Department of International Economic and Social Affairs. ST/ESA/SER.R/III.

United Nations Development Programme. 1997. *Human Development Report 1997.* New York: Oxford University Press.

Van de Kaa, D. J. 1996. "Anchored narratives: The story and findings of half a century of research into the determinants of fertility," *Population Studies* 50(3): 389–432.

Van de Walle, F. 1986. "Infant mortality and the European demographic transition," in A. J. Coale and S. C. Watkins (eds.), *The Decline of Fertility in Europe.* Princeton: Princeton University Press, pp. 201–233.

Watkins, S. C. and A. D. Danzi. 1995. "Women's gossip and social change: Childbirth and fertility control among Italian and Jewish women in the United States, 1920–1940," *Gender and Society* 9(4): 469–490.

Watkins, S. C., N. Rutenberg, and S. Green. 1995. "Diffusion and debate: Controversy about reproductive change in Nyanza Province, Kenya," paper presented at the Annual Meeting of the Population Association of America.

Westoff, C. F. 1992. "Age at marriage, age at first birth, and fertility in Africa," *World Bank Technical Report Paper* No. 169. Washington DC: The World Bank.

Westoff, C. F. and A. Bankole. 1995. "Unmet need: 1990–1994," *DHS Comparative Studies* No. 16. Calverton, MD: Macro International.

Westoff, C. F. and L. Ochoa. 1991. "Unmet need and the demand for family planning," *DHS Comparative Study* No. 5. Calverton, MD: Macro International.

Wilson, C. and P. Airey. 1999. "How can a homeostatic perspective enhance demographic transition theory?" *Population Studies* 53(2): 117–128.

Wrigley, E. A. 1978. "Fertility strategy for the individual and the group," in C. Tilly (ed.), *Historical Studies of Changing Fertility.* Princeton: Princeton University Press, pp. 135–154.

Yemen, Central Statistical Organization. 1998. *Demographic and Maternal and Child Health Survey 1997.* Sana'a.

The Globalization of Fertility Behavior

JOHN C. CALDWELL

BETWEEN THE LATE 1950s and the late 1970s fertility began a persistent major decline in countries containing almost four-fifths of the world's population. The exceptions that did not follow within a further decade were nearly all found in three regions: sub-Saharan Africa, Arab Southwest Asia, and Melanesia. The range of populations involved in the decline was unpredicted and unprecedented. Few developing countries had ever before had a sustained fertility decline, while the West had immediately beforehand been experiencing either stable fertility levels or, because of the postwar "baby boom," rising levels.

It seems likely that such near-simultaneity was the product of the same forces everywhere. Yet this has rarely been suggested. Instead, one set of theories has been developed to explain the Western experience, and a different set has been produced for developing countries. There is very little overlap.

This chapter will focus on this short period of around two decades when decisive fertility decline began or resumed in three types of society: in industrialized or high-income countries, in most of the developing world, and, very significantly but also unnoted in the larger context, in the indigenous minorities in English-speaking, overseas, European-settlement societies. That the decline was significant is shown by the fact that within one-third of a century fertility had fallen by 40 to 60 percent in most of the world's regions and by 40 percent in the world as a whole, almost certainly the first major global decline in history (United Nations 1999).

My central thesis here is that any adequate theory of the onset of fertility decline must address this simultaneity. Any all-embracing theory must take socioeconomic change to be fundamental over long periods, but, for the timing of the onset of periods of fertility decline and the tempo of that decline, theory must also take into account ideologies, attitudes, and the mechanisms of fertility control. I also propose that available methods of fertility control can influence not only fertility but other behavior and attitudes. The argument takes off from that advanced in Caldwell (1999), where the interaction between socioeconomic change, ideologies, and means of fertility control was discussed for the historical West. It also addresses the three propositions put forward by Coale in 1973 (p. 65): for fertility decline to occur, (1) fertility must be within the calculus of conscious choice; (2) reduced fertility must be advantageous; and (3) effective techniques of fertility reduction must be available.

The global fertility decline

Table 1 shows that during most of the 1950s there was little evidence of the coming fertility decline. The major exception was East Asia, where Japan resumed an earlier fertility decline interrupted by militarist pronatalist policies in the 1930s and during World War II, and where China's fertility in the late 1950s was temporarily depressed by the famine at the end of the Great Leap Forward. There were lesser declines in Western Asia as Turkey began to retreat from very high levels of fertility and in Eastern Europe as the new satellite countries of the Soviet Union reacted to the changed political situation (as they were to do again 40 years later) and gained access to legalized abortion. Offsetting these fertility declines were rises in Australasia (Australia and New Zealand), North America, Northern

TABLE 1 Regional fertility declines in the second half of the twentieth century

	Total fertility rate			First quinquennium in which TFR is at specified level compared with 1955–59		Decline in TFR from 1955–60 to 1990–95
Region	**1950–55**	**1955–60**	**1990–95**	**5+% below**	**10+%below**	**(percent)**
Eastern Europe	2.69	2.62	1.61	1960–65	1965–70	49
Northern America	3.47	3.72	2.02	1960–65	1965–70	46
Australasia	3.25	3.51	1.91	1965–70	1965–70	46
Northern Europe	2.32	2.53	1.81	1965–70	1970–75	28
Latin America and Caribbean	5.89	5.94	2.97	1965–70	1970–75	50
Western Asia	6.38	6.25	4.05	1965–70	1970–75	35
Western Europe	2.39	2.50	1.50	1970–75	1970–75	40
Eastern Asia	5.71	5.12	1.88	1970–75	1970–75	63
South-Eastern Asia	6.03	6.07	3.05	1970–75	1970–75	50
Southern Europe	2.65	2.65	1.41	1970–75	1975–80	47
South-Central Asia	6.08	6.06	3.79	1970–75	1975–80	37
Pacific Islands	6.45	6.54	4.59	1965–70	1975–80	30
North Africa	6.82	7.01	3.97	1970–75	1975–80	43
Sub-Saharan Africa	6.52	6.59	5.90	1985–90	1990–95	10

SOURCE: United Nations 1999.

Europe, and Western Europe as the baby boom peaked, and smaller rises with changes attributable to modernization (e.g., shorter breastfeeding intervals, less widowhood) in Africa, Latin America, the Pacific Islands, and parts of Asia.

By 1960–65 fertility was falling in Northern America (in the United States annual rates fell after 1957) as well as Eastern Europe and Western Asia, to be joined in 1965–70 by Australasia (in Australia from 1961), Northern Europe (from 1964), and Latin America and the Caribbean and the Pacific Islands, and in 1970–75 by Western and Southern Europe, the remaining regions of Asia, and North Africa. There was no clear pattern of developed countries being the first to move and being followed by developing countries.

An even more surprising and little-noted change took place during this period, as is revealed in Table 2. The indigenous minority populations of the United States, Canada, New Zealand, and Australia suddenly began steep fertility declines that were soon to halve their birth rates. This was a revealing phenomenon for these were peoples who had failed to adopt the demographic behavior of their co-nationals, the immigrant settler populations, for the better part of a century. One could hardly argue that they had no small-family models or no access to contraception. It could perhaps be argued that fertility control would not be rewarded by the same upward social mobility that rewarded the majority populations, but it would be hard to show that circumstances changed greatly in the 1960s or early 1970s.

The demographic statistics for those countries listed in Table 2 are far from satisfactory but nothing equivalent exists for indigenous minorities in Asia or Latin America. We do know that fertility decline began among the indigenous majority during the 1960s in another settler country of the old British Empire, South Africa (Caldwell and Caldwell 1993: 231). If we take the new Asian states formed from the former Soviet Union as earlier representing indigenous minorities within that country, then it might be noted that such states in Western Asia (Armenia, Azerbaijan, and Georgia) all began their fertility transitions in the 1960s, while in the Central Asian

TABLE 2 Fertility declines among indigenous minorities in developed countries

	Estimated date of		
Indigenous minority	Onset of decline	5+% decline	10+% decline
American Indians	1960	1961	1962
Canadian Indians	1962	1964	1966
New Zealand Maoris	1963	1964	1966
Australian Aborigines	1971	1972	1973

SOURCES: Jaffe 1992: 154–156; Snipp 1996: 26–31; Romaniuc 1987: 72; Kunitz 1994: 135; Khawaja 1985: 164; Australian Bureau of Statistics 1999: 78; Caldwell 2001.

states, with the exception of Kazakhstan (where fertility decline began in 1960–65, possibly because Kazakhs were outnumbered by people of European ancestry), fertility decline was postponed until after 1975.

Explanations for the fertility declines

The theories seeking to explain the onset of fertility declines in the 1960s and early 1970s are usually embedded in underlying socioeconomic change. These forces probably are fundamental, but the theories mostly share two characteristics that warrant concern. First, they do not address the global nature of the fertility decline. Second, they are often unconvincing as to why fertility fell hardly anywhere in the years immediately before 1960 but fell widely soon afterward.

In the historically broadest approach, Davis (1986: 58–59) repeated a message he had proclaimed half a century earlier (Davis 1937): "there is an incompatibility, or tension, between the family on the one hand and the industrial economy on the other. The fundamental principle of the family is ascription of status.... The principle of industrial society is the opposite.... [I]ndustrial societies...inherently discourage procreation." Particularly interesting is the lack of reference to economic imperatives. Westoff (1983: 100) held essentially the same view when he wrote that the long-term Western fertility decline was to be expected, but what had been inadequately explained was the pause in that trend from the 1930s to the 1950s and especially the baby boom, rather than the subsequent resumption of the decline.

Ariès (1980) also saw change in terms of family sociology, but he came closer to explaining why change occurred in the 1960s. His two motivations for the declining birth rate in the West saw late-nineteenth-century parents already in their early adulthood as having little chance of further upward socioeconomic mobility but as being able to aspire to lineage mobility by restricting fertility so as to provide their small families with the education needed for economic and social advancement. As society became richer, parents could achieve this aim on a larger scale by relaxing their strict fertility control, thus causing the baby boom. In the new affluent society that gradually developed after World War II, the possibilities of educational, occupational, and social improvement were widely available to young adults and hence they could place their hopes in themselves rather than in their children, especially if they could remain unmarried or childless or restrict themselves to a very small delayed family. These conditions fell into place with the contraceptive revolution of the 1960s when, according to Ariès, the "child-king" was dethroned. This was essentially also the position of van de Kaa (1987: 5): "The first transition to low fertility was dominated by concerns for family and offspring, but the second emphasizes the rights and self-fulfillment of individuals."

The major economic theorists in the debate, the new household economists originating at the University of Chicago, were closer to these views than is often realized. From the 1960s they built on Becker's theories on the economics of the family. Becker (1991: 155ff) argued that parents in industrialized societies were altruistic toward their children and were willing to spend on their smaller families in order to secure "quality"—read "educated"—children partly for dynastic reasons, which is presumably the upward socioeconomic mobility of the family in the form of their descendants. Willis (1973) expanded Becker's earlier arguments by concentrating on young women and young wives—on "king adults" and not "king children." He wrote of the value of women's time and emphasized that the value of time spent on rearing children instead of working became an ever-greater economic sacrifice as women's real wages rose or as they rose relative to men's wages. In the decades after World War II more wives and more mothers entered the work force. It is difficult to posit that 1960 marked a major fault line, although Schultz (1986: 96) argues that in most industrialized countries the participation of women in the work force rose steeply between 1960 and 1980, as male and female participation rates converged—a result, he maintains, of convergence in educational levels (p. 103). The dating of the rise in women's labor force participation seems a little late to provide the whole explanation for the fertility decline, although one might counter that the rise was weak in Ireland and nonexistent in Greece, where fertility decline began in the late 1970s and early 1980s respectively.

A distinction should be made between explanations of fertility limitation based on women's time (and ultimately on family income) and those that posit the conflict arising from simultaneously being a mother of young children and holding down a full time job. Wulf (1982: 63) summarized the papers reporting on field investigations of low fertility to the 1981 Manila General Conference of the IUSSP by stating that most saw the fertility decline in the West as arising from a change in the role and expectations of women, especially participation in the labor market: "As more and more women anticipate that work outside the home will be a permanent feature of their adult lives, they are forced to make serious and far-reaching decisions about whether and how to combine wage-earning with childrearing. The dilemma that this conflict poses for both men and women is not easily resolved, and we need no more persuasive evidence of its intractable nature than the fact that more and more couples are deciding to forgo childbearing altogether or to limit their family size to two or fewer children." This stance, as will be reported below, receives strong support from a series of investigations carried out in Australia.

Clearly, the economic and social theses can be welded together. Lesthaeghe (1983) argued that economic change was fundamental but that the impact of accompanying ideational changes, increasingly individualistic and secular, should not be underestimated. There was more to the story than the economic balance between costs and benefits of children (p. 412). Easterlin (1973) added a demographic thread. If times are good and jobs are plentiful, as they are likely to be for persons born at times of unusually low fertility such as the 1930s, then there will be early marriages and a readiness to have children. If one has to compete with members of a large cohort such as those born during the baby boom, then marriage rates and fertility levels will fall. It is true that American fertility rates rose to replacement level in the 1990s, but the recovery was modest and has been explained by making up for previously deferred births (Bongaarts and Feeney 1998). The recovery was also less obvious in other countries that had experienced the baby boom.

What is interesting is the modest emphasis placed on contraceptive change even though this was a subject area in which many of the theorists worked. Ryder and Westoff (1967: 3) wrote: "It is our hunch that what has been happening to fertility in the 1960s would have happened in direction if not in degree even if the oral contraceptive had not appeared on the scene, although the tempo of decline most recently can probably be attributed in part to the availability of this highly efficient and apparently highly acceptable method of fertility regulation." But they also noted that "pill use is more likely than not to be a replacement for the condom or the diaphragm, both highly effective contraceptives." In 1971 they pointed out that the fertility decline had started well in advance of the advent of the pill (actually two years earlier) but that much of the tempo of decline could probably be attributed to its use (Ryder and Westoff 1971: 152–153). By the mid-1970s they appear to have moved closer to regarding the American fertility revolution as a contraceptive one, citing the influence of the pill, IUD, and sterilization (Westoff 1975; Westoff and Ryder 1977). Easterlin (1973: 187ff) believed that the pill might have been an important means of allowing young married baby boomers to keep their families small, and Ariès (1980: 649–650) held that effective contraception and abortion permitted couples to place greater emphasis on their own development than on that of their children.

Theories explaining fertility decline in developing countries usually place greater emphasis on contraception but give little more attention to the timing of the decline than do explanations of fertility decline in developed countries. The most comprehensive theory is that of Easterlin (1978), who identifies the demand for children as being determined by tastes, income, and prices within a broader context of the potential supply (actual reproduction—that is, natural fertility eroded by child mortality) and the cost of fertility regulation (both market costs and those of a personal and psychological nature). The timing of fertility decline is presumably determined by the society's economic development and its tastes (which may encompass social change, including change in the costs of fertility regulation). Elsewhere I have hypothesized that in sub-Saharan Africa in the 1970s there was little demand for fertility control and a significant demand for children because the *net* intergenerational wealth flow was upward (Caldwell 1976, 1977, 1982). Subsequent studies of India (Caldwell, Reddy, and Caldwell 1982, 1988) and Bangladesh (Caldwell et al. 1999), where fertility was falling and national family planning programs were operative, concluded that economic and social changes were the underlying factors in inducing fertility decline, with the education of children being an important element, but that family planning programs almost certainly hastened the process. Freedman and Berelson (1976) reached a similar conclusion after a survey of family planning programs.

Some studies have argued that "the additional effect of contraceptive availability or family planning programs on fertility is quantitatively small and explains very little cross-country variation" (Pritchett 1994: 247; see also Demeny 1979). Others have assigned contraception and organized family planning programs a major causal role in the timing and pace of fertility decline (Tsui and Bogue 1978; Chowdhury 1983, Cleland and Wilson 1987; Robey, Rutstein, and Morris 1993; Carty, Yinger, and Rosov 1993; Cleland et al. 1994; Potts 1997). Still others have attributed the tempo, and sometimes the timing, of fertility decline to family planning provision while seeing the decline as part of massive economic development and social change (Mauldin and Berelson 1978; Cutright 1983; Kelly, Poston, and Cutright 1983; Sherris 1985; Guzmán 1994; Bongaarts and Watkins 1996).

None of these studies relates the onset of fertility decline in developing countries to the contemporaneous renewal of fertility decline in industrialized countries. Robey, Rutstein, and Morris (1993: 60), drawing on international demographic and contraceptive surveys, concluded that "recent evidence suggests that birth rates in the developing world have fallen even in the absence of improved living conditions.... Developing countries appear to have benefited from the growing influence and scope of family-planning programs, from new contraceptive technologies and from the educational power of the mass media." They buttress this with the observations that "differences in contraceptive prevalence explain about 90 percent of the variation in fertility rates" and that now more-efficient contraceptives are being used (p. 62). In fact, no one denies that contraception is the mechanism for most fertility reduction; rather, the question is why it is employed. Cleland and Wilson (1987: 28) argued that "the distinction between groups with unchanging fertility and those experiencing transition is the propensity to translate desires into appropriate behaviour." Again, the question is what determines that propensity. Guzmán (1994) concluded that mass fertility control in Latin America in the 1960s was triggered by renewed economic adversity and a simultaneous increase in organized family planning activity.

Explanations for the decline in fertility and its timing among indigenous minorities are even more meager. Jaffe (1992: 155–157) argues that the decline of fertility of the American Indians was achieved by a greater mixing of the minority and majority populations as the former streamed in larger numbers to the cities, enabled to do so by increasing education levels and by the economic boom conditions of the 1950s and 1960s. This is also one of the explanations put forward in Canada, Australia, and New Zealand. In New Zealand, Sceats and Pool (1985: 191) argue that the Maori fertility decline took place in the 1960s because of the new availability of the pill, sterilization, and injectables. More light is thrown on the situation among indigenous minorities by the Australian experience. In 1967 a federal referendum recognized Aborigines as full Australian citizens. Thereafter the Australian Government increased allocations for health services for the Aborigines both under the conservative Liberal/Country Party coalition and from 1973 under the Whitlam Labor Government. Gray (1983: 312–316) concluded that it was very difficult to place the Aboriginal fertility transition within demographic transition theory. Rather he noted that in the first half of the 1970s enthusiastic young white doctors who were determined to raise living standards and improve the position of Aboriginal women worked in Aboriginal health services. The memoirs of six of these doctors revealed that they made the new contraceptive technology available, and that such contraception was acceptable to Aboriginal women, especially older women who had met social obligations by having at least two surviving children. Female-controlled contraception was important in their family situations. In the early 1970s Aboriginal fertility began a steep decline.

Toward an explanation of the global fertility decline

The near-simultaneity of the onset of fertility transition among most of the world's populations is evidence of the globalization of the fertility transition, a situation with major implications for the present and the future. Explaining what happened provides a key to understanding contemporary demographic transition. Any fertility transition theory that fails to address declines in both developing and developed countries and to explain their parallel occurrence is deficient.

What happened, I suggest, is the following. (1) Before the 1950s fertility had consistently declined only in the West and Japan; the Western decline occurred throughout Europe, Northern America, Australasia, and Argentina and Uruguay—usually, together with Japan, referred to as the industrialized countries even though at very different levels of manufacturing. This decline had been achieved over generations, often with methods such as withdrawal that had to be learned and that required cooperative conjugal relationships which were far from universal. (2) During the 1950s and 1960s concern in the West about "population explosion" in the developing world spread from specialists to the public. This in turn had two effects. It undermined the legitimacy of large families in the West as well, and it encouraged the development of new and more efficient contraception to meet developing-world needs—methods that would turn out to meet needs in the West as well. (3) Because children had not been an economic burden in developing countries before the great socioeconomic changes in the decades after World War II, and were still only marginally so in many parts of the world, the methods the West had slowly learned to use for restricting fertility were not—at least in the short term—available. (4) New, easier-to-use forms of fertility regulation became available around 1960 and were instrumental in the fertility transition in developing countries. (5) They were also more effective and more egalitarian than the methods hitherto employed in industrialized countries, and were employed in these countries at just the same time as in developing countries and in places even earlier. (6) The developing countries did not experience the mass concern about population explosion felt in the West, and many countries still do not, but the elites came increasingly to advocate limiting population growth, a perspective that was of key importance in establishing effective national family planning programs. (7) All these changes could not have occurred without unprecedented economic growth and social change both in developed and developing countries. This global socioeconomic revolution would have eventually brought fertility decline even without the new contraception, but not so rapidly. (8) Certain populations did not participate in the fertility declines of the 1960s and early 1970s because of insufficient socioeconomic change or because either the elites or broader communities were not convinced of the need for fertility control. (9) The fertility decline and the means used to achieve it were new material conditions in both the developed and developing world and brought about further socioeconomic changes. (10) The globalization of fertility attitudes and behavior has major implications for future demographic trends and population policies.

These points will now be consolidated. The discussion of change in the West will focus on the Australian experience because of a series of relevant studies and of in-depth investigations linked to surveys (Caldwell et al. 1973; Caldwell et al. 1976; Ruzicka and Caldwell 1977).

Before 1960, persistent fertility decline was almost unknown in the developing world. Small declines occurred in the late 1950s in a few atypical places. One was Sri Lanka, which had long been relatively rich by regional standards, was highly educated, had been a European colony for almost 300 years, and had a significant Christian minority. Even there, the early fertility decline was mostly achieved by delayed marriage (Fernando

1975; Alam and Cleland 1981; Caldwell et al. 1989; B. Caldwell 1999), assisted by rhythm and withdrawal (Caldwell et al. 1987). Sri Lanka appears to have experienced some fertility decline in the economic depression of the 1930s (Sarkar 1957: 95). Fertility decline had already begun in Singapore, an educated city with an active family planning association; in Mauritius, where some of the same conditions applied; in India, where a national family planning program was employing male sterilization; and in Turkey, mostly in Istanbul and the large towns of the west coast.

In the industrialized countries fertility was controlled by a mixture of older and more recent contraceptive methods. In the United States and Australia the majority of couples were using rhythm, withdrawal, and the diaphragm (Caldwell et al. 1973: 59); in Europe the first two and condoms. The European fertility decline had probably been originally achieved employing withdrawal (Santow 1993), although van de Walle and Muhsam (1995) believe that the French probably limited fertility by sexual practices not involving intercourse, and Szreter (1996: 367–439) asserts that in Britain long periods of sexual abstinence were important. Delayed female marriage and spinsterhood were also factors. Even in the English-speaking West the use of contraception was long limited by a suspicion and apprehension of it, which in turn meant that contraceptives were primitive, possibly unsafe, and difficult to obtain (Caldwell 1999).

It is intriguing to remember how pronatalist were public statements in the West of the late 1940s, how limited was public discussion about contraception, and often how difficult it was for individuals to obtain adequate assistance with contraception. The most powerful force in changing this situation was the growing belief, rapidly becoming an ideology, that the deliberate control of fertility in poor, high-growth countries was desirable, even the path of virtue. In September 1948 the *New York Times* published an editorial echoing the sentiments in an FAO report saying so. In 1959 the World Council of Churches endorsed family planning; General William Draper presented a report to the United States Congress recommending that the US offer birth control assistance to developing countries; and the American Public Health Association announced that family planning services should be an integral part of health services. The last had partly been provoked by the successful 1958 battle to allow New York public hospitals to provide contraceptive services (Guttmacher 1966: 461–462). In the 1960s concern over rapid population growth in the developing world intensified in the West, fueled, among other things, by Paul Ehrlich's many television appearances in the United States, Australia, and elsewhere, and by his publication of *The Population Bomb* in 1968.

In Australia a 1971 survey of Melbourne found that 68 percent of women believed that the world was overpopulated, 62 percent believed that governments should take action to prevent the situation from deteriorating further, and 52 percent believed that they would now respond—if they were in a position to do so—to government requests for everyone to limit family size to two children (Australian Family Formation Project 1972: Questions 111–170). A majority believed that "The pill has brought more benefit to women than any other modern invention." The proportion of contraceptive users among married women who believed themselves to be at risk of conceiving rose from 64 percent in 1945–49 to 92 percent in 1970–71 (Caldwell and Ware 1973: 13).

For 40 years we have been asking, in surveys and in one-on-one anthropological investigations in sub-Saharan Africa, rural South India, and rural Bangladesh, both of contraceptive users and of nonusers, whether their parents used contraception or worried about their inability to control family size. The answers have been the same. Their parents had not practiced birth control because they had no access to services. They had never contemplated restricting family size because, without the methods for doing so, it was unimaginable (see Caldwell and Caldwell 1984). Abortion was rare and was not used to limit family size. Again, Sri Lanka was the exception.

This was not our experience alone; it was also that of persons who contributed significantly to the crusade against high fertility in the developing world. In 1948 Frank Notestein, Marshall Balfour, Irene Taeuber, and Roger Evans in a mission to East Asia visited a rural area in north China, where family size had long been controlled through infanticide, and where the mayor and his associates wanted to introduce family planning in their densely populated and land-hungry area. No circumstances could have been more conducive to family planning success. But the group members "knew that there was no method of contraception really suitable to the needs of…[this] community" (Balfour et al. 1950: 83). They concluded: "The main difficulty is that there is no single contraceptive method that is likely to prove of any substantial importance to the peasant population of Asia's mainland. Any such method must be very cheap, simple, safe and effective. So far as we know such a method neither exists nor is on the horizon" (pp. 119–120).

This situation changed around 1960, largely because of altered attitudes in the West. Gregory Pincus requested funding for research on the development of the pill in the 1950s on the grounds that such a contraceptive was needed in the developing world. The pill became available in many developed countries at the beginning of 1960 but was at first too expensive for mass use in developing countries. The Lippes Loop, an intrauterine contraceptive device, was promoted in a number of developing-country settings from 1962 and was a regular part of South Korea's family planning program from 1964 (Kim and Kim 1966: 426). Such older methods as sterilization and abortion became more widely available. In the early 1960s

American doctors were permitted to perform sterilization for family planning reasons (Guttmacher 1966: 455), and in Australia the journal of the Australian Medical Association ceased warning doctors that they might be prosecuted if they carried out such operations. Legal abortion became readily accessible in Eastern Europe in the mid-1950s, in Britain in 1967, in South Australia in 1969, in India in 1972, and in the United States in 1973. From about 1965 suction abortion made the operation simpler and safer. All these developments were hastened by socioeconomic changes and growth in secular and civil rights attitudes in the industrialized countries, but there can be little doubt that the growing clamor for the control of population numbers gave birth control methods respectability.

These methods made possible national family planning programs in the developing world. The first successful national programs, in South Korea and Taiwan, were in the early years largely IUD programs; India's was overwhelmingly a sterilization program, first of males and later of females; China employed its own type of IUD (a metal ring) as well as sterilization; Turkey, Thailand, and Indonesia concentrated on the IUD and pill; the South African program was driven by pills and injectables. As late as 1985, sterilization, IUDs, and hormonal contraception accounted for 83 percent of contraception in developing countries, compared with 48 percent in developed societies (Mauldin and Segal 1988: 341). In Latin America the pill and sterilization were widespread in the 1960s. Nearly everywhere these methods were backed up by abortion, more often illegal than legal. In 1965 an international conference reported on the experience of national family planning programs in 12 countries (Berelson et al. 1966). Nevertheless, it was in developed countries that pill use first took off. In Australia by 1971 pill use was almost double that of all other methods combined (Lavis 1975: 2), and between 1960/63 and 1970/71 current pill and IUD use by married women rose from 14 percent to 46 percent (Caldwell and Ware 1973: 17).

The question remains why the new contraceptives were taken up by family planning programs in a way that the older ones were not. In inexperienced or less motivated hands they probably were more certain of preventing conception. However, in these circumstances there were also more complaints of side effects and higher rates of discontinuation. There are other reasons as well. One that is frequently cited is logistic ease. Sterilization needs only one encounter between the program and client in a lifetime; the IUD one encounter every few years. India long believed that its program was only capable of delivering sterilization.

The major and little-explored reasons may well have been two features of the modern methods: they were not coitus-related and they were medicalized. The diaphragm, condom, douching, foams, and jellies all needed action around the time of coitus, involved partner cooperation, and usually required touching the sexual organs. On the last point many Australian Catholics connected the ban on contraceptives with the dubious nature of sex for pleasure and with their repugnance for the sexual organs. The result was that they had until the early 1970s only one-sixth of the level of use the non-Catholics had of the diaphragm, half of douching, but over three-quarters the level of pill use (Caldwell and Ware 1973: 24). In the 1950s 39 percent of Australian fertility control was through coitally related contraception; by the early 1970s that was down to 7 percent (Caldwell 1982b: 257).

It is hard to overstate the advantage that developing-country family planning programs attained by having a range of methods that required consultation only between a woman and a family planning worker, or only needed the worker to accompany the woman to a clinic or hospital. When international demographic or contraceptive surveys report that spouses have discussed contraception, it usually means little more in rural India than that the husband has suggested or agreed to the "operation" or in rural Bangladesh that his wife can talk to and be influenced by the family planning worker.

The new contraceptives were egalitarian in that they required little effort or social and communication skills. This allowed the gulf in use to narrow not only between developed and developing countries but also between social groups in the West. In the 1950s when use of the diaphragm peaked, twice as many women in Australia with upper secondary or tertiary education were using the method as were less-educated women; there were no educational differentials in the early 1970s in either pill or IUD use (Caldwell and Ware 1973: 26).

Concern with global population growth and an association between that concern and one's own fertility intentions grew steadily in the West from the 1950s to the 1970s. There were reflections of this concern in Latin America, East Asia, and parts of Southeast Asia, but much less so in South Asia and Africa. The strongest reflection in developing countries was among governments and elites, progressively percolating down the social structure. In India this process began in the nineteenth century (Caldwell 1998), but elsewhere it was a characteristic of the second half of the twentieth century (Caldwell 1993; Khuda et al. 1996). Davis (1944) had argued that this process could not begin until postcolonial times because national elites regarded any attempt by colonial governments to introduce family planning as an effort to maintain their own control. Ultimately the diffusion of ideas and attitudes may become a mass movement, at least among women (see Bongaarts and Watkins 1996).

Fertility control has not operated in a vacuum in either the developing or developed world. Vast economic growth, the spread of schooling, urbanization, the changing position of women, and increasing economic and social globalization have been the underlying factors everywhere. So has the movement of women into the paid work force in all developed and many developing countries. Nevertheless, the dating of the advent of new contraceptives and of the onset or renewal of fertility decline makes it hard to argue that the contraceptive revolution did not accelerate fertility decline and, in many cases, hasten its onset. The continued dependence of developing countries on the new forms of fertility control strengthens the argument.

As can be seen in the Appendix Table, sub-Saharan Africa, much of Arab Southwest Asia, and Melanesia did not participate in the fertility declines of the 1960s and 1970s. Sub-Saharan Africa was at that time poor but no poorer than much of Asia (Caldwell and Caldwell 1988). Its people probably were more pronatalist than elsewhere for religious and cultural reasons (Caldwell and Caldwell 1987). Most of the region was newly independent and had no history of nation-states led by elites. Those who did offer leadership were usually convinced that African fertility culture was different and would remain so. The result was that national family planning programs were established only in Kenya and Ghana, where they received weak government support, and in South Africa where the program was put in place by the minority white government. In the Middle East and North Africa explanations must be sought in Arab Muslim attitudes to interventions in Allah's plans, political tensions, and the position of women. In Melanesia the situation resembled that in sub-Saharan Africa.

The battle to contain global population growth changed the developed world in two ways. First, it provided young couples, especially young women, with a justification for deferring births, having small families, or alternatively having no children or not marrying. Second, more effective contraception, backed up by more accessible abortion and followed by sterilization, provided almost certain fertility control. Ruzicka and Caldwell (1977: 334 ff.) summarized the 1975–76 Australian studies as showing the following: (i) Most young adults were satisfied that they now had reasonably certain fertility control that they could use as a basis for planning their lives, and marveled that their parents had made do with such high-risk regulation. (ii) Most couples agreed that continuous contraception was the normal way of life; indeed, in most relationships contraception could not be discontinued unless both partners agreed. (iii) Most respondents agreed that pregnancy should not come straight after marriage (or marriage after the beginning of a sexual relationship), but that time was needed for the partners to mature and to have such experiences as travel, and for each (but especially the wife) to have completed education or training and for the wife to have gained enough work experience and promotion to be able to be re-employed after a birth or a period looking after a young child. Cosford et al. (1976: 109) reported that the same study had shown "just how deeply the tenets of the Women's Movement have spread in the society. There is no longer a significant body of young women, even in the working-class or amongst the Australian-Irish, who do not wonder about problems of identity and role." The 1986 study, held at a time when Australian fertility had fallen well below the long-term replacement level, found that most young couples intended to have at least two children when they married, but successive postponements led many couples into thinking that this was no longer desirable (Caldwell et al. 1988: 123).

These changes occurred within a framework provided by economic growth, more women entering the work force, greater emphasis on the individual, the unrest of the Vietnam War years, the rise of the women's movement, a further sexual revolution, and an increase in nonmarital cohabitation. But the new, safer contraception also provided a basis for this social change, and many aspects of society would have been different without the contraceptive revolution of the early 1960s.

Support for fertility control, which a few decades ago was confined to developed countries and the governing elites of developing countries, is becoming a mass phenomenon in an increasing segment of the developing world. Most sub-Saharan African elites have now joined the consensus, as has the majority of the population in East Asia. This, in a world of ever more comprehensive communications, is likely to lead to an extraordinary degree of globalization of fertility behavior.

Synthesis

The revolution of the early 1960s in attitudes toward population growth, family size, the virtues of reproducing, and the type of contraception used met all three of Coale's (1973) prerequisites, and fertility fell further in developed countries and began to fall in developing ones. Fertility came increasingly within the calculus of conscious choice. There were real or supposed economic advantages in reducing fertility in developing countries and, in the West, major social advantages for women. More effective techniques of fertility reduction became available—with the advantage, particularly in developing countries, that lower levels both of spousal communication and of sustained will were needed to make them effective.

The Appendix Table illustrates an innovational wave of new fertility attitudes and practices that began to gain momentum in the 1960s. Eastern Europe, which had still not become part of the global culture of reproductive attitudes because of communication barriers, was an outlier with fertility behavior influenced mostly by the availability of abortion and the shortages of housing and consumer goods. Similarly, somewhat isolated Malta and Cyprus can be seen as belatedly moving toward the lower fertility levels of the rest of Mediterranean Europe.

In the West the timing of fertility decline was predictable. First came the United States, where the new contraceptives had been invented and where the debates about both population explosion and women's roles had been loudest. Then followed those countries most closely bound up with the

United States through the influences of media and communication: other English-speaking countries of overseas European settlement, Scandinavia, and the Netherlands. The rest of continental Europe lagged further (as they also did in the use of the new contraception). Finally, Mediterranean Europe hardly changed, evidence perhaps of the different position of women. This is particularly ironic given the extremely low fertility that Spain, Italy, Greece, and Portugal were to attain at the close of the twentieth century.

In Asia, again excluding the Soviet Union, change came first to free-market city-states. The larger countries with national family planning programs did not, with the exception of South Korea, achieve 10 percent fertility declines until the 1970s. The same was true of North Africa. In sub-Saharan Africa, only in South Africa with its ruling white minority can the family planning association and government program provision of the new contraceptives be compared with the situation in Asia, and there the onset of the fertility decline occurred in the 1960s. Finally, the fertility of the indigenous minorities fell at much the same time as did that of the majorities in the English-speaking settlement countries, in complete contrast to the situation during the preceding three-quarters of a century, evidence that the first of Coale's three stipulations had been met.

The global fertility decline between 1960 and 1980 is summarized in Table 3, a condensation of the information provided in the Appendix Table. The decline began in countries with almost 80 percent of the world's population. Three-quarters of them lived in countries that had never previously experienced a fertility transition.

Four points of importance should be reiterated.

TABLE 3 Number of countries in various regions and number of indigenous minorities whose fertility had first fallen by 10 percent, by quinquennium

Region	1960–65	1965–70	1970–75	1975–80	Later or not at all
"West"	2 (8%)	8 (31%)	9 (35%)	4 (15%)	3 (11%)
Eastern Europe	5 (25%)	8 (40%)	1 (5%)	0 (0%)	6 (30%)
Asia	1 (3%)	12 (33%)	5 (14%)	6 (17%)	12 (33%)
Arab Southwest Asia and North Africa	0 (0%)	0 (0%)	4 (27%)	4 (27%)	7 (46%)
Latin America and Caribbean	1 (3%)	8 (26%)	10 (32%)	8 (26%)	4 (13%)
Sub-Saharan Africa	0 (0%)	1 (2%)	0 (0%)	1 (2%)	44 (96%)
Pacific islands	2 (25%)	1 (13%)	3 (37%)	0 (0%)	2 (25%)
Indigenous minorities[a]	1 (25%)	2 (50%)	1 (25%)	0 (0%)	0 (0%)

[a]See Table 2.

NOTE: Figures in parentheses indicate percent of countries in region in each quinquennium and in column "Later or not at all."

SOURCE: See Appendix Table.

First, the post–World War II struggle to contain population growth affected the industrialized countries as strongly as the developing countries. In the richer countries low fertility was legitimized as never before. New contraceptives, developed primarily for the poor world, had their earliest impact on the rich world. The development of a near-certainty in fertility control allowed the development of new ways of life, new roles for women, and new types of union. The movement of women into the work force accelerated. The legitimation of low or zero fertility and of the new contraceptives almost certainly quickened changes that would otherwise, driven by economic change, have happened more slowly. Indeed, fertility in the United States first fell in 1958, two years before the advent of the pill, but it would probably not have fallen so soon without the legitimation of low fertility.

Second, the onset of fertility decline among indigenous minorities, after generations of ignoring demographic trends in the majority populations, must owe a good deal to the new contraceptives. None of these minority populations would be disconcerted if their proportions of the total populations rose.

Third, the demographic events of the 1960s and 1970s were at least partly the result of the globalization of fertility attitudes and behavior. The attitudes of the West converted developing-world elites. That and the availability after 1960 of the new contraception began the conversion of the populations at large. Globalization has proceeded apace since 1960. It is partly an awareness of this that has prevented Western countries with below-replacement fertility levels (or even declining population numbers as in parts of Europe) from following the precedents of the 1930s and adopting policies aimed at raising fertility levels. Certainly, any future adoption of such policies is likely to influence the attitudes of developing-country governments.

Fourth, the population activism in the developed world over the last half-century has had as strong a demographic impact on developed as developing countries. The developed countries' crusade was directed outward but they could hardly be insulated from it. Furthermore, the first countries to experience the fertility decline were those that had been most active in its promotion: the United States, the other English-speaking countries of overseas European settlement, Scandinavia, and the Netherlands.

Finally, the central proposition of this chapter is that the simultaneity of the developed- and developing-country fertility transitions after 1960 is so striking that adequate demographic theory must cover both and find reasons for change at that time that cover the experience of both types of societies. It is hard to overlook for inclusion in such theory the new egalitarian contraceptives and the legitimization of small family size and limits to national numbers.

Appendix Table **Quinquennium in which a country first recorded a total fertility rate 10 percent below its TFR in 1955–59**

Region	1960–65	1965–70	1970–75	1975–80	Later or not at all
"West"	Malta United States	Australia Canada Cyprus Denmark Finland Iceland Netherlands New Zealand	Austria Belgium France Germany[a] Luxembourg Norway Sweden Switzerland United Kingdom	Israel Italy Japan Portugal	Greece Ireland Spain
Eastern Europe	Bosnia and Herzegovina Macedonia Poland Slovakia	Albania Belarus Czech Rep. Lithuania Moldava Russia Ukraine Yugoslavia[a]	Croatia		Bulgaria Estonia Hungary Latvia Romania Slovenia
Asia	Singapore	Armenia Brunei Georgia Hong Kong Kazakhstan Korea (South) Macau Malaysia Philippines Sri Lanka Turkey Turkmenistan	Azerbaijan Cambodia China Indonesia Thailand	East Timor India Korea (North) Kyrgyzstan Myanmar Uzbekistan	Afghanistan Bangladesh Bhutan Iran Iraq Laos Maldives Mongolia Nepal Pakistan Tajikistan Vietnam

Arab Southwest Asia and North Africa			Bahrain Egypt Lebanon Tunisia	Kuwait Morocco Qatar U.A.R.	Algeria Gaza Strip Jordan Oman Saudi Arabia Syria Western Sahara Yemen
Latin America and Caribbean	Netherlands Antilles	Bahamas Barbados Brazil Chile Costa Rica Martinique Puerto Rico Trinidad and Tobago	Colombia Dominican Rep. Ecuador El Salvador Guadeloupe Guyana Panama Paraguay Suriname Venezuela	Bolivia Cuba Haiti Honduras Jamaica Mexico Nicaragua Peru	Argentina Belize Guatemala Uruguay
Sub-Saharan Africa		South Africa		Zimbabwe	All other 44 sub-Saharan African countries
Pacific islands	Fiji New Caledonia	Guam	French Polynesia Samoa Vanuatu		Papua New Guinea Solomon Islands
Indigenous minorities	American Indians	Canadian Indians New Zealand Maoris	Australian Aborigines		

[a]Territory as of 1998.
SOURCE: United Nations 1999.

Note

This work has been assisted by Pat Caldwell, Wendy Cosford, Elaine Hollings, and Bruce Missingham. It was funded by a grant from the Population Division of the Rockefeller Foundation.

References

Alam, Iqbal and John Cleland. 1981. "Illustrative analysis: Recent fertility trends in Sri Lanka," *WFS Scientific Reports*, no. 25. Voorburg: International Statistical Institute.

Ariès, Philippe. 1980. "Two successive motivations for the declining birth rate in the West," *Population and Development Review* 6, no. 4: 645–650.

Australian Bureau of Statistics. 1999. *Births 1998*. Canberra.

Australian Family Formation Project. 1972. *The 1971 Melbourne Survey: Distribution of Responses*. Canberra: Department of Demography, Australian National University.

Balfour, Marshall C., Roger F. Evans, Frank W. Notestein, and Irene B. Taeuber. 1950. *Public Health and Demography in the Far East: Report of a Survey Trip, September 13–December 13, 1948*. New York: Rockefeller Foundation.

Becker, Gary S. 1991. *A Treatise on the Family*. Enlarged edition. Cambridge, MA: Harvard University Press.

Berelson, Bernard, Richmond K. Anderson, Oscar Harkavy, John Maier, W. Parker Mauldin, and Sheldon J. Segal (eds.). 1966. *Family Planning and Population Programs: A Review of World Developments*. Chicago: University of Chicago Press.

Bongaarts, John and Griffith Feeney. 1998. "On the quantum and tempo of fertility," *Population and Development Review* 24, no. 2: 271–291.

Bongaarts, John and Susan Cotts Watkins. 1996. "Social interactions and contemporary fertility transitions," *Population and Development Review* 22, no. 4: 639–682.

Caldwell, Bruce. 1999. *Marriage in Sri Lanka: A Century of Change*. New Delhi: Hindustan.

Caldwell, John C. 1976. "Toward a restatement of demographic transition theory," *Population and Development Review* 2, nos. 3–4: 321–366.

———. 1977. "The economic rationality of high fertility: An investigation illustrated with Nigerian survey data," *Population Studies* 31, no. 1: 5–27.

———. 1982a. *Theory of Fertility Decline*. London: Academic Press.

———. 1982b. "Fertility control," in Economic and Social Commission for Asia and the Pacific, *Population of Australia*, Vol. 1. ESCAP Country Monograph no. 9. New York: United Nations, pp. 230–258.

———. 1993. "The Asian fertility revolution: Its implication for transition theories," in Richard Leete and Iqbal Alam (eds.), *The Revolution in Asian Fertility: Dimensions, Causes, and Implications*. Oxford: Clarendon, pp. 299–316.

———. 1998. "Malthus and the less developed world: The pivotal role of India," *Population and Development Review* 24, no. 4: 675–696.

———. 1999. "The delayed Western fertility decline: An examination of English-speaking countries," *Population and Development Review* 25, no. 3: 479–513.

———. 2001. "Aboriginal society and the global demographic transition," *Aboriginal History*, in press.

Caldwell, John C. and Pat Caldwell. 1984. "The family planning programme at the local level: A study of a village area in South India," in Gavin W. Jones (ed.), *Demographic Transition in Asia*. Singapore: Maruzen Asia, pp. 111–124.

———. 1987. "The cultural context of high fertility in sub-Saharan Africa," *Population and Development Review* 13, no. 3: 409–437.

———. 1988. "Is the Asian family planning program model suited to Africa?" *Studies in Family Planning* 19, no. 1: 19–28.

———. 1993. "The South African fertility decline," *Population and Development Review* 19, no. 2: 225–262.

Caldwell, John C., Pat Caldwell, Michael Bracher, and Gigi Santow. 1988. "The contemporary marriage and fertility revolutions in the West: The explanations provided by Australian participants," *Journal of the Australian Population Association* 5, no. 2: 113–145.

Caldwell, John C., Dot Campbell, Pat Caldwell, Lado Ruzicka, Wendy Cosford, Rita Packer, Janine Grocott, and Margaret Neill. 1976. *Towards an Understanding of Contemporary Demographic Change: A Report on Semi-Structured Interviews.* Canberra: Department of Demography, Australian National University.

Caldwell, John C., Indira Gajanayake, Bruce Caldwell, and Pat Caldwell. 1989. "Is marriage delay a multiphasic response to pressure for fertility decline? The case of Sri Lanka," *Journal of Marriage and the Family* 51: 337–351.

Caldwell, John C., K. H. W. Gaminiratne, Pat Caldwell, Soma de Silva, Bruce Caldwell, Nanda Weeraratne, and Padmini Silva. 1987. "The role of traditional fertility regulation in Sri Lanka," *Studies in Family Planning* 18, no. 1: 1–21.

Caldwell, John C., Barkat-e-Khuda, Bruce Caldwell, Indrani Pieris, and Pat Caldwell. 1999. "The Bangladesh fertility decline: An interpretation," *Population and Development Review* 25, no. 1: 67–84.

Caldwell, John C., P. H. Reddy, and Pat Caldwell. 1982. "The causes of demographic change in rural South India: A micro approach," *Population and Development Review* 8, no. 4: 689–727.

———. 1988. *The Causes of Demographic Change: Experimental Research in South India.* Madison: University of Wisconsin Press.

Caldwell, John C. and Helen Ware. 1973. "The evolution of family planning in Australia," *Population Studies* 27, no. 1: 7–31.

Caldwell, John C., Christabel Young, Helen Ware, Donald Lavis, and Anh-Thu Davis. 1973. "Australia: Knowledge, attitudes, and practice of family planning in Melbourne, 1971," *Studies in Family Planning* 4, no. 3: 49–59.

Campbell, Dorothy and Wendy Cosford. 1972. "Population policies and programs," report on a newspaper search project, 1920–1970. Demography Department, Australian National University, Canberra.

Carty, Winthrop B., Nancy V. Yinger, and Alicia Rosov. 1993. *Success in a Challenging Environment: Fertility Decline in Bangladesh.* Washington, DC: Population Reference Bureau.

Chowdhury, Osman H. 1985. "Conditions of fertility decline in developing countries: 1960–1980," *Asian Profile* 13, no. 5: 433–460.

Cleland, John, James F. Phillips, Sajeda Amin, and G. M. Kamal. 1994. *The Determinants of Reproductive Change in Bangladesh: Success in a Challenging Environment.* Washington, DC: World Bank.

Cleland, John and Christopher Wilson. 1987. "Demand theories of the fertility transition: An iconoclastic view," *Population Studies* 41, no. 1: 5–30.

Coale, A. J. 1973. "The demographic transition," in *International Population Conference, Liège, 1973*, vol. 1. Liège: IUSSP, pp. 53–72.

Cosford, Wendy, Margaret Neill, Janine Grocott, Pat Caldwell, and John C. Caldwell. 1976. "Semi-structured interviews of individuals: The Canberra survey and supplementary interviews," in Caldwell et al. 1976, pp. 55–115.

Cutright, Phillips. 1983. "The ingredients of recent fertility decline in developing countries," *International Family Planning Perspectives* 9, no. 4: 101–109.

Davis, Kingsley. 1937. "Reproductive institutions and the pressure for population," *Sociological Review* (July): 289–306. Reprinted as "Kingsley Davis on reproductive institutions and the pressure for population," *Population and Development Review* 23, no. 3 (1997): 611–624.

———. 1944. "Demographic fact and policy in India," *Milbank Memorial Fund Quarterly* 22, no. 3: 256–278.

———. 1986. "Low fertility in evolutionary perspective," in Davis, Bernstam, and Ricardo-Campbell 1986, pp. 48–65.

Davis, Kingsley, Mikhail S. Bernstam, and Rita Ricardo-Campbell (eds.). 1986. *Below-Replacement Fertility in Industrial Societies: Causes, Consequences, Policies,* Supplement to *Population and Development Review* 12.

Demeny, Paul. 1979. "On the end of the population explosion," *Population and Development Review* 5, no. 1: 141–162.

Easterlin, Richard A. 1973. "Relative economic status and the American fertility swing," in Eleanor B. Sheldon (ed.), *Family Economic Behavior: Problems and Prospects.* Philadelphia: Lippincott, pp. 170–223.

———. 1978. "The economics and sociology of fertility: A synthesis," in Charles Tilly (ed.), *Historical Studies of Changing Fertility.* Princeton: Princeton University Press, pp. 57–133.

Ehrlich, Paul R. 1968. *The Population Bomb.* New York: Ballantine Books.

Fernando, Dallas F. S. 1975. "Changing nuptiality patterns in Sri Lanka, 1901–1971," *Population Studies* 29, no. 2: 179–190.

Freedman, Ronald and Bernard Berelson. 1976. "The record of family planning programs," *Studies in Family Planning* 7, no. 1: 1–40.

Gray, Alan. 1983. "Aboriginal fertility in decline," Ph.D. thesis, Australian National University, Canberra.

Guttmacher, Alan F. 1966. "The United States medical profession and family planning," in Berelson et al. 1966, pp. 455–463.

Guzmán, José M. 1994. "The onset of fertility decline in Latin America," in Thérèse Locoh and Véronique Hertrich (eds.), *The Onset of Fertility Transition in Sub-Saharan Africa.* Liège: IUSSP, pp. 43–67.

Jaffe, A. J. 1992. *The First Immigrants from Asia: A Population History of North American Indians.* New York: Plenum.

Kelly, William R., Dudley L. Poston, and Phillips Cutright. 1983. "Determinants of fertility levels in developed countries: 1958–1978," *Social Science Research* 12: 87–108.

Khawaja, Mansoor A. 1985. "Trends and differentials in fertility," in Economic and Social Commission for Asia and the Pacific, *Population of New Zealand,* vol. 1. ESCAP Country Monograph no. 12. New York: United Nations, pp. 152–177.

Khuda, Barkat-e-, John C. Caldwell, Bruce Caldwell, Indrani Pieris, and Pat Caldwell. 1996. "The global fertility transition: New light from the Bangladesh experience," in *Seminar on Comparative Perspectives on Fertility Transition in South Asia, Rawalpindi/Islamabad, 17–19 December 1996: Papers,* vol. 2. Liège: IUSSP.

Kim, Taek Il and Syng Wook Kim. 1966. "Mass use of intra-uterine contraceptive devices in Korea," in Berelson et al. 1966, pp. 425–432.

Kunitz, Stephen J. 1994. *Disease and Social Diversity: The European Impact on the Health of Non-Europeans.* New York: Oxford University Press.

Lavis, Donald R. 1975. *Oral Contraception in Melbourne: An Investigation of the Growth in Use of Oral Contraceptives and Their Effect upon Fertility in Australia, 1961–1971.* Canberra: Department of Demography, Australian National University.

Lesthaeghe, Ron. 1983. "A century of demographic and cultural change in Western Europe: An exploration of underlying dimensions," *Population and Development Review* 9, no. 3: 411–435.

Mauldin, W. Parker and Bernard Berelson. 1978. "Conditions of fertility decline in developing countries, 1965–75," *Studies in Family Planning* 9, no. 5: 89–147.

Mauldin, W. Parker and Sheldon J. Segal. 1988. "Prevalence of contraceptive use: Trends and issues," *Studies in Family Planning* 19, no. 6: 335–353.

McDonald, Peter. 1997. "Gender equity, social institutions and the future of fertility," Working Papers in Demography. Canberra: Research School of Social Sciences, Australian National University.

Potts, Malcolm. 1997. "Sex and the birth rate: Human biology, demographic change, and access to fertility-regulation methods," *Population and Development Review* 23, no. 1: 1–39.

Pritchett, Lant H. 1994. "Desired fertility and the impact of population policies," *Population and Development Review* 20, no. 1: 1–55.

Robey, Bryant, Shea O. Rutstein, and Leo Morris. 1993. "The fertility decline in developing countries," *Scientific American* 269, no. 6: 60–67.

Romaniuc, A. 1987. "Transition from traditional high to modern low fertility: Canadian aboriginals," *Canadian Studies in Population* 14, no. 1: 69–88.

Ruzicka, Lado T. and John C. Caldwell. 1977. *The End of Demographic Transition in Australia*. Canberra: Australian National University.

Ryder, Norman B. and Charles F. Westoff. 1967. "The United States: The pill and the birth rate, 1960–1965," *Studies in Family Planning* No. 20: 1–3.

———. 1971. *Reproduction in the United States*. Princeton: Princeton University Press.

Santow, M. Gigi. 1993. "Coitus interruptus in the twentieth century," *Population and Development Review* 19, no. 4: 767–792.

Sarkar, N. K. 1957. *The Demography of Ceylon*. Colombo: Ceylon Government Press.

Sceats, Janet and Ian Pool. 1985. "Fertility regulation," in Economic and Social Commission for Asia and the Pacific, *Population of New Zealand*, vol. 1. ESCAP Country Monograph no. 12. New York: United Nations, pp. 178–192.

Schultz, T. Paul. 1986. "The value and allocation of time in high-income countries: Implications for fertility," in Davis, Bernstam, and Ricardo-Campbell 1986, pp. 87–108.

Sherris, Jacqueline D. (ed.). 1985. "The impact of family planning programs on fertility," *Population Reports*, Series J, no. 29: 733–771.

Snipp, C. Matthew. 1996. "The size and distribution of the American Indian population: Fertility, mortality, migration, and residence," in Gary D. Sandefur, Ronald R. Rindfuss, and Barney Cohen (eds.), *Changing Numbers, Changing Needs: American Indian Demography and Public Health*. Washington, DC: National Academy Press.

Szreter, Simon. 1996. *Fertility, Class and Gender in Britain, 1860–1940*. Cambridge: Cambridge University Press.

Tsui, Amy Ong and Donald J. Bogue. 1978. "Declining world fertility: Trends, causes, and implications," *Population Bulletin* 33, no. 4.

United Nations. 1999. *World Population Prospects: The 1998 Revision*, vol. 1, *Comprehensive Tables*. New York.

Van de Kaa, Dirk J. 1987. "Europe's second demographic transition," *Population Bulletin* 42, no. 1.

Van de Walle, Etienne and Helmut V. Muhsam. 1995. "Fatal secrets and the French fertility transition," *Population and Development Review* 21, no. 2: 261–279.

Westoff, Charles F. 1975. "The yield of the imperfect: The 1970 National Fertility Study," *Demography* 12, no. 4: 573–580.

———. 1983. "Fertility decline in the West: Causes and prospects," *Population and Development Review* 9, no. 1: 99–104.

Westoff, Charles F. and Norman B. Ryder. 1977. *The Contraceptive Revolution*. Princeton: Princeton University Press.

Willis, Robert J. 1973. "A new approach to the economic theory of fertility behavior," in T. W. Schultz (ed.), *New Economic Approaches to Fertility: Proceedings of a Conference June 8–9, 1972, Sponsored by the National Bureau of Economic Research and the Population Council*. Chicago: Chicago University Press, pp. S14–S64.

Wulf, Deirdre. 1982. "Low fertility in Europe: A report from the 1981 IUSSP meeting," *International Family Planning Perspectives* 8, no. 2: 63–69.

Comment: Globalization and Theories of Fertility Decline

CHARLES HIRSCHMAN

BEGINNING WITH THE pioneering works of Warren Thompson (1929), Kingsley Davis (1945), and Frank Notestein (1953), demographers have been tinkering with demographic transition theory for the better part of the last century. Relative to most of what passes for theory in the social sciences, transition theory is a remarkable achievement. The fundamental thesis that modernization and declining mortality lead, after some lag, to a decline in fertility is the working axiom of most empirical researchers in the field. At the same time, many students and members of the educated public are acquainted with the general idea of demographic transition theory, if not with the theoretical details or empirical applications.

Within the field of demography, however, the status of demographic transition theory is fiercely contested. The many shortcomings of the theory have given rise to a variety of alternative perspectives on both historical and contemporary fertility declines (Cleland and Wilson 1987; Knodel and van de Walle 1979; McDonald 1993). A new theoretical synthesis is likely to emerge in the coming years, but the scope and content of a new theory remain on the distant horizon. In the meantime, researchers continue to study the fertility transitions in many parts of the world that are still incomplete and the others that are just beginning. Considerable work is necessary to examine the many novel ideas and hypotheses from alternative theoretical perspectives that have not been subjected to empirical tests.

In his chapter in this volume, John Caldwell asks whether commonalities might explain the global fertility declines that began in the 1960s and 1970s. The beginnings of sustained fertility declines in Asia and Latin America coincided with the rapid reduction of childbearing in many countries of the industrialized West from the baby boom highs in the 1950s to below-replacement levels by the 1970s. Caldwell also notes the parallel with contemporaneous rapid reduction in fertility among indigenous minorities in the United States, Canada, Australia, and New Zealand. He suggests that the spread of new contraceptive technology (the pill in particular) and ideological shifts contributed to the global declines in fertility during this period.

Without diminishing the value of Caldwell's critical insights, the dilemma for the field is how to move from post hoc interpretations based on selected observations to tests of rival hypotheses. Bivariate correlations or selected associations cannot make or break demographic transition theory, nor can case studies reveal broad-scale historical patterns. The current research literature tells us that many factors, including socioeconomic conditions, cultural receptivity, new technology, ideology, and organized family planning programs, can influence fertility levels and fertility decline in particular situations. The discovery of the relative importance of these factors and how they interact in different times and places will require a less polemical assessment of the strengths and weaknesses of demographic transition theory and a different analytical framework than has guided the field in the past.

Explaining fertility transitions

The classical model of the demographic transition emphasizes socioeconomic development and modernization as causal forces. When only modest correlations between socioeconomic variables and the timing of fertility declines were initially reported, some researchers immediately concluded that demographic transition theory had been proven false. The absence of common socioeconomic thresholds for the onset of fertility declines across societies and the occasional evidence of cultural diffusion of fertility behavior within and across countries are important findings (Cleland 1985; Cleland and Wilson 1987; Lesthaeghe 1983; Lesthaeghe and Surkyn 1988). These results, however, do not necessarily mean that socioeconomic change has no causal role in fertility declines, only that bivariate associations of socioeconomic variables and indicators of fertility can be very low.

Much of the controversy over the appropriate theoretical framework for fertility change arises from assumptions that all fertility transitions follow a similar path and that the same causal variables are present everywhere. The research literature shows, however, that initial fertility levels and the mechanisms of fertility decline have varied widely. Fertility in late-nineteenth-century Europe was already at moderate levels. The European marriage system ensured that average family size was only about 4 to 5 births per couple even without control of marital fertility. Further fertility decline required the adoption of birth control within marriage. This type of fertility transition exemplifies the model in which knowledge of birth control and legitimation for its adoption were the primary prerequisites for sustained fertility declines. Once the demand for smaller family size was present in many European societies, the new information and change in values spread first along paths of cultural and linguistic homogeneity (Anderson 1986; Watkins 1987).

Pretransition fertility levels in the rest of the world were typically much higher than those in Europe, ranging from 6 to 8 births per woman. In contrast to the situation in premodern Europe, there was simply more room in the fertility regimes of Asia, Africa, and Latin America for a wider range of forces to shape reproductive behavior in the early stages of contemporary fertility declines. In these societies, reproduction was also regulated by cultural patterns, but by different means such as infanticide, taboos on sexual intercourse at certain periods, and terminal abstinence from intercourse after becoming a grandparent. The early signs of fertility transition in these societies might result from changes in marriage patterns or spousal separation, and not necessarily from determined efforts to control fertility within marriage. Changes in other proximate determinants of fertility, such as breastfeeding, could also produce sizable fluctuations in fertility prior to the sustained declines that identify a clear case of fertility transition.

Much of the recent empirical and theoretical literature has sought to present a more balanced assessment of causal factors, including socioeconomic development, that can explain fertility declines (Friedlander, Schellekens, and Ben-Moshe 1991; Kirk 1996; Lee, Galloway, and Hammel 1994). In their survey of modern fertility transitions, Bongaarts and Watkins show a very strong relationship between a summary measure of socioeconomic development and fertility declines from the 1960s to the 1980s, although there was no single threshold (1996: Figure 2). Indeed, there was evidence of an increasingly lower socioeconomic threshold for declining fertility in the 1980s relative to the 1960s (ibid.: Figure 3). One of their most intriguing findings is that the level of socioeconomic development is strongly related to the pace of fertility decline even when it is unrelated to the onset of fertility declines (ibid.: Figure 7). Karen Mason (1997) cogently argued that much of the debate on the causes of fertility transitions is over variations in the proximate conditions that influence the timing of fertility declines, and that there is considerable agreement over the long-term historical factors, especially mortality decline, that have led to fertility transitions.

I have previously argued (1994) that the portrayal of demographic transition theory as a universal, unilineal, ahistorical model of modernization and fertility decline is too simplistic. Fertility, and population growth more generally, respond to societal pressures that threaten the survival and well-being of human communities (Davis 1963; Wilson and Airey 1999). Socioeconomic development is surely a major force influencing demographic processes in modern times, but it is not the only source of pressures that may generate demographic, technological, and social change.

Toward a new analytical framework of fertility decline

The study of fertility transitions typically excludes much of the temporal variance in fertility behavior. Fertility transition is identified as a decline from a plateau of "natural fertility" leading to replacement-level fertility within a relatively short time.[1] This framework excludes the declines in fertility that are not sustained and that do not culminate in replacement-level fertility. Because natural fertility levels during the pretransition era can vary by a factor of two (from 4 to 8 births per woman), this ignores a considerable range of variation between and within societies. The logic is, however, that these variations from moderately high to very high fertility are caused by culture and customs that are unrelated to motivations to control fertility.

This peculiar definition originated with specific conditions that prevailed in Western Europe in the late nineteenth century. In this setting, fertility, and population growth more generally, were limited by delayed marriage, moderate levels of celibacy, patterns of overseas migration, and child abandonment in foundling homes (Davis 1963). One of the few intermediate variables not controlled was marital fertility (but, see Friedlander and Okun 1995). As population pressure continued to increase on households striving for upward mobility, a momentous change occurred in the popular *mentalité*, leading to the rejection of traditional and religious authority that circumscribed family limitation within marriage. Given the historical significance of this shift, and given that it led to replacement-level fertility within a short time, it is understandable why other societal efforts to limit population growth were not considered elements of fertility control, but only fluctuations associated with natural fertility.

The definition of controlled fertility—the historic break from natural fertility—relies on conscious planning as evidenced by parity-specific behavior that stopped (or delayed) childbearing after desired family size was reached (Henry 1961). Such behavior is probably necessary to reach replacement-level fertility, but this does not mean that less deliberate means of family-size regulation were not responding to similar pressures. For example, a shortage of agricultural land in densely settled rural areas might have put pressure on families to limit the number of offspring. Initially, families may have responded by out-migration and delayed marriage, and only after these possibilities were exhausted did they adopt parity-specific means to limit births in marriage. Although this last means was distinctive in that it involved conscious planning, a comprehensive analysis of demographic change requires consideration of all means used to reduce population growth in response to social or economic conditions.

This shift in focus is critical for studying the wave of late-twentieth-century fertility transitions, where the plateau of pretransitional fertility might be 6 to 8 births per woman and not the 4 to 5 births per woman that characterized the European case. In circumstances where most women desire fewer children, the simple availability of birth control may lead to a continuous and rapid change in behavior resulting in low fertility. However, in higher-fertility settings, there are many more possible routes to lower fertility than simple reductions in marital fertility. The reproductive responses to social change in many modernizing societies may be numerous, with possibilities for short-term fluctuations, lags and stalls, and even rises in fertility.

Consider a plausible scenario in which the forces of modernization have multiple and contradictory effects on fertility through different mechanisms. The expansion of schooling may influence more women to postpone marriage and childbearing, thereby lowering fertility among women in their teens and 20s (if the postponement is temporary, there may be a subsequent rise as births are "made up"). A decrease in infant and child mortality may also reduce fertility, but through a different mechanism and at a different stage of the reproductive life course. If families reach their desired number of children at an earlier stage than was common in prior generations and this occurs in a context with limited resources for bequests (such as agricultural land), there may be pressures for "stopping" childbearing. Other aspects of modernization may work in the opposite direction. Increased female employment outside the household economy may lead to a decline in breastfeeding and thus shorter birth intervals. The growth of cities without extensive opportunities for stable employment may lead to increased premarital sexual behavior and births. A rapid rise in real incomes (perhaps caused by movement to a frontier region or a rise in export prices for petty commodity producers) may lead to a relaxation of traditional constraints on fertility such as postponed marriage.

Considering the range of possibilities for change in reproductive behavior in societies experiencing modernization, bivariate associations between socioeconomic status and measures of fertility cannot be considered serious tests of theoretical propositions. At a minimum, it is necessary to decompose changes in fertility by age group and marital status in order to observe the likely intervening mechanisms (Hirschman 1985; Hirschman and Guest 1990a). Much more informative are studies that trace the impact of social change on fertility through proximate determinants, such as contraceptive use and breastfeeding (DaVanzo and Haaga 1982).

Empirical research on fertility transitions should incorporate two additional elements in order to meaningfully test hypotheses from demographic transition theory (and alternative theories). First, historical paths of fertility transitions must be tracked over time, rather than relying on cross-sectional comparisons or aggregate temporal trends. Even with all the investment in demographic data collection over the last generation, there are relatively few cases (societies) for which we have comparable, high-quality survey data for several time points. The primary data used by Caldwell and by Bongaarts and Watkins (1996) are aggregate estimates compiled from varied sources and adjusted by the United Nations. Although most research on fertility is based on survey data (collected at one point in time), theories of fertility decline postulate that *changes* in social structure and institutions are the primary determinants of change in individual behavior (Smith 1989).

The other important element of an improved analytical framework would be a clearer specification of the hypothesized impact of independent variables on fertility and family planning behavior. In many empirical analyses, any available socioeconomic variable is considered equivalent to (and interchangeable with) any other. As noted earlier, there could be contradictory influences from the many societal and individual changes experienced during an era of modernization. Even a single variable, such as education, can have a variety of potential impacts on fertility depending on the time period, the unit of analysis, and the intervening mechanisms (Cochrane 1979).

In my own research, I have tried to find appropriate indicators for the widely accepted major structural forces that influence family formation and fertility, namely infant and child mortality, the status and roles of women, and the costs and benefits of children (Hirschman and Guest 1990b; Hirschman and Young 2000). Because these forces are elements of social structure and not necessarily embodied in individual characteristics, this research strategy faces enormous empirical challenges (Casterline, this volume).

Another critical issue is the impact of policy—family planning programs in particular—on fertility. It is ironic that demographers are still debating the impact of public intervention on fertility trends even as fertility is beginning to decline in most countries around the world. The assessment of the impact of family planning programs on fertility has advanced only modestly from the pioneering work of Freedman and Berelson (1976), who reported that countries with stronger family planning effort had more rapid fertility declines, net of socioeconomic development. Although the basic methodology of this approach has been refined over the last two decades, two major flaws remain. The first is that the measurement of family planning effort may well be influenced by fertility declines (expert evaluations of family planning may be based on perceptions of success). The second problem is that family planning programs (especially successful ones) may be endogenous to socioeconomic development. Some empirical studies have found a modest impact of family planning programs on fertility (Gertler and Molyneaux 1994; Prichett 1994), though flaws in these studies have been clearly identified (Bongaarts 1994; Knowles, Akin, and Guilkey 1994).

The problems of evaluating family planning programs are those that affect all assessments of public policy. Without conducting experiments, it is impossible to conclude with certainty that the policy—as opposed to other social forces—has affected the outcome. In an influential study conducted more than three decades ago, Freedman and Takeshita (1969) carried out an experiment to assess whether the presence of a family planning program (and the methods used by the program) had an impact on contraceptive behavior.[2] A social experiment, as opposed to those conducted in laboratories, however, cannot be completely controlled. Information can flow from the experimental area to the control area and actors rarely perform in accordance with the script of experimental design. Studies of clinic-based data—the other major source of program evaluation studies—are invariably clouded by the problem of "selectivity." These problems have led many in the field of program evaluation (not just in family planning assessment) to conclude that little is to be gained from additional refinements in evaluation methodology.

Considerable room exists for advances in the assessment of family planning programs (and other public policies) in research on the fertility declines that have occurred over the last few decades. One possibility for innovative research is to combine population data from censuses and surveys with geo-coded data on the locations, activities, and budgets of institutions, such as health clinics and hospitals. Using statistical techniques that model the patterns of temporal and spatial change, researchers could use these data to measure the diffusion of influence on fertility from clinics and hospitals (and other institutions). Modeling spatial patterns of diffusion presents great methodological and statistical challenges (Rosero-Bixby and Casterline 1993). Since information can spread in a nonlinear fashion and population migration is an alternative means for the geographic spread of social change, it would be necessary to assemble data over very large areas for long time periods. Although the appropriate models of spatial change and diffusion have not yet become part of normal science in demography, there is a high likelihood of payoff from the exploration of the emerging methods of spatial statistics from other disciplines.

As more evidence of emerging fertility transitions is reported from Africa and South Asia, public interest in "population problems" and demographic science is likely to decline. It is tempting to claim that the "crisis" of rapid population growth will persist because of population momentum and that the speed of the transition is still of critical concern. But many other "crises" are competing for attention on the public agenda, and the news of progress in reducing population growth means that attention will shift to other issues.

Even as public attention shifts away from studies of fertility transitions, it is important for demographers to continue with the incomplete work on our empirical and theoretical studies of fertility decline. The extraordinary efforts in data collection and the development of new methods of measurement over the last generation have brought impressive results. But scientific progress comes slowly, and promising theoretical syntheses are always subject to debate and repeated empirical studies before their acceptance. My guess is that there will be a widely accepted theory of fertility transition before the world reaches zero population growth, but that it will be a close race. We are too close to both goals to allow any slackening of effort.

Notes

1 Coale (1973: 57) observes that the origin of the European marriage system in the Middle Ages—the shift away from universal and early marriage—could be labeled the Malthusian transition and that the declines in marital fertility in Europe, beginning in the 1870s, could be labeled the neo-Malthusian transition.

2 Other family planning experiments have been conducted in Bangladesh (Phillips et al. 1982), Egypt (Kelley et al. 1982; Stycos et al. 1988), and Ghana (Binka et al. 1995).

References

Anderson, Barbara A. 1986. "Regional and cultural factors in the decline of marital fertility in Europe," in Ansley J. Coale and Susan Cotts Watkins (eds.), *The Decline of Fertility in Europe*. Princeton: Princeton University Press, pp. 293–314.

Binka, Fred N., Alex Nazzar, and James F. Phillips. 1995. "The Navrongo Community Health and Family Planning Project," *Studies in Family Planning* 26: 121–139.

Bongaarts, John. 1994. "The impact of population policies: Comment," *Population and Development Review* 20: 616–620.

Bongaarts, John and Susan Cotts Watkins. 1996. "Social interactions and contemporary fertility transitions," *Population and Development Review* 22: 639–682.

Caldwell, John C. 1982. *Theory of Fertility Decline*. London: Academic Press.

Cleland, John. 1985. "Marital fertility decline in developing countries: Theories and the evidence," in John Cleland and John Hobcraft (eds.), *Reproductive Change in Developing Countries: Insights from the World Fertility Survey*. Oxford: Oxford University Press, pp. 223–252.

Cleland, John and Christopher Wilson. 1987. "Demand theories of the fertility transition: An iconoclastic view," *Population Studies* 41: 5–30.

Coale, Ansley J. 1973. "The demographic transition," in *International Population Conference, Liège 1973*, Vol. 1. Liège: International Union for the Scientific Study of Population, pp. 53–73.

Cochrane, Susan. 1979. *Fertility and Education: What Do We Really Know?* Baltimore: Johns Hopkins University Press.

DaVanzo, Julie and J. Haaga. 1982. "Anatomy of fertility decline: Peninsular Malaysia, 1950–1976," *Population Studies* 36: 373–393.

Davis, Kingsley. 1945. "The world demographic transition," *The Annals of the American Academy of Political and Social Science* 237: 1–11.

———. 1963. "The theory of change and response in modern demographic history," *Population Index* 29: 345–366.
Freedman, Ronald and Bernard Berelson. 1976. "The record of family planning programs," *Studies in Family Planning* 7(1): 1–40.
Freedman, Ronald and John Y. Takeshita. 1969. *Family Planning in Taiwan: An Experiment in Social Change*. Princeton: Princeton University Press.
Friedlander, Dov and Barbara S. Okun. 1995. "Pretransition marital fertility variation over time: Was there deliberate control in England?" *Journal of Family History* 20: 139–158.
Friedlander, Dov, Jona Schellekens, and Eliahu Ben-Moshe. 1991. "The transition from high to low marital fertility: Cultural or socioeconomic determinants?" *Economic Development and Cultural Change* 39: 331–351.
Gertler, Paul J. and John W. Molyneaux. 1994. "How economic development and family planning programs combined to reduce Indonesian fertility," *Demography* 31: 33–63.
Henry, Louis. 1961. "Some data on natural fertility," *Eugenics Quarterly* 8: 81–91.
Hirschman, Charles. 1985. "Premarital socioeconomic roles and the timing of family formation: A comparative study of five Asian societies," *Demography* 22: 35–59.
———. 1994. "Why fertility changes," *Annual Review of Sociology* 20: 203–233.
Hirschman, Charles and Philip Guest. 1990a. "The emerging demographic transitions of Southeast Asia," *Population and Development Review* 16: 121–152.
———. 1990b. "Multilevel models of fertility determination in four Southeast Asian countries: 1970 and 1980," *Demography* 27: 369–396.
Hirschman, Charles and Yih-Jin Young. 2000. "Social context and fertility decline in Southeast Asia: 1968–70 to 1980–90," in C. Y. Cyrus Chu and Ronald Lee (eds.), *Population and Economic Change in East Asia*. Supplement to *Population and Development Review* 26: 11–39.
Kelley, Allen C., Atef M. Khalifa, and M. Nabil El-Khorazaty. 1982. *Population and Development in Rural Egypt*. Durham, NC: Duke University Press.
Kirk, Dudley. 1996. "Demographic transition theory," *Population Studies* 50: 361–387.
Knodel, John and Etienne van de Walle. 1979. "Lessons from the past: Policy implications of historical population studies," *Population and Development Review* 5: 217–245.
Knowles, James C., John S. Akin, and David K. Guilkey. 1994. "The impact of population policies: Comment," *Population and Development Review* 20: 611–615.
Lee, Ronald D., Patrick R. Galloway, and Eugene A. Hammel. 1994. "Fertility decline in Prussia: Estimating influences on supply, demand, and degree of control," *Demography* 31: 347–373.
Lesthaeghe, Ron. 1983. "A century of demographic and cultural change in Western Europe: An exploration of underlying dimensions," *Population and Development Review* 9: 411–435.
Lesthaeghe, Ron and Johan Surkyn. 1988. "Cultural dynamics and economic theories of fertility change," *Population and Development Review* 14: 1–45.
Mason, Karen Oppenheim. 1997. "Explaining fertility transitions," *Demography* 34: 443–454.
McDonald, Peter. 1993. "Fertility transition hypotheses," in Richard Leete and Iqbal Alam (eds.), *The Revolution in Asian Fertility: Dimensions, Causes, and Implications*. Oxford: Clarendon Press, pp. 3–14.
Notestein, F. W. 1953. "Economic problems of population change," in *Proceedings of the Eighth International Conference of Agricultural Economists*. New York: Oxford University Press, pp. 13–31.
Phillips, James F. et al. 1982. "The demographic impact of the Family Planning–Health Services Project in Matlab, Bangladesh," *Studies in Family Planning* 13: 131–140.
Pritchett, Lant H. 1994. "Desired fertility and the impact of population policies," *Population and Development Review* 20: 1–55.
Rosero-Bixby, Luis and John B. Casterline. 1993. "Modelling diffusion effects in fertility transition," *Population Studies* 47: 147–167.

Smith, Herbert L. 1989. "Integrating theory and research on the institutional determinants of fertility," *Demography* 26: 171–184.

Stycos, J. Mayone et al. 1988. *Community Development and Family Planning: An Egyptian Experiment*. Boulder: Westview Press.

Thompson, Warren. 1929. "Population," *American Journal of Sociology* 34: 959–975.

United Nations. 1999. *World Population Prospects: The 1998 Revision*. New York.

Watkins, Susan Cotts. 1987. "The fertility transition: Europe and the third world compared," *Sociological Forum* 2: 645–673.

Wilson, Chris and Pauline Airey. 1999. "How can a homeostatic perspective enhance demographic transition theory?" *Population Studies* 53: 117–128.

PART TWO

INSTITUTIONAL FACTORS BEARING ON FERTILITY TRANSITION

Government and Fertility in Transitional and Post-Transitional Societies

GEOFFREY MCNICOLL

THE STUDY OF human fertility, informed by a welter of household survey data, is focused on family and individual behavior and on the ("proximate") biological and behavioral components into which reproduction can be analyzed. There is a complementary view of fertility that, in contrast, has been relatively neglected. This is fertility seen as part of the core generic problem of societal management—where the focus is not on micro-level conditions, preferences, and decisions but on the fertility consequences, whether recognized or not, of how a society organizes and governs itself. This alternative perspective is my subject.

In some respects, it is a return to the interests of the classical population theorists. There is much good sense about it in Malthus. Subsequently, explanations of demographic change increasingly left the state in the background. For example, demographic transition theory ties fertility decline to economic and social, not political, development. When admitted, government roles are confined to the programmatic—although they are sometimes then acclaimed. Only in post-transition regimes, with societies facing drastically *low* fertility, is the state routinely brought back in.

There was some justification for this narrow and selective attention to government. The milestones of the development process were indexes of economic and social attainment: income, literacy, health, and the like. Fertility was a natural addition to the list. The indexes moved not in lockstep, but in a ragged group (see Chenery and Syrquin 1975). In contrast, political circumstances—form of government, administrative reach, delimitation of the private sphere—seemed more variable. Even in the more economically advanced societies, material progress and low fertility apparently could be attained under widely different political regimes. This justification such as it was, however, has been eroding for some time. The dismal experience of "failed" states in the third world, the spectacular collapse of Communism in the second, and the general retreat from statism in the first, have suggested a closer connection between political structures and economic outcomes than had formerly been accepted. A political connection to demographic outcomes might exist as well.

Government is not, of course, a simple thing. It is both an endogenous element in the social system and a quasi-exogenous agent of change. Neither aspect captures the whole: government is more than a mere creature of interest groups in the society, but much less than an independent, rational entity engaged in the design and execution of public policy. And government is itself a constellation of interests and capabilities, with vaguely defined and mutually incompatible objectives, its perceptions and procedures influenced by a particular historical experience. Fertility sometimes appears prominently on its radar screen, eliciting alarm and forceful action; more often it is no more than a remote blur. Government response to fertility levels that are seen as too high or too low is typically hesitant, clumsy, and often, no doubt, futile. At the same time, fertility may be strongly influenced inadvertently by government actions taken with no demographic intent.

My aim in this chapter is to explore the scope and nature of government influence on fertility, whether deliberate or inadvertent. I start with a sketch of fertility change as a "natural" accompaniment of social and economic development. Government stays in the margin of such an account, at various stages a propagandist on population matters and a manager of family planning programs—shifting, in low-fertility settings, to promoter of vaguely family-friendly legislation and welfare-state institutions. It is portrayed at one extreme as distantly (and toothlessly) signaling its preferred demographic regime, at the other as actively modifying fertility outcomes to accord with a declared social interest—though doing so with full respect for individual preferences. Neither portrait is helpful. In any state, the scope and nature of the government's influence on fertility is set by major features of the polity, irrespective of policy intentions in the matter. And in addition to programs explicitly directed at changing fertility—the effectiveness of which governments are prone to overestimate—there is a wide range of other government actions that probably impinge on fertility. These considerations are discussed in the second and third sections below. I will deal mainly with government influence on fertility over the conventional course of development in the modern period (for simplicity, the twentieth century), but touch also on the post-transition situation of very low fertility. Finally, I consider whether any of the foregoing potentially contributes to the desideratum of an enriched fertility theory—in particular, whether a political perspective can potentially offer a more seamless view of fertility determination, without the sharp disjunction between a theory of transition and a (yet-to-emerge) theory of low fertility.

Fertility change: A background sketch

Consider the process of fertility transition embedded in a society, economy, and culture, but, for the time being, leaving government aside.

Society and fertility: The classical picture

The "classical" account of fertility decline refers to the economic and social transformation wrought by industrialization and urbanization. There are new resources and technologies, some of them yielding improved survivorship rates; shifts in the legal and political order; changing values about family and authority; even anticipations based on awareness of change elsewhere. Perhaps most important, there is an opening up of the social and economic "space" around families and individuals—wider cultural horizons and greater opportunities for mobility, both social and geographic. People seek to maintain or improve their relative positions in a society that is now characterized by new status-linked consumption patterns and new requirements for investment in human capital. New labor market opportunities, especially for women, and rising consumption and investment demands, when translated into effects on the utilities and costs of children, prove strongly antinatalist. In effect, people find that the game has changed around them and they have no alternative but to play by the new rules.

Judith Blake (1972b) has given a cogent depiction of the Western fertility transition in these terms. She was of course writing in a well-cultivated vein of thinking on the subject, dating back to Malthus and virtually a commonplace by the end of the nineteenth century. The fertility link is captured in Arsène Dumont's awkward metaphor of "social capillarity." F. W. Taussig (1911: Ch. 53), in a textbook that was the Samuelson of its day, attributed fertility decline to "awakened ambition of the individual...":

> The causes of the declining birth rate are to be found in the intellectual and material forces which have so wonderfully stirred the people of western Europe during the last century: the spread of education, newspapers and books; cheap movement by railway and steamship; the stirring of stagnant populations by the new modes of employment, by large scale production and the factory system, by the changes through emigration.

Marital fertility was dropping "because parents are solicitous not only to maintain, but to raise, the social and economic position of their children." In the United States, "the influence of free institutions and of free opportunities is to lessen, possibly to destroy, the caste-like character of social classes.... [T]he leaven of social and economic ambition slowly but surely affects them. It makes well-nigh certain a relaxation of the rate of growth in population" (ibid.).

There may have been something structurally special about Northwest European families (and East Asian families—see Greenhalgh 1988) that facilitated this mobility–fertility connection. South Asian and African fertility transitions, some have argued, have been impeded by the weakness of the nuclear family as a solidary or budgetary unit. Economic opportunity itself, however, is a powerful incentive for sloughing off extended kin-ties as their social security value lessens.

In some accounts of fertility transition, development is identified with a progressive relaxation of social control over families and individuals. There may indeed be a perception within the society of increasing freedom in personal and social behavior, associated with decay of the kind of informal neighborhood surveillance that is a feature of community life in traditional settings and with the opening of new routes of social mobility. But the shift is away from a geographic dimension of control, not from the fact of control. Spatial relocation and long-distance communication allow a reassignment of group affiliations and obscure the resulting patterns of behavioral conformity; the patterns are still there. Thus, prosperous low-fertility societies are not characterized by a high variance in completed family size but by a tight clustering of size options. In effect, the family has been reconfigured to mean one or two children—or none—with social pressures realigned accordingly. Family sizes above three become almost deviant. Only in a few outlier subcultures is group support for high child numbers to be found, with that behavior becoming one marker of their peculiarity. A satisfactory theory of fertility transition must encompass the factors behind this reconfiguration.

It is difficult to describe this perspective on social change without appearing to make "society" into a conscious, deliberating entity. That is of course absurd. The social pressures bearing on demographic behavior are enmeshed in inherited institutional forms conveying societal interests (and perhaps, as some would argue, biological interests) in survival and continuity, and are likely to be barely recognized. Moreover, they are not just features of premodern or developing countries, vanishing with prosperity; they are realities of social life. Blake (1972a) was specifically including the post–World War II United States when she wrote:

> [R]eproduction and replacement, like other societal functions, require an organized allocation of human and material resources. Societies have resolved this problem of resource allocation by means of diffused control mechanisms (rather than a government planning board, for example), but the mechanisms are nonetheless quite palpably there. And they involve the individual in an articulated and coercive set of constraints.

Her worry at the time was with the "coercive pronatalism" built into a familistic culture but unrecognized in discussions of population policy. In the last quarter-century, the "palpable mechanisms" that once held fertility well above replacement in the developed world seem to have corroded, leaving others that validate one-child families and childlessness.

Social groups do have a place in the classical picture: fertility is in some measure determined by and within them. They are the locus of values and sanctions that influence the various constituent behaviors in family formation and may in effect be repositories of particular arrays of knowledge and myth. In some cases they might appropriately be seen as subcultures. I do not mean to exaggerate the extent of conformism here, or to downplay the role of individual agency. Individual decisions are ultimately what matter, and individual interests, particularly economic interests, will nearly always have a significant effect on them. Group norms are themselves constructed and reconstructed from overlays of actual behaviors and their accompanying rationalizations, and in consequence are never as rigid or as current as sometimes painted. Moreover, individuals can to some degree adjust their normative surroundings by shifting or reweighting their membership affiliations. A familiar example is the formal constancy but diminishing effect of certain religious prescriptions on sexual morality, as adherents choose other sources of moral legitimation in that domain. However, the scope for such adjustments is itself a societal characteristic, constricted in authoritarian settings and expanding along with the growth and elaboration of civil society.

Microeconomics, cognition, and fertility

The economic account of fertility decline covers much of the same ground but is somewhat starker. The direct costs of children increase as parents recognize the growing importance of human capital in the new dispensation, requiring much greater expenditure per child—and with fewer options to spread the burden over kin. Child care, like other nonmarket, time-intensive activities, is seen to have a rising opportunity cost. At the same time, distant economic returns from children in the form of support in old age look insecure. Families and individuals contemplating their reproductive lives conclude that they can do better with fewer children. Improvements in the knowledge and affordability of effective birth control ease the behavioral change.

The economic modeling literature presents stylized pictures of the process. One-period household models show how fertility decisions (and mortality outcomes) might be expected to change with increases in the value of time, working through changes in wages and labor participation and investment in health and education. This microeconomic picture can be given a time dimension by drawing on parallel work on overlapping-generation growth models, which relate fertility levels to the intergenerational transfers that are needed to meet consumption needs in childhood and old age. (See Willis 1998 for a synthesis of this research.) But such models, powerful as they are conceptually and, to a lesser degree, empirically, do not exhaust the subject of fertility determination. In many cases, indeed, it can be argued that the model, once it has been set out, and providing its assumptions on family structure remain valid, can be "folded up" as a taken-for-granted component of the larger picture (see Ben-Porath 1974). Attention can then turn elsewhere: to the dynamics of change in the social structure—as in the classical view outlined earlier—and to the perceptions and valuations of the factors entering individual decisions.

These perceptions and valuations warrant further mention. Not bothering to specify them or to consider how they might be formed is partly economists' shorthand—taking it as self-evident, for example, that price effects are filtered through a preconceptual and informational penumbra—but partly too it is economists' disciplinary conviction that such complications do not count for much.

Can the cultural or "ideational" environment be an autonomous source of behavioral change? Anyone but a thoroughgoing materialist would concede that fertility determinants are both material and ideal, however contentious are views about the balance and the degree of separability between them. On the side of cultural determination, the process of secularization and growing individual autonomy is seen as a major factor driving the so-called first demographic transition in the West, with external systems of authority and morality losing force (see Lesthaeghe 1983). The second transition—the continued drop in the fertility of already prosperous societies to well below replacement levels—is linked to the spread of postmaterialist values (Inglehart's term), notably the goal of individual self-fulfillment (see Lesthaeghe 1995; van de Kaa 1996). Of course, cultural change has an institutional manifestation: the former systems of morality were not ethereal beliefs but actual structures of power—a confluence exemplified by the Inquisition and *auto da fé*. The process of change can be seen as the slow emergence of the concept of a private domain—an arena of beliefs and behaviors that are allowed to be outside the concern of external authority. By and large, family life came to lie within this domain. As tolerance of diversity expanded in postindustrial times, de facto privacy was accorded to a still-wider range of formerly public individual behavior—though the private domain was nonetheless transparent to market forces, making for convergent fertility outcomes.

This makes an appealing picture of liberal development, but is something of a caricature. What counts as private is always subject to contestation, particularly where it involves sex and reproductive behavior. And beyond explicit interventions, behavior in the private sphere is still subject to social and cultural pressures from the surrounding society.

To recognize cultural influence is not to elevate "ideational factors" and diffusion as a preferred explanation of fertility change. As investigations of technological change make clear, there are always many more ideas around than are ever turned into practical application. What determines the matter is the *market* for ideas: receptivity to change (where path dependence may enter) and, to some degree, fortuity. An application can always be traced back to an idea; hence the idea must have diffused. But that is hardly adequate as theory. Inadequacy is the greater in a situation where the ideas at issue are not just about contraceptive methods but about family life, gender roles, social mobility, economic opportunity, and much else.

In recent work on fertility determinants, economic and ideational factors play oddly symmetric roles in explanation. Proponents of each would deny that social change is in part an autonomous process, seeing it instead either as a reflection of deeper-seated economic forces or as the outcome of ideational change generated by the diffusion of new ideas, particularly from a Western or globalized culture. Purists on each side see the other as the opposing contender in the explanatory stakes, with no other horses running. For fertility, the result is two mutually incompatible interpretations of the same reality, both of them tending to be asociological. Empirically, ideationists aver, economic explanation has failed, in that survey-based measures of economic status appear to be weak predictors of individual fertility outcomes. Ideational change, not yet subjected to an analogous (equally dubious) test, for the time being retains its a priori plausibility unpunctured. Tertium non datur.

Each of the various sets of factors in this sketch no doubt contributes something to the explanation of fertility. I am not concerned with deciding how much—efforts to identify additive effects are suspect—let alone with banishing any of them. Rather, this view of the process of fertility change serves as a background against which to explore the influence of the state and serves to remind us that there are underlying forces and processes of change in a society that are often, and perhaps nearly always, more significant for the course of fertility than are the actions of government.

Varieties of the modern state and their significance for fertility

Along with its economy, social institutions, and cultural patterns, a society of any size and complexity inherits a polity—a political-administrative structure that is the institutional manifestation of the state. This overall regulatory regime and system of public administration provides a legal-administrative setting for civil society, economic activity, and family life. Together, these inherited features define a framework of roles and statuses within which individual behavior is played out. In particular, that framework sustains a demographic regime: the set of routine behaviors surrounding cohabitation, marriage, childbearing, and "health-seeking," and their antecedents or supports in patterns of socialization, organization, and economic activity.

In modern times governments of any stripe claim and are generally assumed to represent the interests of their societies. The minimalist requirement of government extends little beyond the maintenance of social order. That entails defense against external threat and preservation of stability and predictability in economic relationships—at the least, security of person and property, a system of adjudication, and a capacity to enforce contracts. This was a theme of the classical economists, and is echoed by modern libertarians. Minimalism in a sense also exists when there is thoroughgoing administrative *in*capacity, as in the case of the failed or so-called quasi-state. Most actual governments, of course, are far from minimalist. At the interventionist extreme, they may attempt to minutely regulate social and economic life through surveillance and sanction. In modern social democracies, a more benign but still meticulous regulatory regime has acquired the sobriquet of the nanny state. Countries are arrayed across this spectrum, and over time have relocated themselves.

Cutting across the libertarian–nanny state axis is what might be termed the administrative-legal dimension. Early in the development process—and often well before it—national governments discover the need for an effective administrative order. Usurping familial and community authority, they strengthen local officialdom, sometimes coopting traditional or elected village leaders as public servants. For a firmer backbone, they may introduce a second, parallel hierarchy of military command or state-party cadres. Governance is by fiat. Over time, as described earlier, the processes of social and geographic mobility, accelerated by economic growth, undermine the spatially defined hierarchy of local and regional public administration, replacing it with a national legal order.

We can describe the position or path of change of a given society in terms of these two axes: one measuring the scope and intensity of state intervention, the other, the balance between administrative and legal authority. A typical trajectory for a developing country over the last half-century might see an early espousal of state intervention, followed by a partial retreat, and at the same time a steady shift from fiat to codified civil law. The position at a given time has significant implications for fertility behavior and for the nature and efficacy of fertility policy (see McNicoll 1997 for a fuller discussion). As a simple illustration, consider the four situations generated by low and high combinations of values along each axis.

—*Minimalist state/rule by fiat.* Distancing of the state from local affairs here is more likely to reflect administrative incapacity than libertarian principle. Governments try to impose authoritarian control but their efforts are erratic and often predatory and economically damaging. Regional underadministration leaves a power vacuum that is filled by tax-farmers or mafia-type entities (see Putnam 1993). In extreme cases there may be a more radical institutional decay and breakdown of social order (see R. Kaplan 1996). Fertility outcomes under these conditions bear little or no relation to societal interests. For families in such settings efforts to create and maintain informal security alliances take precedence over any long-run economic-demographic calculations. Fertility policy measures are irrelevant.

—*Intrusive state/rule by fiat.* An authoritarian state with effective administrative outreach through an Interior Ministry or equivalent agency can apply that apparatus in support of line-ministry activities deemed of particular significance for, say, national security or development. Dealing with high fertility has sometimes been seen as such an activity, accorded quasi-security status. It was arguably so in 1970s' China, with antinatalist measures supported by a mobilized Communist Party apparatus; in Indonesia in the same decade, with support from a militarized local government system (and sporadically from the military itself); and in Emergency-era India (1975–77), with general backing from the civil service and local government. In some other circumstances, authoritarian states have sought to *raise* fertility. There is no doubt that fertility can be influenced to some degree by close range administrative pressures: neighborhood-level social pressures once did as much. However, passive noncompliance—one of the "weapons of the weak" (Scott 1985)—may be an effective counterforce, overcome only at high political cost. We can note also that locally based authority tends to erode over the course of development and this route then ceases to be available.

—*Intrusive state/rule of law.* This combination would typically be associated with modern welfare states, where social and economic development is likely to have already brought about low fertility. Elaborate social policy objectives are pursued through family law, personnel-policy requirements imposed on employers, and tax expenditures. Very low fertility may be flagged as a problem but in most welfare states raising fertility has not assumed a prominent place in the social policy agenda beyond measures promoting a benign family-friendliness. (I return to this topic below.) This administrative combination is not associated only with social democracy. Although conservatism broadly seeks the dominance of society over the state, *social* conservatives are willing to have the state's legislative backing for their particular moral agenda—one that embraces familism. In low-fertility situations, they would likely push for pronatalist outcomes through fiscal or ideational means, but would also permit pro-family policies to be embodied in law and public administration.

—*Minimalist state/rule of law.* The administrative patterns that best promote economic development are usually held to be those that expand economic freedom within a framework of secure property rights. (The recipe is sufficient rather than necessary: rapid economic growth can be attained in the absence of political freedom and even—as in China—with curtailed demographic freedom.) The presumption is that the market economy fosters rapid economic growth, in turn bringing about fertility transition as a virtually certain byproduct: the same ingredients, such as achievement-orientation and the shaking up of tradition, will initiate or hasten fertility decline. The often-derided dictum of the 1974 Bucharest population conference, that "development is the best contraceptive," left open the option of a heavy state role. The paraphrased stance of the US delegation to the Mexico City conference a decade later was that "capitalism is the best contraceptive." Even more excoriated at the time, this view has gradually found much wider acceptance. The same recipe may of course underlie the very low fertility of post-transition societies. For economic conservatives, however, low fertility would not be any cause for intervention; rather, it would be accepted as the result of the free choice of individuals.

The last two of these combinations describe issues of law and public administration that are important in fertility determination in low-fertility situations. Welfare state institutions and the intergenerational transfers they accommodate require strong administrative support, not least to maintain the revenue side of the state budget. The globalization pressures that have pushed the partial dismantlement of those institutions by disadvantaging countries with very high governmental shares of gross domestic product have restrained the redistributionist inclinations of the state. Child allowances are among the transfers that have been squeezed (see the later discussion of public transfers). Of course, a government may be philosophically disinclined to privilege families and their reproductive role, preferring to deal solely with individuals: that stance has a hard-nosed consistency to it, but would be a curious relinquishment of policy interest in the society's future. A similar indifference to fertility levels might be found during a period in which major international institutional changes are underway—for example, as currently in the development of the European Union, with emergence of a supranational labor market and centralization of some areas of social policymaking. Eventually, however, the prospect of a substantial, continued population decline is likely to elicit a strong political response, necessarily with significant legal and administrative implications.

Structural factors behind government influences on fertility are not only on the side of the state. For any specified degree of state intrusiveness and authoritarianism, societies differ in governability—in how easy or difficult it is for the government to give effect to a given policy. Cultural differences in people's innate pliability may exist, but the more appreciable factors at work most likely have to do with social organization such as class structure, religious or language communities, or emergent nationality. Ethnic and linguistic group boundaries may be particularly impenetrable to government intervention when perceived group interests are at stake, as they often would be in efforts to modify fertility.

Varieties of state actions influencing fertility

As the discussion above suggests, by virtue of its mere existence the state cannot *not* influence fertility. There is no position of "neutrality" from which to measure its positive or negative pressures on reproduction. Discussions of government roles in fertility change, however, are usually concerned with more explicit means of behavioral influence than through the structure and scope of government as a whole. They are concerned with cases in which governments deliberately set out to change fertility, or in which they pursue economic and social policies that have fertility change as a desired byproduct—one that provides part of the rationale for undertaking them. Unfortunately, the efficacy of policy measures, pro- or antinatalist, is itself contentious. Of course, intentions do not necessarily yield intended results, and it is the determinants of outcomes rather than of intentions that are of interest here: we need also to cover inadvertent fertility-affecting measures.

In classifying potential routes of governmental influence on fertility, a two-way scheme—direct versus indirect, or explicit versus implicit—is clearly inadequate. Intentions may matter, or they may not: that issue should not be decided a priori. A better classification would be based on substantive considerations: the hypothesized route of influence and the conceptualization of the process of social change presumed to be operating. On those grounds I would propose the following as the main categories of state action that impinge on fertility behavior and outcomes:

—The state develops, funds, and manages programs that seek to influence family-size outcomes through information, advocacy, economic inducement, or political pressure.

—The state has a part in determining access and opportunity in the society—social mobility, returns to effort, distributional equity—particularly through the social stratification and gender systems, thereby affecting the fertility calculus of individuals and families.

—The state designs and undertakes public-sector expenditures, both infrastructure investments and transfer payments keyed to age or family status, that affect the private economics of fertility.

—The state wields the symbols of national identity and cultural continuity that take the place of local beliefs and traditions, setting individual expectations and behavior in a wider national and even global cultural framework.

I discuss these four roles or sets of influences seriatim in the following sections.

The state and fertility regulation

Social regulation of fertility (or its near-equivalent, of surviving children) is no doubt as old as society, and interference in the matter by government merely formalizes that interest. The perennial government objective has been to boost population numbers, with fertility seen as a perhaps more secure source of recruitment than immigration and conquest. Sporadic efforts to design pronatalist rewards and sanctions have been made by authoritarian rulers at least since Augustus—the implication being that left to themselves many fewer women would choose a life of untrammeled childrearing.

Government antinatalist efforts by comparison are recent. They required a credible prospect of Malthusian scarcity or, in its later form, appreciation of a serious demographic drag on development. Deferred by the industrial revolution, this prospect took firm shape only with the sharp acceleration in population growth set off by the twentieth-century mortality declines. Actual government programs to limit that growth by propagation of birth control date only from the 1950s. As experience was gained and some experimentation undertaken (Taichung, Mysore, etc.), initial caution was replaced by enthusiasm and energy.

From the start, birth control programs had another antecedent in addition to Malthusian worries. This was the campaign for women's rights, autonomy, and reproductive health, begun in Western countries in the nineteenth century. From that tradition came much of the ideology that imbued the family planning movement, in particular its strong voluntaristic ethos and the cross-national similarities in its rhetoric and design. It gained vigor in the Cairo Program of Action.

These antecedents did not have to be found in the country setting up the program: in the early years programs were often imposed on a passive and bemused officialdom and populace by enthusiastic foreign donors when the government itself was neither persuaded of the demographic need nor in favor of the program's implicit ideology (see Warwick 1982). In other cases, the voluntarism entailed in the program's actual implementation was less than claimed—in some instances, much less (see McNicoll 1997). But such cases might well have been more numerous had there not been these strong international linkages: had each country designed a program that accorded with its own perception of the urgency of the problem and the population groups to be targeted, and managed it in the manner of its own political and administrative practices in other domains. The administrative muscle employed in China, India, and Indonesia in the 1970s, mentioned earlier, supports this proposition.

From the standpoint of fertility theory rather than of population policy, the programs have three potential routes of fertility influence. The first, proclaimed loudest, is through meeting existing "needs" (read demand at zero cost) for modern contraception, in essence by lowering information costs and the supply price. The second route is through altering preferences, mainly about contraception and the family, in ways that make birth control more acceptable and promote desires for low fertility. This, an ideational change among individuals and couples, working through diffusion processes and bandwagon effects, is thought to be achieved by the advocacy of government leaders, by face-to-face contact with extension agents, and by exposure to media themes and messages. The third route is through political and administrative pressure, sometimes backed by economic sanction, either to gain program "acceptors" or directly to achieve a particular demographic outcome—a one- or two-child family, say.

China's birth control program, as it evolved in the 1980s and 1990s following the Dengist reforms that reestablished a privatized agrarian economy, exemplifies the second and third routes. It apparently has largely succeeded in persuading people that fertility has significant social as well as private consequences and thus is a legitimate matter for state intervention. It prescribes limits on child numbers and levies fines for noncompliance. The pressure has varied over time and across regions and has been partly vitiated by increasing geographic mobility and other changes that defeat the meticulous monitoring of reproduction that the system requires. Increasing economic differentiation among families erodes the egalitarianism of the policy goal. However, the system in practice is far from rigid: for instance, the quite substantial specified fines, say for a third or fourth birth, may in practice be bargained down, given that the village cadres who must collect them are themselves members of the community—see Zhang (1998). Vietnam's program reportedly has some similar characteristics (Goodkind 1995).

Fully voluntary birth control programs restrict themselves mainly to the first route, with cautious forays into the second. What have they achieved? After decades of experience, that remains a contested matter with sharply disparate readings of the evidence (for example, Pritchett 1994 and Potts 1997). Multivariate analysis has not settled the question: the identification of "program effort" as an independent factor in fertility decline is itself disputed. "Effort," in the alternative reading, is in part elicited by an increasing demand for birth control (Demeny 1979; Schultz 1994) and thus is not properly identified as a "supply" variable. To reach a useful answer requires specifying the counterfactual of what would have happened in a program's absence. Presumably there would rarely have been complete passivity in the face of an onslaught of births (the assumption behind some calculations of program effect). Gauging what would have happened is a necessarily speculative exercise, though one familiar enough to historians. In some societies a perceived collective interest in lower fertility might have generated harsh local-level control measures; in others, a rapidly growing demand by couples for effective contraception may have been met by the private sector; still other societies may have turned to traditional practices regulating marriage and birth intervals. Evaluating the decision to channel birth control energies and resources into government-run programs would thus call for case-by-case assessment. No doubt there would be many cases where such a decision was warranted. However, there might also be situations in which a program, by preempting measures relying more on homegrown responses, in effect yielded a negative number of births averted.

Lant Pritchett (1994: 24) calculates that at low per capita incomes the present discounted cost of a child is 100 times larger than the cost of avoiding a child through birth control. The same multiple was once used (by Stephen Enke, and later by President Johnson) as a compelling argument for investing in family planning programs—offering a remarkably cheap way of improving economic conditions. But that supposes that parents are ignorant about contraception or helpless to act in the matter without government support, a doubtful notion from a more innocent age. ("'Coitus interruptus' has so far not been approved by the Planning Commission or the Government," wrote Gyan Chand, former chief economist in India's cabinet secretariat in 1954, "but the Census Commissioner has referred to it in his Report and with approval" [Chand 1954: 103].) For Pritchett, the implication of the multiple is rather that manipulating birth control costs through family planning programs is unlikely to count for much in childbearing decisions.

Explicit government antinatalist measures extend beyond birth control programs. They include limitations on marriage: once, in many societies, requiring permission from local authorities based on a couple's economic circumstances, now merely specification of a minimum age. (It is often overlooked that such limitations are an accepted exercise of state authority; family planning voluntarism starts later.) Fertility effects are commonly claimed as a partial justification for expanding maternal and child health programs and programs seeking to improve the position of women. Belief in these joint effects is a prominent assumption of the "Cairo agenda," which promotes women's rights and reproductive health mainly on their own merits but with a supposed demographic payoff as well.

*Pro*natalist programs under modern conditions of low fertility rely mainly on tax and other material incentives. Apparent effects are sometimes detectable, more often in the tempo of fertility than in lifetime births, but overall the impact of such measures has been fairly marginal (see Demeny 1986b, 2000; McIntosh 1986). Of course, material incentives that are large in proportion to family income could certainly be effective, but the budgetary cost entailed would be politically prohibitive. Direct parental expenditures on raising a child to age 18 in the United States today, for middle-income families, total substantially above $100,000 (see Espenshade 1984:

his 1981 estimate is $80,000, equivalent to $140,000 at 1998 prices). A proportionality argument parallel to Pritchett's on birth control can be made about interventions to raise fertility in low-fertility societies: against the actual costs of children, the kinds of monetary incentive offered to parents in most pronatalist programs are trivial.

If the political feasibility constraint is relaxed, a case can be made for a much higher subsidy of parenting. Ronald Lee and Timothy Miller (1997), in research undertaken for a study of US immigration, find that the net present value of the "fiscal impact" of an average American birth (that is, the discounted sum of the year-by-year local and federal taxes paid by that person and his or her descendants, less the year-by-year government expenditures imputed to that person) is of the order of $200,000 in 1994 dollars—at a 3 percent discount rate (at 2 percent, the value is roughly doubled; at 4 percent, halved). Accepting such a calculation, and the assumptions it requires (not only on the discount rate but on productivity growth, congestion costs, and environmental impact), massive government birth subsidies could be justified. The sensitivity of the result to those assumptions, however, is a reason for caution in using the procedure as a means for valuing alternative demographic futures. Of course, societies do not expect to have to collectively purchase their descendants, and in contemplating any actual subsidy program the problem of selectivity—of who is bearing and raising the "purchased" children, and hence, to some extent, what is their "quality"—is a critical but highly sensitive question.

If children cannot be bought at affordable cost, what alternative approaches to sustaining fertility can be found? In authoritarian regimes pronatalism may have a forceful edge—the 1966 Romanian prohibition of abortion, virtually doubling the birth rate for the next two years, is often pointed to; Iranian policies in the early 1980s were in some respects parallel. But it is hard to coerce additional births. Promotional campaigns and symbolic rewards call to mind Stalin's "hero mothers" and are unlikely to influence a cynical populace. Kingsley Davis (1937), seeing no way to maintain population replacement under the usual family pattern of modern societies, foresaw a need for the professionalization of parenthood. Various proposals have been made for how to do so, most of them far-fetched or overtly dystopian (often appropriately cast as fiction). Taussig (1911) scornfully decried the "phalansteries and barracks" he associated with the birth planning of full-blown socialism, drawn in that case from Charles Fourier's heated imagination—though something of the sort was actually to be attempted, albeit briefly, in Maoist China.

Overall, this experience offers scant encouragement for a government role in fertility management at low-fertility levels. Andrew J. Cherlin (1988: 24) writes, of the United States, that "fundamental family trends such as changes in divorce, marriage, and birthrates are little affected by government social or economic policies.... [A]ny feasible child care program or family allowance in the United States would be unlikely to influence the birthrate very much in either direction." Frank F. Furstenberg, Jr. (1995: 253) concurs: "our ability to engineer family behaviour is limited at best."

Programs concerned with fertility do not of course have to be about simple numbers of births. The potential social interest in demographic outcomes extends to other characteristics of children. It also involves ethical judgments about appropriate aims and means of birth control. Thus governments might seek to override parental desires for sons over daughters that can be exercised through prenatal sex determination and selective abortion, for moral reasons or so as not to be faced with seriously unbalanced sex ratios in the next generation. More generally, governments set ground rules for abortion, which increasingly must take account of ascertainable knowledge of the genetic makeup of the fetus. Notwithstanding the past excesses of eugenics, it is hard to argue that the manifest public interest in "child quality" should deal only with environment and never with heredity. (Eugenics is the central concern of China's 1994 Law on Maternal and Infant Health Care, which has drawn much less attention than China's one-child policy—see "The new Chinese Law..." 1995.) Governments will inevitably be drawn again into this issue as technologies develop that enable parents to interpose their own eugenic wishes at an ever-finer-grained degree of genetic detail.

The state, social mobility, and fertility

When state and society are used as contrasting terms, *society* refers to those social groups and affiliations that are not part of or beholden to the state and its agencies. The contrast is not one of potential authoritarianism versus benign civility: behavioral control may be stringent or lax on either side. As Joel S. Migdal (1988) and subsequently many others have noted, strong states and weak societies often go together. And as not a few examples of political and social disorder and economic retrogression remind us, state and society can be simultaneously weak.

I noted earlier the strong emphasis that theorists of fertility decline put on opportunity, especially for economic and social mobility. The argument is that much of the fertility-reducing effect of economic development results from the breakdown of rigid stratification and gender systems as new technologies and institutions open new routes of upward mobility—and pose new threats to those disinclined to respond. These systems can also be transformed or disrupted by *political* change: indeed that is a major source of challenge to their rigidity. Blake (1972b) saw eighteenth-century France as a notable case in point, with the early onset of fertility decline a consequence of the political forces shaking up a traditional, ascriptive stratification system. This began well before the technological advances of the agricultural and industrial revolutions.

Major land reforms are an evident source of change in stratification systems. The clearest examples are the post–World War II reforms in Taiwan and South Korea, in which landlords were bought out by the government (and the money assets they gained soon inflated away), leaving a new class of owner-smallholders in some respects resembling European peasant proprietors—with the same inclinations toward low fertility. China is a more drawn-out and much bloodier version of the same story. The violent suppression of China's landlord class in the early 1950s was followed by an economically damaging series of collectivizations, culminating in the disastrous communes. Fertility decline was thereby deferred and eventually had to be jump-started (in the 1970s) by coercive programmatic and administrative measures. Convergence to the Taiwan–Korea agrarian pattern in economy and demography finally came with the Dengist reprivatization of 1978—albeit leaving land still formally in collective ownership—releasing the energies and innovativeness of peasant proprietorship. (See Greenhalgh 1990 for an incisive analysis of this experience.)

Are there more-routine kinds of state action that affect opportunity and mobility? State organization and funding of education is an evident candidate here, at least at the secondary and tertiary levels. The distributional effect may be lessened by the fact that the beneficiaries typically are disproportionately drawn from the higher socioeconomic classes (see Knodel and Jones 1996). For behavioral change, however, it is likely that what matters more than the odds of admission to, say, secondary schooling is the *competition* that is generated for access to a potential path to greater autonomy or upward mobility. Even if the odds are weighted against successful achievement, the prospect of access may still be a strong motivation for restricting fertility. Drastically low odds, of course, will preclude change: the system, its public funding notwithstanding, will then preserve the status quo, socioeconomic and demographic.

The gender systems of many societies are believed to contribute to high fertility by restricting women's extrafamilial roles and opportunities. Such systems tend to be resilient, sustained through the acculturation and socialization of children within the family unit and, more tangibly, from the strength of the interest groups that benefit—men generally, and sometimes older women. In the short term gender systems are not easily disrupted by government, certainly not by constitutional declarations of equality or by endorsement of the provisions of international covenants like the Universal Declaration of Human Rights. Governments are not wholly without influence, however, particularly by promoting equality in educational access. Extension programs may be another means of generating change. For instance, a family planning program may work not only through gains in effective control by women over their reproductive lives but also, in some circumstances, through the role models represented by female outreach workers. (Discussing the program in rural Bangladesh, Simmons et al. [1988: 37] hypothesize that "the presence of the female worker is beginning to amount to an institutional innovation counteracting those elements in the system of patriachy and *purdah* that render women passive in decisions about their fertility.") Over the long term and largely independent of government, stronger corrosive forces weakening traditional gender systems are exposure to "modern" views of sex roles and the family and the entry of women into the formal labor market.

The state, public transfers, and fertility

As an oppositional pair, *state versus market* is perhaps even more familiar than *state versus society*. Both pairs imply arguments for curtailment of state power. In one case, the state is assumed to have some innate expansionary tendencies that impede the development of civil society. In the other case, the state is seen as damaging economic development either by intruding into fields beyond its competence or by engaging in rent-seeking activities. But whereas civil society, as we saw, is not a requirement for vigorous economic performance or for progress in demographic transition, the narrower economic liberty of the free market does appear to be a requirement. The debate on state versus market has been decisively won by the market.

For fertility transition this is less a facilitating role for the state than abnegation of a potentially impeding role—though recognizing, as discussed above, that an effective market economy calls for skilled, if minimalist, governance. Contrary instances, where the state's role has been economically disastrous, are of course quite common—where the government has snuffed out economic progress and with it any near-term prospect for social development. E. L. Jones (1988) presents a whole array of such cases, spread over several centuries of world history. Africa offers some more-recent instances. Rent-seeking proves an irresistible temptation to ruling elites, leading to predatory or extortionate transfers that ultimately kill the economic goose. Economic collapse is accompanied by social disorder—or potential disorder that elicits harsh repression. Both development and demographic transition are pushed back to square one.

What the state does *within* its share of the economy may also have a distributional effect, with a potential influence on fertility. It finances and manages the public component of physical and social infrastructure. It directs public expenditures toward (or away from) social services benefiting the poor. And, to a substantial and increasing degree, it makes transfer payments among population groups defined by age or family status. Such expenditures and transfers—and expectations about them—may significantly modify the economics of fertility as seen by parents or prospective parents.

In large measure, public expenditures on infrastructure and social services belong to the general story of economic growth and fertility transition rather than to the narrower relationship of government and fertility. The public sector has played a dominant role in infrastructure investment in most developing countries, but that may now be lessening. Many social services, especially public health and education, have been conventionally assigned to government, but in practice have substantial and growing private-sector components. The public/private division in both cases is of interest mainly in discussing efficiency. The distributional effects of these expenditures—through detailed policies on subsidies, cost-recovery, rules of access, and so on—may or may not be important for fertility: research has not given a clearcut answer (Ahlburg 1996). Poverty alleviation efforts, of course, need no such justification.

Public transfers among age groups are more clearly fertility-related. (For general discussions, see Lee 1994 and Willis 1994, 1998.) The fact of childhood- and old age–dependency over the human lifecourse necessitates an institutional means of managing inter-age transfers. The family is in part a device to meet these consumption needs. In isolated groups like hunter-gatherers, a Darwinian argument would predict net positive transfers from parents to children—which empirical evidence seemingly bears out (H. Kaplan 1994). In agrarian societies, the evidence is more mixed, but under certain patriarchal regimes there appears to be a net benefit to elderly survivors from having a larger family (the premise of the "Caldwell hypothesis" on fertility transition). Whatever the biological factors involved, fertility decisions at the margin are potentially affected. The state intrudes into this domain when it defines a public interest in health and education and, perhaps later, in the welfare of the elderly, and when it specifies how families and children are to be treated in the tax code. Public expenditures in these areas may add to or substitute for private expenditures, in either case altering the (private) fertility calculus. Typically, it is argued, by socializing some part of childrearing costs while leaving old-age support to the family, the state in effect promotes high fertility. In aging, mature economies, the position may be reversed: private childrearing costs now are high, reflecting both the need for heavy, partly private educational investments and the magnitude of parental opportunity costs, while old-age dependency costs are substantially socialized through pay-as-you-go pension schemes. Net public-sector transfers hence go decisively toward the old, discouraging childbearing—"reproductive shirking," Willis (1994: 148) calls it.

Transfers in a society become institutionalized as entitlements and are politically costly to change. In effect they become expectations against which economic decisions are taken. Removal of popular subsidies or introduction of user fees for public services, often demanded of countries in economic difficulties as part of structural adjustment programs, are familiar causes of civil disorder. In the same way, fertility-related transfers—likely to be unrecognized as such—acquire entrenched support and become givens in a society, like the built-in pronatalism that Judith Blake pointed to (see above) or the bias against young families and in favor of the elderly that Samuel Preston (1984) documents. In a study of Egypt's fertility, Philippe Fargues (1997) notes that the onset of the steep fertility decline after 1985 coincided not with any development in population policy or program but with measures of economic liberalization that curtailed state subsidies to consumption and necessitated sharply increased family expenditures on health and education.

Recent decades have seen a substantial and virtually worldwide shift from state to market in many areas of life, a process that still continues. Daniel Yergin and Joseph Stanislaw (1998), after describing this shift, discuss the circumstances under which it might halt or be reversed. They identify five "tests" that will shape people's views of the market economy and "provide signposts to the future frontier between state and market" (p. 382). They are: (1) does the market deliver sufficient jobs, consumer goods, and environmental amenity? (2) does it provide requisite fairness of opportunity and rein in greed? (3) does it leave scope for cultural variation and maintenance of national identities? (4) can it cope with an increasing role in environmental protection? and (5) can it cope with emerging demographic patterns, notably population aging? The last of these is by no means least. Population aging will accentuate pressures to raise taxes to finance transfers to the elderly, increasing the government's share of the economy. Moves toward vesting and privatizing pension schemes, begun or foreshadowed in many countries, will likely provide at best a partial offset. The material reality of the transfers is still from wage earners to the retired, with government a necessary overseer.

The state, ideational change, and fertility

The cultural counterpart of the centralization of authority in the early part of political development is the ideological creation of the nation-state. Regional cultural distinctiveness does of course remain—especially when associated with ethnicity—but the state endeavors to monopolize the symbols of nationhood. Nationbuilding, especially when arrived at late, can be a fairly deliberate and self-conscious process, entailing selective borrowing from history to support a legitimating and heroic past and creation of the necessary accoutrements for international distinctiveness (flag, anthem, ceremony, and the like). Even in long-established polities, supposedly time-honored customs and practices often turn out to be of relatively recent design, as studies of the "invention of tradition" have demonstrated.

The state thus constructed wields these various symbols to create a potent source of identity that overlays and may eventually all but extinguish local and kin-based loyalties. The process is what Clifford Geertz (1963) termed the integrative revolution. The classic discussion of it is by Benedict Anderson (1991). Those earlier affiliative ties were the routes of social pressure on fertility, serving to maintain elaborate family systems, to reinforce gender roles, to redistribute childrearing costs, and to blur the economic autonomy of households. The corresponding loyalties evoked by the nation-state may be strong but are amorphous, as are the pressures they accommodate. "Development" typically assumes the status of an ideological goal, justifying the state's imposition of sacrifice in the interest of longer-term gain, and perhaps explaining its award of monopolies or the absence of such appeals to private interest as elections. National security becomes a parallel goal, with its own ideological counterpart to the raft of policies and practices it purports to justify.

Two exceptions to this developmental pattern should be noted. In one, exemplified by Iran following the 1979 revolution, the state enforces a neotraditional religious morality and consciously excludes many of the trappings of modernity. However, this is comparatively rare and plausibly a state cannot long preserve that exclusion. In another, more common exception, integration stalls, with ethnic or cultural groupings inventing their own claims to nationhood, often with acute awareness of demographic relativities within the state's boundaries.

The relevance for demographic behavior comes from the shift in cultural frame of reference from the local to the national level, a cognitive counterpart to the expanded options for geographic and social mobility. The change is not the emergence of a "calculus of conscious choice," defining escape from some prerational stage of existence (a farfetched notion), but a rearrangement of the considerations that enter fertility decisions. The nation-state is not of course the end point in this process. Cultural autonomy and distinctiveness at the national level are continually eroded by international influences as part of the phenomenon of globalization, only partly offset by nationalist and nativist cultural regeneration.

Compared to these major forces, deliberate government efforts to induce lower fertility by ideational change seem unlikely to amount to much. "Political will" is popularly taken to be a significant factor in the success or failure of birth control programs, especially as it is manifested in the speeches of political leaders. No doubt the head of state or other authoritative figure can do much to energize program implementation and, for policies entailing service delivery, perhaps improve quality of service. That sort of gain, after all, is a routine mark of skilled leadership. But how much parallel scope is there to inspire change in reproductive behavior itself—even, at a minimally ambitious level, to motivate people to become program clients? In China, Maoist campaigns to encourage emulation of individuals who supposedly displayed exemplary obedience to state and Party dictates soon gave way to the familiar economic incentives and sanctions of Dengist realism. But perhaps China's authoritarianism makes it a poor example. Bangladesh might be taken as an alternative case. It is sometimes held up as showing fertility decline without development: a kind of "look, no hands!" achievement, the outcome, in some accounts, of pure ideation (or ideation-cum-family planning). More prosaic factors, however, are likely to have been implicated: principally, the marketization of exchange, involving the shift from social capital toward physical and human capital, with their very different rules of investment. The erosion of networks of social support and social control is invisible in economic indexes, but may amount to a radical transformation of the economic environment, requiring families and individuals to consider new strategies of economic and demographic life. Those changes, though not directly fostered by the state, indirectly owe much to the government's economic management and public administration.

Modern communications potentially raise new possibilities for state ideational influence. Free-to-air television can serve as a route by which a government's perception of the social interest—say, in family planning—can reach its citizens, through soap operas and similar items of popular culture. With the further spread of communications technology, that influence is diluted. Demographically, however, the messages of the globalized media—on consumerist values, images of the family, attitudes toward individual achievement and gender roles, and views of sexual morality—may be even more powerfully antinatalist.

In advanced market economies, governments would mostly shy away from accepting any explicit state role in ideational change. Their proclaimed task is to reflect rather than lead the views of their electorates, especially on matters deemed politically sensitive. Family policy is certainly such an area. At some point, however, low fertility, whether through its population aging effect or through the prospect of a radical diminution in numbers, will demand a state-level response. For the family, the ideal of lineage continuity may have all but vanished, but at the national level, despite talk of the "end of the nation-state," the belief in continuity remains. (The usual "ending" arguments have the nation-state being slowly superseded by supranational instruments and institutions on the one hand and subnational or cross-border entities on the other. For a skeptical and countervailing view, see Canovan 1996.) While population numbers can be sustained by immigration probably for generations to come, very high immigration rates would be called for. Even in pluralistic societies, the demographic turnover implied by this course would itself pose a challenge to national identity. Perhaps the concept of national identity will become fluid enough to tolerate the requisite pace of change under high immigration (McNeill 1984 sketches such a future). Or perhaps the threat to identity will help to regenerate familistic beliefs and lead to a resurgence of fertility. Or perhaps as-yet-unforeseen changes in the global political or natural environment will make our current expectations about the "problem" of low fertility seem insignificant or ridiculous. But probably more likely is that, accepting that ideational change lies largely outside its capacity to influence, the state will concern itself with what it plausibly *can* do to affect its fertility, through efforts to redesign social institutions.

Government as designer

In this mapping of state influences on fertility, specific anti- or pronatalist measures made up only one category. The others had to do with the nature of the government's presence and activities, where intentional fertility effects were incidental—merely reflecting the presumption that development will promote a fertility decline. Replacement fertility was reached in the West without any explicit state intervention—indeed, in the face of government opposition—and there is no reason to suppose that the same forces are not operating to bring about fertility declines elsewhere in the world. The novel factor of the last half-century, of course, is the advent of modern contraception, easing the uncertainties and health risks that had always attended birth control practices beyond abstinence. Combined with these new technologies—and hence confounded with them in interpretation—has been the role of government extension programs in promoting their use. Although this role is a frequent cause for self-congratulation, assessments of its effect are exaggerated, perhaps greatly, by use of an inappropriate standard of comparison: government versus nothing. Explicit government efforts to *raise* birth rates in low fertility situations have been conspicuously ineffective.

In many spheres other than fertility, governments are quite ambitious about engineering change. They seek to design whole future urban environments, patterns of industrial organization, and social institutions. The routine expectation that such things are the appropriate bailiwick of government disguises the radical nature of what is being attempted—though the outcome may actually fall far short of the intent. What is the analogue in the population arena? Can the insights derived from the experience of fertility change thus far suggest the kind of institutional innovations that will help to bring about a socially desired path of fertility in the future?

Few would question the legitimacy of a state interest in the matter, at least where demographic trends are far from the socially optimal. Simone Veil (1978: 315), for instance, declares it in straightforward terms: "Avoiding a long-term weakening of a country brought about by a dangerously low birth rate and, inversely, avoiding excessive population growth when it becomes an obstacle to economic development and to the well-being of the population must certainly be among the basic goals of all governments." But if we are to take seriously such a role for the state, it is likely that we must look at more profound kinds of intervention than the programmatic.

In the case of the remaining high-fertility countries, establishment of a secure social order ("just laws impartially administered") and conditions for economic growth (people's "industrious exertions...allowed to have free scope") may well be a sufficient design for fertility reduction, with some family planning programmatic backup to give added confidence in the outcome by ensuring the availability and affordability of modern contraception. (The quotes are from Malthus 1820: ch. 4.) More precise ingredients must come from case-specific institutional analysis—all too rare in a field that celebrates the uniformity of its research protocols. It is not an easy task, but it is notable that the recipe is virtually the same as for promoting broad-based economic development. The required changes do not necessarily yield substantial gains in income in the early years—hence it is possible to observe fertility declining without very much apparent economic growth, as in the case of Bangladesh mentioned above. While administrative pressures can be deployed to lower fertility in the absence of development, the social cost is high and there is some risk of impeding future development.

Turn now to the developed countries. Although their demographic transitions were earlier completed under a wide range of economic and political regimes, these countries have eventually converged to market economies and democratic polities. In those circumstances the market works perhaps too well in undermining societal (and biosocial?) pronatalist pressures and traditions, legitimating in their place a starker economic calculation. Families, and increasingly individuals, must weigh the rich nonmonetary returns from parenthood against the high and ever-rising direct and opportunity costs of children in income and leisure time. The balance, on average, seems to lie below, perhaps much below, a two-child fertility level. The state can attempt to alter that balance through the familiar variety of direct and indirect subsidies of child costs, but these measures, as we noted, are expensive. Moreover, to be significant across the income distribution they have to be quite regressive: richer parents expect to raise more-costly children. Budgetary or tax expenditures to finance the levels of subsidy needed for effectiveness are likely to prove unaffordable (large windfall gains—subsidies needlessly granted to families who would anyway have chosen to have above-average numbers of children—are inescapable) or politically unfeasible, given the international competitive pressures on countries to align tax regimes and lower the government share of the national economy.

Given the usual family division of labor and the usual custodial arrangements under single parenthood, women incur the major time costs of childrearing. They experience more directly the role conflict between parenting and labor force participation. Gøsta Esping-Andersen (1996: 26) sees the problem of "how to harmonize women's employment with family formation" as "one of the greatest challenges for the future welfare state." Jean-Claude Chesnais (1996) points to the contrasting levels of compatibility between work and family in Italy and Sweden in accounting for the ultra-low fertility in the former compared to merely low fertility in the latter. Peter McDonald (2000) makes an analogous argument in terms of the differing degrees of "gender equity" found in the workplace and in the social institutions bearing on the family. Of course the market itself may offer a partial corrective, if demographic conditions lead to heightened competition in the "family-friendliness" of personnel policies. Corporate acceptance of flexible working hours and provision of child care may well be a rational practice. However, such measures would probably not reach a large proportion of the labor force.

Is a pronatalist design of society even possible in the democratic, market-oriented societies to which much of the world seems to be converging in the post-transitional period? Marc Linder (1997) is skeptical. At the end of a dense, insightful commentary on the social and population policy literature, he sets out "desiderata of an intergenerational demographic solidarity." He sees the problem as one of developing a "sustained psychological identification" of individuals with a collectivity that has a past and a future—"a task that is difficult enough in a tabula rasa microcommunity such as a kibbutz, where the generational existential context is palpable, but becomes almost impossibly heroic even in a relatively homogeneous nation" (p. 313). Let alone, he adds, for a country as "quasireligiously opposed to planning" as the United States (p. 314).

That is perhaps too defeatist, requiring the inherently implausible planning of an ideational change. James Coleman (1993), in his presidential address to the American Sociological Association, took a far more sanguine view of the problem. The societal shift away from what he terms "primordial social organization" centered on the family is held to be irreversible, along with the erosion of the social capital it embodied. However, he argues that the new social system emerging is not foreordained: it is being constructed, and there is scope for ensuring that its institutions are rationally designed. The hope would be for "a future in which social control no longer depends principally on coercion, constraint, and negative sanctions, under the oppressive blanket of closed communities, but instead depends principally on positive incentives and rewards for performance" (p. 14).

One consequence of the loss of social capital just mentioned has been a "vacuum in child rearing." The state increasingly strips that function away from parents—through daycare and schools—but does not properly replace it: the state's concerns are more with the imparting of skills than with raising good citizens. Coleman proposes a design of incentives to reaffirm parents' rights in their children in a way that maximizes not the child's welfare (which easily becomes parents' welfare) but the child's value to society—a strong interest of the state. The device is to vest a share of the realized increase in that value in the parents or other caregivers. A more elaborated model describing a similar institutional innovation, seen as a pronatalist measure as well, was earlier proposed by Paul Demeny (1987). In it, some portion of the social security taxes paid by the children (under a pay-as-you-go system) would be earmarked for their parents. And much the same suggestion is made by Shirley Burggraf (1997).

The particular merits of this kind of proposal (it surely would have difficulties too: Peter Uhlenberg 1997 finds it entirely unfeasible) are less important for my purpose here than its representing a class of intervention that could potentially pass democratic muster. The comparative modesty of such interventions and the test applied to them of public acceptability in a civil society would save them from the trenchant criticism advanced by J. C. Scott (1998) of many overweening state efforts in social engineering in recent decades, efforts that have frequently gone seriously awry.

Demeny (1986a: 487) ended his 1986 presidential address to the Population Association of America by posing the "daring questions" that demographers shy away from: "What kind of society would we like to be part of? What kind of arrangements should that society have concerning demographic matters?"—the latter defining "the desirable demographic constitution of contemporary societies." Coleman's 1993 address ended with a very similar challenge to sociologists to engage in normative thinking about the design of society. With such evident problems ahead, there is an urgent task for social scientists in exploring those constitutional issues.

Enriching fertility theory

Government, I have argued, is routinely omitted from fertility theory except in a few formulaic categories: manager of family planning programs, legislator on marriage and birth control methods, the fount of "political will," and so on. I have sketched the actual range of plausible governmental influence on fertility, extending across virtually the entire spectrum of fertility determinants and fertility levels. How should fertility *theory* be expanded to acknowledge these relationships?

A short answer would be that fertility theory should pay more attention to institutional and cultural dynamics, where government actions are generated and where, sporadically and to a limited degree, they have their greatest effect. Thus, beneath the veneer of a poor-country government "adopting" a population policy and setting up a family planning program there may be a real political process unfolding in which the impetus for collective action on high fertility gains ground. Or, just as likely and just as consequential, there may be no such process: fertility instead is left to the benefit–cost calculations of individuals and families—informed, however, by a changing social and economic environment that itself is influenced by government actions. Stripping away that veneer (and with it the hermetic language of latent demand, unmet need, wanted and unwanted births, and program effort) makes the problem of behavioral explanation in fertility not a sui generis exercise for adepts but one with close parallels in other spheres of behavior where economic, social structural, and ideational factors routinely intermingle. It also leaves the high-fertility case far closer to that of low fertility.

There are of course longer answers too. The dimensions of state influence on fertility I have examined define a view of fertility determination in both transitional and post-transitional societies. In that view, the individual perceptions and choices that lead to particular fertility outcomes are conditioned by a broad array of characteristics of the social and economic environment. The information and incentives offered by programmatic interventions in support of anti- (or pro-)natalist ends are one of these characteristics. Others where the state is potentially influential are the legal and administrative systems, the opportunity structure of the society, the direction and scale of intergenerational transfers in the public and private economies, and the sense of cultural continuity and intergenerational solidarity that people feel. In the course of development, these characteristics are transformed, generating—or modulating—the familiar transition from high to low fertility. There is no unique path of development, so no single pattern of fertility transition. Moreover, when low fertility is reached, these conditioning factors do not then cease to operate: fertility is still responsive to them.

This is a "demand" approach to fertility, but not an individualistic approach. All it assumes at the individual level is that the components of fertility behavior are not more or less "rational" than most other behaviors. (Biological factors might be a somewhat more significant ingredient.) Fertility is consequential for societies, and societies have developed elaborate ways of influencing it. With exogenous mortality declines and the institutional changes wrought by development, however, those social influences on fertility may erode or may have effects that in the new circumstances detract from societal welfare. Fertility is typically too high during development, too low after it: a problem for public policy. A necessary first step in searching for possible remedies is to identify where government already bears on fertility, intentionally or not. Commonly, in high-fertility situations, explicit birth control programs are seen, if not as the only means of government intervention, at least as the most direct and probably most efficacious means. But that may not be so, as the discussion above would tend to suggest. In low-fertility situations, governments may think they have no effective recourse to sustain near-replacement fertility, and that too I questioned.

In modeling we can counterfactually alter government policy settings at will. That is hardly a realistic exercise. Indeed, if that could be readily done in practice, we might suspect that the policy at issue had little bite. In many respects the state can be regarded as a largely endogenous element in understanding fertility—high, declining, and low. Moreover, as I noted at the outset, government is not a simple entity. The committees, agencies, and offices it comprises each have political or bureaucratic interests in survival and well-being in addition to their policy or program goals—the latter in part reflecting a response to (or anticipation of) changing community wishes. The context within which fertility is determined is in turn modified by these interests, policies, and programs. Thus the management or oversight of, for example, family law and related tax issues, public-sector intergenerational transfers, labor market policy, and the organization and financing of health and education—all matters that are potentially highly relevant to fertility outcomes—are spread over the bureaucratic map. Intricate as it may be, fertility theory will remain critical in designing societal responses to the problems of population growth and decline.

Modern societies, it is often argued, will all converge toward democracy and the free market, circumstances in which much of the repertoire of public policy responses to low fertility may be deemed illegitimate. It is quite likely that all will eventually face a situation of sustained population attrition. The task of fertility theorizing would not then vanish—indeed, the social interest in the demographic future might well be intensified—but theoretical concerns with government influence on fertility, rooted as they are in the diversity of polities, could properly be allowed to wane.

Note

Comments on an earlier version of this chapter by Ronald Lee and Noriko Tsuya are acknowledged.

References

Ahlburg, Dennis A. 1996. "Population growth and poverty," in Dennis A. Ahlburg et al. (eds.) *The Impact of Population Growth on Well-Being in Developing Countries.* New York: Springer-Verlag.

Anderson, Benedict. 1991. *Imagined Communities: Reflections on the Origins and Spread of Nationalism.* London: Verso.

Ben-Porath, Yoram. 1974. "The micro-economics of fertility," *International Social Science Journal* 26: 302–314.

Blake, Judith. 1972a. "Coercive pronatalism and American population policy," in Commission on Population Growth and the American Future, *Aspects of Population Growth Policy*. Washington, DC. (Research Reports, volume 6.)

———. 1972b. "Fertility control and the problem of voluntarism," in *Scientists and World Affairs*: Proceedings of the 22nd Pugwash Conference. Reprinted in *Population and Development Review* 20 (1994): 167–177.

Burggraf, Shirley P. 1997. *The Feminine Economy and Economic Man: Revising the Role of Family in the Post-Industrial Age*. Reading, MA: Addison-Wesley.

Canovan, Margaret. 1996. *Nationhood and Political Theory*. Cheltenham, UK: Edward Elgar.

Chand, Gyan. 1954. *Some Aspects of the Population Problem of India*. Bihar: Patna University.

Chenery, Hollis and Moshe Syrquin. 1975. *Patterns of Development, 1950–1970*. New York: Oxford University Press.

Cherlin, Andrew J. (ed.) 1988. *The Changing American Family and Public Policy*. Washington, DC: Urban Institute Press.

Chesnais, Jean-Claude. 1996. "Fertility, family, and social policy in contemporary Western Europe," *Population and Development Review* 22: 729–739.

Coleman, James S. 1993. "The rational reconstruction of society," *American Sociological Review* 58: 1–15.

Davis, Kingsley. 1937. "Reproductive institutions and the pressure for population," *Sociological Review*. Reprinted in *Population and Development Review* 23 (1997): 611–624.

Demeny, Paul. 1979. "On the end of the population explosion," *Population and Development Review* 5: 141–162.

———. 1986a. "Population and the invisible hand," *Demography* 23: 473–487.

———. 1986b. "Pronatalist policies in low-fertility countries: Patterns, performance, and prospects," in Kingsley Davis et al., eds., *Below-Replacement Fertility in Industrial Societies: Causes, Consequences, Policies*. New York: Cambridge University Press.

———. 1987. "Re-linking fertility behavior and economic security in old age: A pronatalist reform," *Population and Development Review* 13: 128–132.

———. 2000. "Policy interventions in response to below-replacement fertility," in *Below Replacement Fertility*. New York: United Nations. (Population Bulletin of the United Nations, Special issue nos. 40/41.)

Espenshade, Thomas J. 1984. *Investing in Children: New Estimates of Parental Expenditures*. Washington, DC: Urban Institute Press.

Esping-Andersen, Gøsta. 1996. *Welfare States in Transition: National Adaptations in Global Economies*. London: Sage Publications.

Fargues, Philippe. 1997. "State policies and the birth rate in Egypt: From socialism to liberalism," *Population and Development Review* 23: 115–138.

Furstenberg, Frank F., Jr. 1995. "Family change and the welfare of children: What do we know and what can we do about it?" in Karen Oppenheim Mason and An-Magritt Jensen, eds., *Gender and Family Change in Industrialized Countries*. Oxford: Clarendon Press.

Geertz, Clifford. 1963. "The integrative revolution: Primordial sentiments and civil politics in the new states," in Clifford Geertz, ed., *Old Societies and New States: The Quest for Modernity in Asia and Africa*. New York: Free Press.

Goodkind, Daniel M. 1995. "Vietnam's one-or-two-child policy in action," *Population and Development Review* 21: 85–111.

Greenhalgh, Susan. 1988. "Fertility as mobility: Sinic transitions," *Population and Development Review* 14: 629–674.

———. 1990. "Land reform and family entrepreneurship in East Asia," in Geoffrey McNicoll and Mead Cain, eds., *Rural Development and Population: Institutions and Policy*. New York: Oxford University Press.

Jones, E. L. 1988. *Growth Recurring: Economic Change in World History*. Oxford: Oxford University Press.

Kaplan, Hillard. 1994. "Evolutionary and wealth flows theories of fertility: Empirical tests and new models," *Population and Development Review* 20: 753–791.

Kaplan, Robert D. 1996. *The Ends of the Earth: A Journey at the Dawn of the 21st Century*. New York: Random House.

Knodel, John and Gavin W. Jones. 1996. "Post-Cairo population policy: Does promoting girls' schooling miss the mark?" *Population and Development Review* 22: 683–702.

Lee, Ronald D. 1994. "The formal demography of population aging, transfers, and the economic life cycle," in Linda Martin and Samuel Preston, eds., *The Demography of Aging*. Washington, DC: National Academy Press.

Lee, Ronald D. and Timothy Miller. 1997. "The life-time fiscal impacts of immigrants and their descendants," draft of Chapter 7 of *The New Americans*, a report of the National Research Council Panel on Economic and Demographic Consequences of Immigration (National Academy Press, 1997).

Lesthaeghe, Ron. 1983. "A century of demographic and cultural change in Western Europe: An exploration of underlying dimensions," *Population and Development Review* 9: 411–435.

———. 1995. "The second demographic transition in Western countries: An interpretation," in Karen Oppenheim Mason and An-Magritt Jensen, eds., *Gender and Family Change in Industrialized Countries*. Oxford: Clarendon Press.

Linder, Marc. 1997. *The Dilemmas of Laissez-Faire Population Policy in Capitalist Societies: When the Invisible Hand Controls Reproduction*. Westport, CT: Greenwood Press.

Malthus, T. R. 1820. *Principles of Political Economy*. Reprinted in *The Works of Thomas Robert Malthus*, ed. E. A. Wrigley and David Souden. London: Pickering, 1986, Vol. 5.

McDonald, Peter. 2000. "Gender equity, social institutions and the future of fertility," *Journal of Population Research* 17: 1–16.

McIntosh, C. Alison. 1986. "Recent pronatalist policies in Western Europe," in Kingsley Davis et al., eds., *Below-Replacement Fertility in Industrial Societies: Causes, Consequences, Policies*. New York: Cambridge University Press.

McNeill, William H. 1984. "Human migration in historical perspective," *Population and Development Review* 10: 1–18.

McNicoll, Geoffrey. 1997. "The governance of fertility transition: Reflections on the Asian experience," in Gavin W. Jones et al., eds., *The Continuing Demographic Transition*. Oxford: Clarendon Press.

Migdal, Joel S. 1988. *Strong Societies and Weak States*. Princeton: Princeton University Press.

Potts, Malcolm. 1997. "Sex and the birth rate: Human biology, demographic change, and access to fertility-regulation methods," *Population and Development Review* 23: 1–39.

Preston, Samuel H. 1984. "Children and the elderly: Divergent paths for America's dependents," *Demography* 21: 435–457.

Pritchett, Lant H. 1994. "Desired fertility and the impact of population policies," *Population and Development Review* 20: 1–55.

Putnam, Robert D. 1993. *Making Democracy Work: Civic Traditions in Modern Italy*. Princeton: Princeton University Press.

Schultz, T. Paul. 1994. "Human capital, family planning, and their effects on population growth," *American Economic Review* 84: 255–260.

Scott, James C. 1985. *Weapons of the Weak: Everyday Forms of Peasant Resistance*. New Haven: Yale University Press.

———. 1998. *Seeing Like a State: How Certain Schemes to Improve the Human Condition Have Failed*. New Haven: Yale University Press.

Simmons, Ruth, Laila Baqee, Michael A. Koenig, and James F. Phillips. 1988. "Beyond supply: The importance of female family planning workers in rural Bangladesh," *Studies in Family Planning* 19: 29–38.

Taussig, F. W. 1911. *Principles of Economics*. New York: Macmillan.

"The new Chinese Law on Maternal and Infant Health Care." 1995. *Population and Development Review* 21: 698–702.

Uhlenberg, Peter. 1997. Review of Shirley P. Burggraf, *The Feminine Economy and Economic Man*. *Population and Development Review* 23: 662–663.

Van de Kaa, Dirk J. 1996. "Anchored narratives: The story and findings of half a century of research into the determinants of fertility," *Population Studies* 50: 389–432.

Veil, Simone. 1978. "Human rights, ideologies, and population policies," *Population and Development Review* 4: 313–321.

Warwick, Donald J. 1982. *Bitter Pills: Population Policies and Their Implementation in Eight Developing Countries*. New York: Cambridge University Press.

Willis, Robert J. 1994. "Economic analysis of fertility: Micro foundations and aggregate implications," in Kerstin Lindahl-Kiessling and Hans Landberg, eds., *Population, Economic Development, and the Environment*. Oxford: Clarendon Press.

———. 1998. "Economic transformation and fertility," paper presented at the Conference on Global Fertility Transition, Bellagio, Italy, 18–22 May.

Yergin, Daniel and Joseph Stanislaw. 1998. *The Commanding Heights: The Battle Between Government and the Marketplace That Is Remaking the Modern World*. New York: Simon and Schuster.

Zhang Weiguo. 1998. "Economic reforms and fertility behaviour: A study of a northern Chinese village," Ph.D. dissertation, Institute of Social Studies, The Hague.

Gender and Family Systems in the Fertility Transition

KAREN OPPENHEIM MASON

THAT THE TYPE of family system in a society influences the timing of onset and rapidity of fertility transition is a longstanding tenet; likewise that changes in family systems can precipitate fertility transitions (e.g., Caldwell 1982). That gender systems can influence fertility decline is also widely recognized. Indeed, in recognition of the thesis that women's status or empowerment is a primary feature of gender systems, such systems have recently been elevated to an unprecedented position in ideas about fertility decline. For example, the Program of Action of the United Nations International Conference on Population and Development, held in Cairo in 1994, concluded that

> [I]mproving the status of women...is essential for the long-term success of population programmes. Experience shows that population and development programmes are most effective when steps have simultaneously been taken to improve the status of women. (United Nations 1995: para 4.1)

Thus, gender systems are viewed as interacting with population programs to determine their success. Some would see gender systems as a critical factor in that success.

In this chapter, we review the evidence on the role of gender and family systems in fertility transition and trace the implications for future trends in fertility. First, we discuss how prevailing family and gender systems in pretransitional societies affect the "readiness" of the population to begin the fertility transition. We then discuss how changes in traditional family and gender systems are related to the onset and speed of the transition. Finally, we discuss how family and gender systems are related to post-transitional changes or variations in fertility.

A family system is a set of beliefs and norms, common practices, and associated sanctions through which kinship and the rights and obligations of particular kin relationships are defined. Family systems typically define what it means to be related by blood, or descent, and by marriage; who should live with whom at which stages of the life course; the social, sexual, and economic rights and obligations of individuals occupying different kin positions in relation to each other; and the division of labor among kin-related individuals. A gender system is a set of beliefs and norms, common practices, and associated sanctions through which the meaning of being male and female and the rights and obligations of males and females of different ages and social statuses are defined. Gender systems typically encompass both a division of labor and stratification of the genders. Because all family systems are organized around gender, and because all gender systems delineate the family and kin roles of males and females, the two systems are intertwined but not coterminous in most societies. It thus makes sense to concern ourselves with the implications of both types of system for fertility transitions and post-transitional variation in fertility.

The following theoretical assumptions underlie this chapter. We regard fertility transitions as path-dependent social processes responsive to a variety of initiating conditions rather than as mechanistic responses to a single set of conditions. In this view, there is no single "master determinant" of fertility transitions. Instead, there are conditions that encourage or discourage transitions or hasten or retard their pace once initiated, but only when they coincide with other conditions (Lesthaeghe 1998). The role of gender and family systems in initiating or determining the pace of transitions is thus likely to be interactive; it will be strong only when certain other conditions are present. Our aim is to outline the possible roles of family and gender systems in fertility transitions.

Pretransitional systems

We first consider how prevailing family and gender systems in pretransitional settings influence a population's readiness to undergo a fertility transition—that is, how quickly its members are likely to respond to other initiating conditions such as a decline in infant and child mortality. Following Mason (1997), we focus on three intermediate factors likely to be important for the readiness to enter the transition: (1) the number of surviving children that family systems can accommodate or find valuable; (2) the onset and speed of mortality decline; and (3) the availability and costs of postnatal forms of family-size control. The importance of the number of surviving children that parents or other kin value is obvious. If the family and gender systems can accommodate a large number of surviving offspring, then the pressures for instituting birth limitation will be weaker than in systems where only a small number of offspring can be comfortably accommodated. The onset and speed of the decline in infant and child mortality also have obvious importance for fertility declines. Indeed, many observers view the decline of mortality as the single most important precondition for the decline of fertility. Family or gender systems that retard mortality decline also, presumably, tend to retard the fertility transition. Finally, as argued by Davis (1963), Skinner (1997), and Mason (1997), whether couples have postnatal methods for reducing the size of the family also can influence the onset of the fertility transition. Family and gender systems that condone or encourage the use of postnatal methods of family-size adjustment are more likely to accommodate mortality decline without resort to birth limitation than are systems that do not condone or encourage the use of adjustments. Thus, the extent to which such adjustments are used or are available is likely to condition the population's readiness to undergo the fertility transition.

Ideal or acceptable number of surviving children

Although several authors have recently argued that all family systems are geared to only a small number of surviving children (Cleland 1998; Wilson and Airey 1999), there is reason to question this assumption. Family systems that emphasize the lineage over the household or conjugal unit (found, historically, predominantly in sub-Saharan Africa) and that are hierarchically structured[1] appear to have a higher maximum acceptable family size than do those that emphasize the household or that lack a significant degree of internal stratification (Lesthaeghe 1980). Especially in sub-Saharan Africa, where labor was historically the most important economic resource (in contrast to Europe and Asia, where land tended to be equally or more important: Goody 1973, 1976; Boserup 1985), lineage elders had strong economic and political incentives to maximize numbers of surviving male descendants because these descendants strengthened the lineage and thus the power of its leaders (Lesthaeghe 1980). The burden of caring for large numbers of descendants could also be shared across the lineage rather than falling on the shoulders of one conjugal unit.

At the same time, the widespread practice of polygyny and a tendency to establish separate male and female budgets meant that many of the costs of rearing descendants were borne by women, not by the men who controlled the lineage. Precisely because women were responsible for the support of their children and hence needed their labor power, they, too, desired a large number of offspring (Caldwell 1982: chapter 2). Thus, even though traditional African lineage-based family systems have undergone enormous change during the past century (Lesthaeghe 1980), in their premodern form they appear to have made it highly desirable from the point of view of most actors to have large numbers of surviving children. This may help to explain why the countries of sub-Saharan Africa have been among the last to undergo the fertility transition (Mason 1997).

Another reason that lineage-based family systems may undergo their fertility transitions later than non-lineage-based systems is because of the lineage-wide economic obligations that are characteristic of these family systems (Caldwell 1982; see also Stack 1970 for a description of a similar family system in the United States). Because men in these systems are as firmly obligated to share their resources with their nephews and grandnephews as with their sons and grandsons, pressures toward economic equality within the lineage in turn reduce the possibility of pursuing a strategy of investing in child quality as a substitute for child quantity. Thus, as long as lineage or kin network-wide obligations remain intact, members who are economically most fortunate face enormous pressures to share their wealth within the lineage, rather than investing it in their own children. Under these circumstances, a strategy of having only a few high-quality children becomes less possible than in family systems that limit economic obligations to the immediate family or household.

A case can also be made for variation in optimal family size across other types of family systems. Patrilineal systems emphasizing the joint, multi-generational household of the type historically considered ideal in China and India appear to have accommodated more children (sons in particular) than did family systems based on the stem or conjugal household, such as those widespread in Western Europe and North America in the eighteenth and nineteenth centuries. Especially when population densities were lower than they are today, families in China and India appear to have valued having several surviving sons while the conjugal household families of Western Europe had a low tolerance for more than one or two. Thus, although average family size in China and India rarely exceeded that found in Western Europe, and although such practices as infanticide, sale of infants, and abandonment were more firmly established in China than in Europe, the potential value of sons as part of the joint household's labor force appears to have been greater in China and India than it was in Europe. Thus, type of family system appears to have conditioned the readiness for fertility decline by influencing the numbers of children or sons that families could comfortably accommodate or positively valued.

The literature on gender systems suggests that a high degree of gender (and age) stratification within families or kinship systems is associated with a large desired number of children. Caldwell (1982) and Folbre (1983) argue that men in patriarchal family systems disproportionately benefit from children while women disproportionately bear the costs of rearing them. Although this idea appears to have held for certain traditional sub-Saharan African family systems, it is more questionable in family systems where men have major financial responsibilities for children (Cain 1982). Consistent with this point are the generally small aggregate differences between women and men in their fertility desires even in the most gender-stratified settings (Mason and Taj 1987). A tendency for women to want large numbers of children when they must support them by themselves has, however, been reported not only in sub-Saharan Africa, but in other developing regions as well, for example in the Caribbean and parts of Latin America (Blake 1961; Birdsall and McGreevey 1983; Bunster B. 1983; Caldwell and Caldwell 1987; Merrick and Schmink 1983; Safilios-Rothschild 1980). Thus, even if gender stratification does not increase the number of children that families desire or can accommodate, conditions that require women to bear a heavy economic burden may do so under certain premodern conditions.

Child survival

One of the most common perceptions in the demographic literature is that restrictions on women's freedom of movement, decisionmaking autonomy, access to information, and control of material resources undermine their effectiveness in caring for their children and ensuring child survival (as well as undermining their own health and longevity, which are important for the survival of their children as well). Caldwell (1986) was among the first writers to present evidence for this idea, and many other studies have provided additional evidence (e.g., Basu 1992; Caldwell, Reddy, and Caldwell 1983; Das Gupta 1990; Khan et al. 1989). Also commonly cited in the literature is a tendency, in societies that deny women independent economic roles, for parents to favor sons over daughters, something that may result in excess female mortality in childhood (Cain, Khanam, and Nahar 1979; Das Gupta 1987; but cf. Sastry 1997; Hill and Upchurch 1995; Kishor 1993). Extreme inequality between women and men appears to lower child-survival probabilities. Thus, insofar as fertility transitions depend on a prior decline in child mortality (as Chesnais 1992 argues is normally the case), gender systems that maintain high levels of economic and social inequality between women and men seem likely to retard the onset of fertility decline.

Although some family systems have traditions that enhance child survival by lengthening interbirth intervals—two common examples are prescribed postpartum sexual taboos and lengthy visits of new mothers to their natal homes—these traditions seem unlikely to bring about a decline in mortality. Indeed, a breakdown in these traditions may result in a temporary rise in infant or child mortality by reducing interbirth intervals. In family systems that are built around multi-generational, patrilineal households, child mortality levels may be elevated because mothers lack the power to decide about child nutrition and medical treatment; decisions are instead taken by the mother-in-law with the result that treatment is often delayed and the child dies (Caldwell, Reddy, and Caldwell 1983). In sum, gender stratification tends to reduce child survival, at least insofar as child survival depends on parental decisions and investments rather than on public health systems or programs.

Use of postnatal controls on family size

Postnatal controls on family size, in addition to intentional child neglect and outright infanticide, include child fostering, sending children to other households to act as domestic servants, marrying them off at an early age, and sending them to work in the city (Davis 1963; Mason 1997; Skinner 1997).

The costs of certain postnatal controls are lower in family systems organized around multi-generational households or lineages than in those organized around the conjugal household. Multi-generational households facilitate child marriages because the young couple is incorporated into a preexisting household where they live under the supervision of the husband's or wife's parents. Households that have too many surviving children can use early marriage as a way to reduce internal family pressures, just as those that have too few can use early marriage as a way to bring additional hands into the household.[2] Lineage organization lowers the costs of a different form of postnatal control on number of offspring, namely fostering and adoption. Because all collateral offspring within a lineage of a given gender and birth order are genealogical equivalents (just as same-sex siblings are in the American kinship system), family systems based on lineage organization often circulate children across households by fostering them or adopting them out (Bledsoe 1990; Goody 1982). Although such fostering or adoption can be done to meet the needs of the household into which children are sent or to meet the perceived needs of the child (e.g., for schooling), it also is done to meet the needs of the household from which the children originate. Thus, early marriage, fostering, and adoption facilitate demographic smoothing across households. By giving high-fertility households a safety valve, these practices reduce the pressures to practice birth limitation.

Highly stratified gender systems may also reduce the costs of postnatal family-size controls by encouraging the neglect or outright killing of female offspring (especially those of higher birth orders). Some highly gender-stratified societies proscribe infanticide, but in some settings (e.g., north India, China, and Korea: Miller 1981; Park and Cho 1995) the devaluation of daughters created by gender stratification resulted historically in an inflated level of mortality among girls during the first five years of life. The neglect or killing of daughters is a postnatal control on family size (and composition). Where neglect or infanticide is practiced, the pressures for adopting prenatal controls on family size—that is, birth limitation—may be weaker.[3]

As argued in Mason (1997), differences in family structure and gender stratification between Europe, Asia, and sub-Saharan Africa may help to explain the historical sequence of fertility transitions across these regions. Indeed, the fact that Europe not only was characterized by conjugally oriented family systems, but also was less gender stratified than much of East and South Asia and sub-Saharan Africa, may help to explain why Europe pioneered the fertility transition. The nature of gender and family organization is obviously not the only important factor for the onset of fertility transitions. If that were the case, then fertility should have declined in Southeast Asia before declining in East Asia, which was not the case.[4] When other economic, social, and cultural conditions are comparable, however, then the nature of family and gender systems may indeed affect a population's readiness to undergo the fertility transition.

The onset and speed of the fertility transition

We now discuss how changes in gender and family systems influence the intermediate variables that in turn determine whether or when a fertility transition occurs and the speed with which it progresses. The intermediate variables we consider are the demand for children, the supply of them, and the costs of using fertility limitation (where costs refer to all factors of convenience, supply, price, and social acceptability). In other words, we are interested in the characteristics of family and gender systems that tend to lower the demand for or supply of children, or that lower the costs of birth limitation.

Demand for children

One of the central ideas in the economics of fertility is that married women's entry into the labor market reduces the demand for children by increasing the opportunity costs associated with them (Willis 1973; Lindert 1978; Turchi 1975). When wives work and earn money, each additional child they bear represents time lost from the marketplace and hence earnings forgone. Economists argue that this loss of potential earnings increases the pressures for women to remain in the labor force and simultaneously lowers the demand for children. Thus, the increased entry of married women into the formal labor force that tends to occur in the later stages of industrial development—and which itself represents a change in the family's gender organization—should in turn reduce the demand for children. A related idea is that increases in female education will lower the demand for children because increases in education raise the wages that women can command in the labor force. The value of their time will consequently be higher and so, too, will be the opportunity costs associated with each child.

One implication is that gender systems that restrict women's educational and employment opportunities are likely to delay the onset of the fertility transition by minimizing opportunity costs. Economists normally do not incorporate gender systems into their models, but anything that reduces women's wage levels and earning opportunities will, in principle, also reduce the value of their time and hence make childbearing and rearing less costly. Thus, gender systems can play a role in the demand for children as countries begin to undergo economic modernization.

The evidence that female education is inversely related to fertility is overwhelming, especially at the individual level (Jejeebhoy 1995). The more schooling women have, the fewer children they bear. Opportunity costs are only one possible factor in this association (Cochrane 1979; Jejeebhoy 1995). Indeed, in underdeveloped rural areas with few opportunities for women to engage in paid work, the inverse association between female schooling and fertility almost certainly does not reflect educational variation in opportunity costs (e.g., Sathar and Mason 1993). Nevertheless, in some settings the strong inverse relationship between female education and fertility no doubt reflects the higher opportunity costs that occur when women become relatively well educated and have opportunities to put their schooling to work in the marketplace.

Evidence about the connection between female employment and fertility is mixed (Cleland 1985; Rodríguez and Cleland 1980). The individual-level relationship between women's employment and fertility is highly variable across settings, leading some authors to conclude that female employment does not as a rule tend to reduce the demand for children (e.g., Cleland 1985). Country-level analysis, however, has found an inverse relationship between the rate at which women work in the formal sector of the market and the fertility rate, a relationship consistent with the idea that when gender or family systems prevent women from working, pressures for fertility decline will be relatively low (Kasarda 1971). Thus, although the evidence is mixed, in relatively more-developed or rapidly developing settings female employment in the formal labor force is often linked to reduced levels of fertility, presumably because of a reduced demand for children. Gender systems that restrict women's ability to attend school or earn money may consequently slow the pace of the fertility transition by keeping the demand for children higher than it might have otherwise been.

A more subtle way in which gender stratification may retard the fertility transition is through parents' educating their sons and daughters unequally.[5] One reason that economic modernization is thought to precipitate fertility transition is because of increased pressures to educate children, which result in what economists term the child quality-for-quantity tradeoff. The pressures to substitute child quality for child quantity are presumably strong only where pressures for equity among children within a given family are strong, that is, where investments in all children are expected to be more or less equal. Where gender stratification is strong, parents may feel little pressure to educate their daughters and may therefore pursue a strategy of relatively high fertility combined with educating sons only. Joint-household or lineage-based family systems may also encourage moderate-to-high fertility combined with the selective education of children because of the aforementioned pressures on more fortunate family members to share their wealth. There is much anecdotal evidence of joint households in South Asia or lineages in sub-Saharan Africa that decide to educate only the brightest male child in the hopes that he will obtain a high-earning job and share his income with those who invested in his schooling. Under these conditions, families are less likely to respond to the rise of modern economic systems and the increased importance of schooling for success by limiting numbers of births.

Supply of children

Fertility often rises shortly before the onset of the fertility transition, and this sudden increase in the supply of children has been speculated to put a stress on family resources that in turn triggers an interest in fertility limitation (Dyson and Murphy 1985). Do gender or family systems play a role in such pretransitional increases in fertility? Family systems that regulate fertility through practices intended to increase birth spacing, such as postpartum abstinence, can experience increased fertility if these practices are eroded or abandoned under pressures of modernization. Pretransitional fertility increases do not, however, appear to be restricted solely to family systems that promote these practices (Dyson and Murphy 1985).

In Western Europe in the eighteenth and nineteenth centuries, where women's lives were relatively unrestricted and marriage ages relatively high, industrialization appears to have reduced age at marriage: the working classes no longer had to wait to inherit the family farm before marrying because they could obtain industrial employment (Tilly and Scott 1978). This may have led to an increase in fertility, which eventually may have contributed to the fertility transitions in this region. Whether this convergence of historical events can be viewed as a reflection of a gender system that treated women more equitably than did many of the gender systems found in Asia and sub-Saharan Africa is, however, unclear because it was not just women's ability to assume paid employment but men's as well that appears to have lowered the age at marriage.

Costs of fertility regulation

Gender systems affect the costs of fertility regulation, that is, how easily women can learn about, get access to, and come to view as safe and morally acceptable the means to limit childbearing within marriage (Mason 1993). Family systems may also influence the costs of fertility regulation, although primarily because they influence gender relations. For example, family systems organized around multi-generational extended family households may discourage the adoption of family limitation because they tend to maintain greater control over women of reproductive age than do conjugally based family systems.

The hypothesis is that the greater the extent to which gender or family systems grant women freedom of movement, encourage their education or familiarity with the world outside the home, and give them control over material resources, the greater the extent to which women will be able to learn about and adopt family-limitation methods (Mason 1993). This relationship does not hold in all settings. For example, during the historical fertility transitions in Europe and North America, the primary methods of fertility limitation were controlled by men: withdrawal, abstinence, and the condom. In this context, women's freedom of movement, literacy, awareness of the world, and control of resources are unlikely to have been factors in their access to fertility-limitation methods, although they may have been important for their exposure to new ideas about the moral acceptability of using these methods within marriage. In contrast, where the cultural climate gave women the moral authority to enforce sexual abstinence, as Daniel Scott Smith (1974) argues was the case in the American middle class during the first half of the nineteenth century, women's autonomy may have been instrumental in their willingness to take the radical step of deliberately limiting childbearing within marriage.

In modern developing countries where fertility limitation is achieved predominantly through mechanical and chemical forms of contraception or through sterilization, women's freedom of movement, awareness, and control of resources may determine how quickly they learn about contraception, how able they are to seek out contraceptive supplies, and whether they can afford the transportation and direct costs involved in obtaining them. Women's autonomy has been advanced as an explanation of one of the most rapid fertility transitions of the twentieth century, that of Thailand (Knodel et al. 1987). Women's freedom of movement and control of resources, however, are neither necessary nor sufficient to guarantee that contraception is adopted. In Bangladesh, where family planning service delivery programs have been designed to overcome women's seclusion and lack of resources, contraceptive use has been adopted quite rapidly. Also, even when the predominant means of limiting births are female methods (the pill, IUDs, injections, implants), men may decide whether or not the couple practices contraception. All other things equal, however, less-stratified and less-restrictive gender systems are likely to lower the costs to women of adopting family limitation by making them more able to learn about and obtain birth control.

Family systems that are relatively unstratified by gender or age and that emphasize the conjugal unit may reduce the costs of fertility limitation through another mechanism, namely by encouraging communication and diffusion of information, new attitudes, and beliefs between husband and wife. An older demographic literature argued that a high level of communication between husbands and wives facilitates discussion about fertility goals and contraceptive methods, thereby increasing the likelihood of adopting fertility limitation and the effectiveness of attempts to limit births (Beckman 1983). Although the causal relationships in this area are often hard to disentangle—does good communication lead to contraceptive use or are couples who are interested in practicing contraception motivated to discuss it?—at least limited evidence supports the communication hypothesis. Diffusion theory also suggests the relevance of husband–wife communication.[6] Family and gender systems that promote the separation of married couples from the parental generation and encourage close cooperation and communication between them may help speed fertility transition by increasing the diffusion of innovation from husband to wife or vice versa.

In sum, there is some evidence that more egalitarian gender and family systems that emphasize the conjugal unit as the primary focus of family life promote fertility transitions by lowering the costs of fertility regulation. The evidence is consistent with the historical sequence in which fertility transitions have occurred in major world regions: first in Europe with its strong emphasis on the conjugal family and relative equality between the genders within the family; then in Asia and Latin America with more gender-stratified or complex family systems; and finally in sub-Saharan Africa with the most highly elaborated, corporate family systems. Neither family systems nor gender systems can be considered master determinants of fertility transitions, but in interaction with other factors they appear to play important roles.

Post-transitional fertility variations

Although fertility transitions tend to homogenize fertility rates across provinces and countries (Watkins 1991), post-transitional populations nevertheless show considerable variation in fertility levels. In particular, while some post-transitional populations have total fertility rates close to the long-term replacement level of approximately 2.1 children per woman, others have far lower rates—1.5 children per woman or less (Population Reference Bureau 1997). These latter countries face the prospect of extreme population aging and population decline, and building up a negative-growth momentum. On its face, the rise of these negative-growth demographic regimes is consistent with transformations in gender and family systems in many post-transitional societies. Gender and family systems in Europe and North America have become more egalitarian and conjugally oriented (Lesthaeghe 1995; Mason, Tsuya, and Choe 1998). Insofar as these changes encourage late marriage and childbearing or the limitation of fertility within marriage, the development of ultra-low fertility regimes is not surprising.

A closer look at the evidence, however, raises doubts about the nature of the links between gender and family change and post-transitional variations in fertility. (Recognizing that the forces that create fertility transitions need not be identical with those that determine post-transitional variation in fertility raises further doubts.) As Chesnais (1996) and McDonald (2000) have noted, fertility is higher in the Scandinavian countries, which generally have moved farthest in terms of gender equality and the simplification of the family, than in Italy or Spain, which are more conservative Roman Catholic countries where gender and family forms reflect an older set of traditions.[7] Other comparisons suggest a similar paradox. For example, fertility in the United States is far higher than in Japan, even adjusting for the presence in the US of a large higher-fertility Hispanic population of recent origin. Yet there is far greater gender equality and emphasis on the conjugal family in the United States than in Japan.

What is the explanation for this seemingly paradoxical set of differences among countries? The explanations provided by Chesnais and McDonald are similar and emphasize what McDonald calls incomplete institutionalization. In all of the post-transitional countries of Europe, Chesnais and McDonald suggest, women's roles have changed markedly. In most countries, women are nearly as well educated as men and participate in the labor force in large numbers, often on a life-long basis. Women also conceive of themselves as independent earners, not just as wives and mothers, an attitude that may be reflected in a rise in divorce rates in many countries. Chesnais and McDonald suggest that where governments accommodate this change in women's roles and orientations and provide the social supports that enable women to remain independent while rearing children, women are indeed able to have the two children that most people in post-transitional societies consider ideal. Where little or no accommodation has been made to the change in women's roles, however, women face conflicts between maintaining their independence and having children. The result is postponement of marriage and childbearing and a tendency to have only one child. Thus, both Chesnais and McDonald attribute post-transitional variation in fertility to the extent to which state institutions have accommodated changes in the gender system. A similar argument could made vis-à-vis changes in the family system. Were family roles to change in a way supportive of wives' career activities—for example, through equal sharing of housework and childrearing by husband and wife—this too might sustain replacement-level childbearing.

The evidence marshaled to date in support of the Chesnais/McDonald hypothesis has been limited. Nevertheless, it is worth asking what this hypothesis portends for the future of population growth in the countries that are now entering or will soon enter the post-transitional phase of the demographic transition. We speculate that many of these countries will join the "new" post-transitional countries such as Japan, Singapore, South Korea, Hong Kong, and Taiwan in having below-replacement fertility, especially if they are developing economically. Economic development and demographic modernization appear to work in tandem to increase women's participation in the modern economic sector. As fertility declines, the availability of young male labor shrinks and the population of aged dependents grows. The time that women have available for extra-domestic activities also increases greatly, not only because of decreased fertility but also because of enhanced longevity. In this situation, the entry of young women into the labor force becomes increasingly attractive to employers and to young women and their families.

The rise of consumerism that accompanies development and exposure to global economic and communications networks often has the effect of destabilizing family relationships, with a consequent rise in divorce (Bumpass and Mason 1998). These conditions in turn move the gender system toward the form it has taken in Western Europe and North America. Thus, unless governments support women's independence with programs to make motherhood and employment compatible, women in these countries may well follow the path taken by their counterparts in Europe and the most developed parts of East Asia: late marriage, late childbearing, and low marital fertility. Because many formerly developing countries have a strong tradition of relying on families to provide social security and social welfare, the development of programs designed to accommodate women's new attitudes and goals seems unlikely (Ogawa and Retherford 1997). It remains to be seen whether changes in family roles wrought through women's political activism can achieve the same end as it has in the United States and parts of Europe. Also, the below-replacement demographic regimes that we argue are likely to emerge in many countries as they complete the demographic transition may be a temporary phenomenon. But there is no guarantee that they will be. Thus, an important policy item for many governments whose populations are close to completing the fertility transition—or whose populations are well into the post-transitional phase—is to consider how to ensure that an egalitarian shift of gender systems does not lead to extreme population aging and negative growth.

Notes

1 A lineage refers to all of the living descendants of an identifiable individual who can trace their relationship to him or her through a series of male or female ascendants. Most lineage-based family systems are patrilineally organized, that is, descent is traced through the male line, meaning that children belong to their father's lineage rather than to their

mother's. A minority of lineage systems are matrilineally organized, that is, ties are traced through females and children belong to the lineage of their mother. Matrilineal descent systems are *not* matriarchal, i.e., the lineage is controlled by men, not by women, even though it is their sisters' children who are their descendants, rather than their own children. Although family systems in parts of South and East Asia are also organized around lineages, they tend to emphasize the household much more strongly than the lineage per se, which rarely has the corporate character it traditionally had in sub-Saharan Africa.

2 One of the more extreme examples of this use of early marriage is the *sim pua* or "little bride" system traditionally practiced in parts of China (Wolf and Huang 1980). In this system, a girl was sent to the household of her prospective husband in early childhood, even infancy, and was reared by her mother-in-law, thereby providing the latter with help long before reaching sexual maturity and consummating the marriage. This system enabled poor households to slough off unwanted baby girls while satisfying the needs of households hungry for an enhanced domestic labor force.

3 Indeed, insofar as the goal is to reduce the number of daughters, not just the total number of children, prenatal controls have had an important disadvantage: until recently, they did not permit sex selection of offspring.

4 Family systems in Southeast Asia tend to be far more conjugally oriented or more likely to be based on a stem-family principle than those in East and South Asia, which emphasize the multi-generational extended family household as the ideal.

5 I am grateful to Mark Montgomery for this suggestion.

6 The diffusion hypothesis is discussed in Bongaarts and Watkins (1996), Cleland (1985, 1998), Cleland and Wilson (1987), and Freedman and Takeshita (1969).

7 Although the Scandinavian countries have adopted explicit policies designed to promote equality of women and men, they nonetheless remain gender stratified (Hoem 1995). These countries appear to have moved much further through the "second demographic transition" than the countries of southern Europe, however (Lesthaeghe 1995).

References

Basu, Alaka. 1992. *Culture, the Status of Women and Demographic Behaviour: Illustrated with the Case of India*. Oxford: Clarendon Press.

Beckman, Linda J. 1983. "Communication, power, and the influence of social networks in couple decisions on fertility," in Rodolfo A. Bulatao and Ronald D. Lee (eds.), *Determinants of Fertility in Developing Countries*, Vol. 1. New York: Academic Press, pp. 856–878.

Birdsall, Nancy and William Paul McGreevey. 1983. "Women, poverty, and development," in Mayra Buvinić, Margaret A. Lycette, and William Paul McGreevey (eds.), *Women and Poverty in the Third World*. Baltimore: Johns Hopkins University Press, pp. 3–13.

Blake, Judith. 1961. *Family Structure in Jamaica: The Social Context of Reproduction*. Glencoe, IL: Free Press.

Bledsoe, Caroline. 1990. "The politics of children: Fosterage and the social management of fertility among the Mende of Sierra Leone," in W. Penn Handwerker (ed.), *Births and Power: Social Change and the Politics of Reproduction*. Boulder, CO: Westview Press, pp. 81–100.

Bongaarts, John and Susan Cotts Watkins. 1996. "Social interactions and contemporary fertility transitions," *Population and Development Review* 22(4): 639–692.

Boserup, Ester. 1985. "Economic and demographic interrelationships in sub-Saharan Africa," *Population and Development Review* 11(3): 383–397.

Bumpass, Larry and Karen Oppenheim Mason. 1998. "Family processes and their implications for families in the future," in Karen Oppenheim Mason, Noriko O. Tsuya, and Minja Kim Choe (eds.), *The Changing Family in Comparative Perspective: Asia and the United States*. Honolulu: East-West Center, pp. 237–250.

Bunster B., Ximena. 1983. "Market sellers in Lima, Peru: Talking about work," in Mayra Buvinić, Margaret A. Lycette, and William Paul McGreevey (eds.), *Women and Poverty in the Third World*. Baltimore: Johns Hopkins University Press, pp. 92–103.

Cain, Mead. 1982. "Perspectives on family and fertility in developing countries," *Population Studies* 36(2): 159–175.

Cain, Mead, Syeda Rokeya Khanam, and Shamsun Nahar. 1979. "Class, patriarchy, and women's work in Bangladesh," *Population and Development Review* 5(3): 405–438.

Caldwell, John C. 1982. *Theory of Fertility Decline*. London: Academic Press.

———. 1986. "Routes to low mortality in poor countries," *Population and Development Review* 12(2): 171–220.

Caldwell, John C. and Pat Caldwell. 1987. "The cultural context of high fertility in sub-Saharan Africa," *Population and Development Review* 13(3): 409–437.

Caldwell, J. C., P. H. Reddy, and Pat Caldwell. 1983. "The social component of mortality decline: An investigation in South India employing alternative methodologies," *Population Studies* 37(2): 185–205.

Chesnais, Jean-Claude. 1992. *The Demographic Transition: Stages, Patterns, and Economic Implications: A Longitudinal Study of Sixty-Seven Countries Covering the Period 1720–1984*, translated by Elizabeth Kreager and Philip Kreager. Oxford: Clarendon Press.

———. 1996. "Fertility, family, and social policy in contemporary Western Europe," *Population and Development Review* 22(4): 729–739.

Cleland, John. 1985. "Marital fertility decline in developing countries: Theories and the evidence," in John Cleland and John Hobcraft (eds.), *Reproductive Change in Developing Countries: Insights from the World Fertility Survey*. Oxford: Oxford University Press, pp. 223–252.

———. 1998. "Potatoes and pills: An overview of innovation-diffusion contributions to explanations of fertility decline," paper prepared for the National Academy of Sciences Workshop on Social Processes in Fertility Transitions, Washington, DC, 28–30 January.

Cleland, John and Christopher Wilson. 1987. "Demand theories of the fertility transition: An iconoclastic view," *Population Studies* 41(1): 5–30.

Cochrane, Susan Hill. 1979. *Fertility and Education: What Do We Really Know?* Baltimore: Johns Hopkins University Press.

Das Gupta, Monica. 1987. "Selective discrimination against female children in rural Punjab, India," *Population and Development Review* 13(1): 77–100.

———. 1990. "Death clustering, mothers' education and the determinants of child mortality in rural Punjab, India," *Population Studies* 44(3): 489–505.

Davis, Kingsley. 1963. "The theory of change and response in modern demographic history," *Population Index* 29(October): 345–366.

Dyson, Tim and Mike Murphy. 1985. "The onset of fertility transition," *Population and Development Review* 11(3): 399–440.

Folbre, Nancy. 1983. "Of patriarchy born: The political economy of fertility decisions," *Feminist Studies* 9: 261–284.

Freedman, Ronald and John Y. Takeshita. 1969. *Family Planning in Taiwan: An Experiment in Social Change*. Princeton: Princeton University Press.

Goody, Esther N. 1982. *Parenthood and Social Reproduction: Fostering and Occupational Roles in West Africa*. Cambridge: Cambridge University Press.

Goody, Jack. 1973. "Bridewealth and dowry in Africa and Eurasia," in Jack Goody and S. J. Tambiah, *Bridewealth and Dowry*. Cambridge: Cambridge University Press, pp. 1–58.

———. 1976. *Production and Reproduction: A Comparative Study of the Domestic Domain*. Cambridge: Cambridge University Press.

Hill, Kenneth and Dawn M. Upchurch. 1995. "Gender differences in child health: Evidence from the Demographic and Health Surveys," *Population and Development Review* 21(1): 127–151.

Hoem, Britta. 1995. "The way to the gender-segregated Swedish labour market," in Karen Oppenheim Mason and An-Magritt Jensen (eds.), *Gender and Family Change in Industrialized Countries*. Oxford: Clarendon Press, pp. 279–296.

Jejeebhoy, Shireen. 1995. *Women's Education, Autonomy, and Reproductive Behaviour: Experience from Developing Countries*. Oxford: Clarendon Press.

Kasarda, John D. 1971. "Economic structure and fertility: A comparative analysis," *Demography* 8(3): 307–317.

Khan, M. E., Richard Anker, S. K. Gosh Dastidar, and Shashi Bairathi. 1989. "Inequalities between men and women in nutrition and family welfare services: An in-depth enquiry in an Indian village," in John C. Caldwell and Gigi Santow (eds.), *Selected Readings in the Cultural, Social and Behavioural Determinants of Health*. Canberra: Australian National University, Health Transition Centre, pp. 175–199.

Kishor, Sunita. 1993. "'May God give sons to all': Gender and child mortality in India," *American Sociological Review* 58(2): 247–265.

Knodel, John, Aphichat Chamratrithirong, and Nibhon Debavalya. 1987. *Thailand's Reproductive Revolution: Rapid Fertility Decline in a Third-World Setting*. Madison: University of Wisconsin Press.

Lesthaeghe, Ron. 1980. "On the social control of human reproduction," *Population and Development Review* 6(4): 527–548.

———. 1995. "The second demographic transition in Western countries: An interpretation," in Karen Oppenheim Mason and An-Magritt Jensen (eds.), *Gender and Family Change in Industrialized Countries*. Oxford: Clarendon Press, pp. 17–62.

———. 1998. "On theory development: Applications to the study of family formation," *Population and Development Review* 24(1): 1–14.

Lindert, Peter H. 1978. *Fertility and Scarcity in America*. Princeton: Princeton University Press.

Mason, Karen Oppenheim. 1993. "The impact of women's position on demographic change during the course of development," in Nora Federici, Karen Oppenheim Mason, and Sølvi Sogner (eds.), *Women's Position and Demographic Change*. Oxford: Clarendon Press, pp. 19–42.

———. 1997. "Explaining fertility transitions," *Demography* 34(4): 443–454.

Mason, Karen Oppenheim and Anju Malhotra Taj. 1987. "Differences between women's and men's reproductive goals in developing countries," *Population and Development Review* 13(4): 611–638.

Mason, Karen Oppenheim, Noriko O. Tsuya, and Minja Kim Choe (eds.). 1998. *The Changing Family in Comparative Perspective: Asia and the United States*. Honolulu: East-West Center.

McDonald, Peter. 2000. "Gender equity, social institutions and the future of fertility," *Journal of Population Research* 17(1): 1–16.

Merrick, Thomas W. and Marianne Schmink. 1983. "Households headed by women and urban poverty in Brazil," in Mayra Buvinić, Margaret A. Lycette, and William Paul McGreevey (eds.), *Women and Poverty in the Third World*. Baltimore: Johns Hopkins University Press, pp. 244–271.

Miller, Barbara D. 1981. *The Endangered Sex: Neglect of Female Children in Rural North India*. Ithaca, NY: Cornell University Press.

Ogawa, Naohiro and Robert D. Retherford. 1997. "Shifting costs of caring for the elderly back to families in Japan: Will it work?" *Population and Development Review* 23(1): 59–94.

Park, Chai Bin and Nam-Hoon Cho. 1995. "Consequences of son preference in a low-fertility society: Imbalance of the sex ratio at birth in Korea." *Population and Development Review* 21(1): 59–84.

Population Reference Bureau. 1997. *World Population Data Sheet, 1997*. Washington, DC.

Rodríguez, Germán and John Cleland. 1980. "Socio-economic determinants of marital fertility in twenty countries: A multivariate analysis," in *World Fertility Survey Conference 1980, Record of Proceedings*, vol. 2. London: World Fertility Survey, pp. 337–414.

Safilios-Rothschild, Constantina. 1980. "A class and sex stratification theoretical model and its relevance for fertility trends in the developing world," in Charlotte Höhn and Ranier Makensen (eds.), *Determinants of Fertility Trends: Theories Re-examined*. Liège: Ordina Editions, pp. 189–202.

Sastry, Narayan. 1997. "Family-level clustering of childhood mortality risk in Northeast Brazil," *Population Studies* 51(3): 245–261.

Sathar, Zeba A. and Karen Oppenheim Mason. 1993. "How female education affects reproductive behavior in urban Pakistan," *Asian and Pacific Population Forum* 6 (Winter): 93–103.

Skinner, G. William. 1997. "Family systems and demographic processes," in David I. Kertzer and Tom Fricke (eds.), *Anthropological Demography: Toward a New Synthesis*. Chicago: University of Chicago Press, pp. 53–95.

Smith, Daniel Scott. 1974. "Family limitation, sexual control, and domestic feminism in Victorian America," in Mary Hartman and Lois W. Banner (eds.), *Clio's Consciousness Raised: New Perspectives on the History of Women*. New York: Harper & Row, pp. 119–136.

Stack, Carol B. 1970. *All Our Kin: Strategies for Survival in a Black Community*. New York: Harper Colophon Books.

Tilly, Louise A. and Joan W. Scott. 1978. *Women, Work, and Family*. New York: Holt, Rinehart and Winston.

Turchi, Boone A. 1975. *The Demand for Children: The Economics of Fertility in the United States*. Cambridge, MA: Ballinger Publishing Co.

United Nations. 1995. "Program of Action of the 1994 International Conference on Population and Development (Chapters I–VIII)," *Population and Development Review* 21(1): 187–213.

Watkins, Susan Cotts. 1991. *From Provinces into Nations: Demographic Integration in Western Europe, 1870–1960*. Princeton, NJ: Princeton University Press.

Willis, Robert J. 1973. "A new approach to the economic theory of fertility behavior," *Journal of Political Economy* 81(2, Part II): S14–S64.

Wilson, Chris and Pauline Airey. 1999. "How can a homeostatic perspective enhance demographic transition theory?" *Population Studies* 53(2): 117–128.

Wolf, Arthur and Chieh-shan Huang. 1980. *Marriage and Adoption in China, 1845–1945*. Stanford: Stanford University Press.

Comment: A Gender Perspective for Understanding Low Fertility in Post-Transitional Societies

HARRIET B. PRESSER

EXISTING DEMOGRAPHIC RESEARCH on gender is not as extensive or as finely tuned as one might like. While we have come a long way since the mid-1970s, when a session titled "The status of women: A concern for demographers?" was considered highly controversial at the Annual Meeting of the Population Association of America—many demographers at that time answering in the negative—we have still just scratched the surface (Presser 1997). It is increasingly recognized that we need to move beyond crude "status of women" measures, often operationalized by education and labor force status, and think about how to better analyze and incorporate the multi-dimensional and multi-level nature of gender systems in our research so that we can relate them to family systems and demographic processes, and thus better understand the complex interrelationships.[1] In my view, such an effort calls for more middle-range theory and more creative thinking about the concepts we seek to operationalize. This applies to research on both industrialized and developing countries.

I devote my discussion to industrialized countries. Specifically, I propose a new perspective on the relevance to fertility behavior of gender and family systems in postindustrial societies—a perspective less grandiose than transition theory but more in touch with social-psychological processes that relate to both macro- and micro-level events. This perspective pertains to the greater ability that recent cohorts of women have to control the timing of events over the life course, the resulting greater sense of entitlement to leisure time this generates for women, and how both aspects of time relate to the timing and number of births women have.[2]

In elaborating on this perspective, I address some issues with which demographers are familiar: changing birth control technology, the timing of first births, and the marital or nonmarital context in which children are born and reared. But I place these familiar topics within a less familiar context by relating them to changing notions about the concept of time. I believe that situating demographic processes—including gender and family systems—in this context offers a fruitful direction for better understanding low fertility in post-transitional societies. Moreover, the implication of this perspective is that fertility in such societies may become even lower in the near future.

I start from a macro perspective by discussing changes in birth control technology. Fertility was low in Western countries during the 1920s and 1930s when the highly effective modern contraceptives, such as the pill, were not available and voluntary sterilization for contraceptive reasons was rarely practiced. So it is not a necessary condition that birth control technology be highly effective to bring about, in the aggregate, low levels of fertility. Strong motivation among many not to have a (another) child, along with the use of traditional methods plus illegal abortion for unplanned pregnancies, or pervasive sexual abstinence, can bring this about. Modern birth control methods, however, make it easier to control fertility with less motivation; thus a lower level of motivation (or lower intensity of "demand for children") is needed to sustain, *in the aggregate*, low fertility. I emphasize "in the aggregate" because, before the availability of modern methods like the contraceptive pill—and when methods (condoms, diaphragms, withdrawal) were generally used at the time of coitus—it was still difficult for individual women and men to effectively control the timing and number of their births.

The introduction of the contraceptive pill (which preceded the legalization of abortion "on demand" in most countries) changed this situation. I would argue that this single development led to a significant transformation in the way women in general felt about being "on call" for unintended childbearing and childrearing throughout their reproductive span. The widespread reliance on legal abortion in countries that did not adopt the pill (e.g., Japan) had a similar effect. Before the availability of the pill and legal abortion, timing failures were more extensive, and this sustained a "contingency" orientation over women's life course. The pill and legal abortion significantly reduced this uncertainty.[3] Thus, improvement in birth control technology was a critical source of empowerment, enabling women to feel in greater control not just of reproductive timing, but of their educational and employment activities as well. Children, however timed, generally are disruptive of such activities, but with the availability of the pill and legal abortion the timing of this disruption could be planned much more effectively.[4] Moreover, the technological ability to effectively control reproductive timing undoubtedly helped broaden labor force opportunities for women by weakening the rationale of employers that women were unpredictable, temporary workers, and thus not worthy of well-paying jobs. The elimination of such "contingency thinking" at the macro as well as the micro level was, in my mind, what made the pill truly revolutionary.[5]

What difference did this shift from contingency thinking to being in control of birth timing make for fertility behavior in post-transition societies and what is the relevance of gender and family systems in this regard? This volume contains detailed evidence of sustained below-replacement fertility in many postindustrial societies and theories about postmodernism and ideational change. The implicit if not explicit focus is on changes in family-size desires, but not on changes in the desired timing of first births. I would argue that the two need to be distinguished—and more attention needs to be given to the determinants of delayed childbearing, as well as to changes in women's sense of entitlement to child-free time for themselves, which the pill and legal abortion have helped bring about.

Clearly, effective fertility control gave women—and men—the ability to have sex without fear of having a child, an illegal abortion, or a "shotgun wedding." The greater separation of sex from reproduction not only delayed marriage and first births but, by diminishing the stigma of sex outside of marriage, diminished the stigma of reproduction outside of marriage, thereby making fertility less contingent on marriage—or even cohabitation. The growing separation of fertility and co-residence of parents, particularly in the United States, means that increasingly large numbers of mothers are becoming sole parents without the benefit of two incomes. This trend suggests that questions of time with children relative to questions of economic affordability may be gaining ground in fertility decision-making in postindustrial societies. The salient tradeoffs then become the desire for children versus the desire for leisure, and the desire for children versus the importance of childrearing with a father/husband present.

An important distinction here is the number of hours for free time versus work, unpaid and paid combined, rather than the number of hours women are engaged in paid employment versus all other time—the more usual dichotomy studied in relation to childbearing behavior. What is missing in discussions of the effect of work on fertility in postindustrial societies is the unpaid work component. Most childcare is not leisure, especially when children are of preschool age (although sometimes coded as leisure by researchers). Moreover, when others provide childcare to enable women to work outside the home, this does not provide women with more leisure; it just adds to the total number of hours, paid and unpaid, worked—and thus minimizes free time.

In the common scenario in postindustrialized countries, women postpone childbearing and consequently have more years to experience, and feel entitled to, time of their own for activities other than work or schooling. With generally higher education and higher employment status than their mothers, how do women in these countries feel about the demands of day-to-day childrearing that come with the first child? And what is the changing nature of gender relations when men feel no less entitled to having time of their own while women increasingly expect men to participate more in childrearing—at least women who have children within marriage? If we understand these dynamics, we will come a long way toward better understanding—and better predicting—fertility in postindustrial contexts, at both the individual and aggregate level.[6]

As I have noted elsewhere (Presser 1986), most women and men want to be parents. But it takes only one child to make us a "parent." We may "desire" two or more children, but the marginal social—as distinct from economic—cost of the second child compared to the first is for many women greater, not less, relative to the benefit. By social cost, I mean specifically the value of personal time: time for child-free leisure activities (e.g., travel, entertainment, reading, being with friends, being able to sleep late). I contend that women, who generally assume day-to-day childrearing responsibilities, are becoming more like men in their sense of entitlement to personal time, and that this trend encourages many women to postpone, forever, second births—even in the absence of marital instability. We need to operationalize this sense of entitlement in our research,[7] both for men and women, so that we can better understand the relationship between first-birth timing and completed family size—as well as the growing tensions in gender negotiations over time use within families.

In this context, I briefly note my view about the controversy in the United States concerning the "overworked American" that Juliet Schor (1991) has written about. Her analysis of census data shows that Americans are employed more hours than in the past. John Robinson and Geoffrey Godbey (1997), in contrast, use data from time diaries since 1965 to show that Americans are not working longer hours: they just feel they are, since they experience more stress. And it is women, more than men, who seemingly over-report work hours in census data as compared to reporting in time diaries.

I would argue that this perception of greater stress among women comes largely from having changed one's sense of entitlement to personal time as a consequence of postponed childbearing. Moreover, the shock most women experience after the birth of their first child, when they realize how demanding of their time a young child is (not to minimize the pleasures), may also facilitate the postponement (possibly forever) of a second child. Taking care of young children means being "on call" around the clock for their emotional and physical needs in a child-controlled way (Presser 1995). The demands on one's time, along with the sense of personal responsibility to meet these demands, make this an unusual form of work and help to explain men's resistance to getting more involved. This impediment to women's growing sense of entitlement to time of their own, along with the increasing pressure, especially among the middle class, to invest in the social and educational activities of children, may well play a significant role in discouraging additional births.

A focus on leisure may also help us to understand some perplexing relationships between employment and fertility in industrialized countries. For example, the Netherlands has experienced a decline in fertility to below replacement levels, yet Dutch women have a low attachment to the labor force despite high educational attainment. Although about 40 percent of women are employed, about 75 percent are working part-time, most of them less than 20 hours per week. The labor force is highly sex-segregated. Why the decline in fertility among Dutch women as the proportion working part-time is growing? One can point to the lack of institutional childcare relative to, say, Sweden, but my impression based on many discussions with Dutch women in 1994–95 was that they generally do not want to work more hours. The opportunity structure for jobs commensurate with their education is not very good, and gender relations are highly traditional. This traditionalism is reinforced by state policy, which assures married women with minimal work experience that, if divorce should occur, they can survive economically by having access to a considerable share of their ex-husband's income. On the basis of my discussions, I am convinced that Dutch women feel strongly about their entitlement to leisure and perhaps increasingly so. I see the process as follows: in a society that constrains high-status opportunities for women in the labor force but educates them highly, women postpone childbearing and increase their taste for leisure.[8]

Japan is another country that confounds demographic expectations by having very low fertility while most women are only marginally attached to the labor force. The notable postponement in age at marriage for both sexes over recent decades (facilitated by widespread condom use and legal abortion, rather than the pill) has led to higher education for women and increased freedom of activity outside the home prior to marriage. This has undoubtedly led to a greater sense of entitlement to time of one's own. Then, upon marriage and subsequent childbearing, life changes dramatically for most Japanese women. As Tsuyo and Mason (1992) have documented, the majority do not consider marriage a primary source of happiness. The daily "on call" demands of childcare and the growing expectations placed on mothers for generating "quality" children are probably highly relevant in explaining low levels of fertility in Japan.

A growing sense of entitlement to time of one's own among women would, I believe, also help explain low fertility in countries such as Italy, with late age at marriage, and—like Japan—low fertility outside marriage and traditional gender roles after marriage (along with heavy reliance on legal abortion). Francovich (1998) shows that Italian men tend to live with their parents until they are about to marry, in their late 20s or early 30s. Mothers undoubtedly provide housekeeping services for many of these men, including preparing meals. Men then marry women who are generally only a few years younger and who have been relatively independent for many years. The expectation that such women take on traditional gender roles following marriage undoubtedly leads to tensions between spouses, and perhaps discourages couples from having more than one child.

We might also gain from studying differentials within societies in women's and men's sense of entitlement to leisure time. This may be relevant to why, in societies like the United States, with a notable postponement in age at first marriage and first birth and less traditional gender roles than countries like Italy and Japan, out-of-wedlock childbearing and rearing are substantial and on the rise. (Two-fifths of all US first births are now out of wedlock; Bachu 1998.) While middle-class American women are participating in the trend toward later marriage and childbearing, nonmarital childbearing remains far more characteristic of lower-class women. Why take on the considerable time burden of childrearing in a context of financial hardship? I suspect the answer is, in part, that there is a marked class difference in the sense of entitlement to leisure, which may be related to class differences in women's age at first birth and class differences in women's views about the need to have children in order to achieve a meaningful life. The minimal stigma attached to single parenthood in countries like the United States is undoubtedly also relevant.

To conclude, demographic theories need to consider the concept of time as well as timing, be more middle-range in theoretical perspective, and be more gender oriented. Future fertility studies of postindustrialized countries should include measures relating to entitlement to time of one's own, both for women and men, and examine class differences within societies. This should provide a better understanding of how gender and family systems relate to the process of fertility behavior, and why, as I anticipate, fertility in postindustrialized societies, while fluctuating, may fall below current levels in the near future.

Notes

1 For a collection of papers on this topic, see Presser and Sen (2000).

2 This is different from the more traditional way in which economists view time, where the "cost of time" is at issue.

3 There are, of course, health concerns related to the pill. Such concerns were pervasive when the dosages of estrogen and progestin were much greater than they are today; see Seaman (1969).

4 Scrimshaw (1981: 260) has made a similar argument, stating that "With the pill, family planning—in the true sense of the phrase—was finally possible. Women and men had the option of developing careers and *then* starting their families, of *planning* children to

fit with career and financial development, or even of having no children at all" (emphasis in original).

5 It is arguable whether the so-called sexual revolution also facilitated by the availability of the pill has been as beneficial to women.

6 We should also consider that if men were to substantially increase their participation in childrearing, *their* fertility desires might decrease even if this would make childrearing less time-demanding for women.

7 The desire for future leisure *on the job* by high school seniors in the US was measured over time: between 1976 and 1991 the extent to which this was very important increased for both sexes, but more for females than males (Marini et al. 1996).

8 In contrast to Jean-Claude Chesnais (1996), I do not view Sweden as representing "the equality model," given that the country has the most sex-segregated labor force of all Western countries. It is debatable whether Sweden's family policies in this context are a better model than a less sex-segregated labor force without such generous family policies. The ideal, of course, would be both generous family policies and minimal occupational sex segregation.

References

Bachu, Amara. 1998. "Trends in marital status of U.S. women at first birth: 1930 to 1994, Population Division Working Paper No. 20. Washington, DC: U.S. Census Bureau.

Chesnais, Jean-Claude. 1996. "Fertility, family, and social policy in contemporary Western Europe," *Population and Development Review* 22(4): 729–739.

Francovich, Lisa. 1998. "Male cohabitation and marriage in Italy: First results according to the 1995–96 Fertility and Family Survey," paper presented at the IUSSP Seminar on Men, Family Formation, and Reproduction, Buenos Aires, 13–15 May.

Marini, Margaret Mooney, Pi-Ling Fan, Erica Finley, and Ann M. Beutel. 1996. "Gender and job values," *Sociology of Education* 69(1): 49–65.

Presser, Harriet B. 1986. "Changing values and falling birth rates: Comment," *Population and Development Review* 12 (Supp.): 196–200.

———. 1995. "Are the interests of women inherently at odds with the interests of children or the family?" in Karen Oppenheim Mason and An-Margritt Jensen (eds.), *Gender and Family Change in Industrialized Countries*. Oxford: Clarendon Press.

———. 1997. "Demography, feminism, and the science–policy nexus," *Population and Development Review* 23(2): 295–331.

Presser, Harriet B. and Gita Sen. 2000. *Women's Empowerment and Demographic Processes: Moving Beyond Cairo*. Oxford: Oxford University Press.

Robinson, John P. and Geoffrey Godbey. 1997. *Time for Life: The Surprising Ways Americans Use Their Time*. University Park: Pennsylvania State University Press.

Schor, Juliet. 1991. *The Overworked American: The Unexpected Decline of Leisure*. New York: Basic Books.

Scrimshaw, Susan C. M. 1981. "Women and the pill: From panacea to catalyst," *Family Planning Perspectives* 13(6): 254–256, 260–262.

Seaman, Barbara. 1969. *The Doctors' Case Against the Pill*. New York: Avon.

Tsuyo, Noriko O. and Karen Oppenheim Mason. 1992. "Changing gender roles and below-replacement fertility in Japan," paper presented at the IUSSP Seminar on Gender and Family Change in Industrialized Countries, Rome, 27–30 January.

Population Policies, Family Planning Programs, and Fertility: The Record

AMY ONG TSUI

IN 1976 OUT OF 156 COUNTRIES, both developing and developed, 40 had policies to lower their levels of fertility; 14 countries sought to raise fertility. In 1996 of 179 countries, 80 had policies to lower and 23 to raise fertility. Currently two-thirds of developing countries—covering the majority of the developing world's population and its childbearing couples—have national population policies or programs. In parallel with the shift in government views, fertility levels have declined in developing countries. Total fertility rates (TFRs) decreased from an average of 5.4 children per woman of childbearing age in 1970–75 to 3.5 in 1990–95 (United Nations 1998b). While fertility rates have not declined as sharply in the African region (6.7 to 5.8), they have fallen by about half in both Asia (5.7 to 3.0) and Latin America and the Caribbean (6.0 to 3.1) in this period. Presently 35 percent of the countries in the world have TFRs at or below 2.1 (U.S. Census Bureau 1998).

A question of longstanding interest to many in the population field has been: What role have national population policies and family planning programs played in fertility transitions? It is possible that population policies and programs are related to fertility in only spurious or insignificant ways. Fertility levels in developing countries may have declined for entirely different reasons. If so, this fact would consign national expressions of support for lower fertility and provision of means to achieve them to only bit parts in a larger script of global social change.

Substantial social and economic gains have occurred in the developing world, seen in trends since World War II in literacy and schooling, urbanization, nutrition, industrialization, and household incomes. Mass communication media in print and electronic form have carried and diffused information, images, and messages into households and policy circles. Intrinsically connected to these changes are the dramatic declines in infant and child mortality levels, occurring throughout the developing world and conditioning subsequent fertility declines. Age at marriage has increased, and motivations to limit the size of families and adopt means to achieve this goal have risen.

Over the same period, the development of modern contraceptive methods has meant that safe and effective means of controlling fertility have become available for widespread individual use without significant medical supervision. The ability to separate coitus from conception has become a reality for millions of sexually active individuals. If population programs have been a major factor in fertility decline, there should be evidence that they extended the contraceptive option to a substantial proportion of eligible populations in the developing world.

Last, what are the implications if the null hypothesis—that population policy interventions addressing fertility had little or no effect—cannot be rejected in the end? At present, contraceptive service delivery is being actively expanded by many national governments. With each decade, the sustained declines in fertility are accompanied by sustained rises in contraceptive practice using modern methods. These trends tend to reinforce in the minds of program managers the perceived linkage and value of their efforts. If it is eventually agreed that these programs have been largely ineffectual, what are the likely consequences for future fertility policies and interventions? How would this affect the expected benefits and influence of pronatalist policies and action? To inform ongoing and future initiatives, the assessment of the effectiveness of developing-world population policies and programs remains a valuable exercise.

This assessment reviews the plausibility of causal linkages between population policies and programs and fertility transitions in developing countries. The next section reviews the evolution of population policy since 1960. A third section addresses the design, content, and effort levels of population programs. The fourth section presents the behavioral trends accompanying the fertility transitions in recent decades, while the fifth details a cross-national trend analysis that attempts to link social, programmatic, and fertility change. The sixth section proposes considering other disciplinary perspectives and methods to examine organizational systems and processes of population programs. The final section discusses implications of current social trends for the future of family planning programs.

Population policy since 1960

India adopted a national population policy in 1951, the earliest country to do so, followed by Pakistan, the Republic of Korea, China, and Fiji during 1960–62. The majority of other developing countries did not legislate national policies articulating demographic concerns until the late 1960s and early 1970s.

The United Nations played a major role in increasing global awareness of population problems and the need to integrate population policy into general economic and social development policies and programs (United Nations 1993). At the first World Population Conference in 1954, primarily a forum for scientific exchange, a debate on the role of population in development emerged between Western capitalist countries and those with centrally planned economies. Third world countries identified themselves with the latter group, an alignment that reappeared at the 1965 Belgrade and 1974 Bucharest World Population Conferences. The 1984 International Conference on Population in Mexico City marked a reversal of positions. The United States delegation adopted a revisionist posture, declaring population growth to have a neutral role in development. At the same time, the majority of African delegations reversed their previous pronatalist positions and became uniform in expressing concern over the consequences of rapid population growth. The Mexico City conference served as a watershed in global sentiment about the linkage between population and development; subsequently the issue has become less divisive for most developing and developed countries. At the 1994 International Conference on Population and Development in Cairo, delegates turned their attention to micro-level rationales for population's role in development by reaffirming the right of couples and individuals to choose the number and timing of children and to have access to the information and means for doing so. At the same time they broadened these rights to include those securing sexual and reproductive health.

Consistent with the history of positions taken at international population conferences, governments have articulated through successive rounds

TABLE 1 Governments' views on fertility level, intervention policy, and access to contraceptive methods, 1976–96 (percent of countries)

View	1976	1983	1986	1989	1993	1996
No. of countries	156	168	170	170	170	179
Fertility level						
Too low	12	13	14	12	12	13
Satisfactory	53	50	46	45	44	40
Too high	35	37	40	44	45	47
Policy to influence fertility						
Raise	9	14	12	12	12	13
Maintain	14	14	11	11	14	9
Lower	26	29	32	38	41	45
None	51	43	45	39	33	34
Contraceptive access						
Limited	7	4	4	4	2	1
Not limited						
No support	22	19	11	12	10	12
Indirect support	15	17	14	12	7	7
Direct support	55	60	72	72	82	79

SOURCE: Brennan 1997: Tables 1–3; UN 1998a: Tables 3–5.

of the UN Population Inquiry their growing support for reduced fertility levels and for policy interventions, specifically those addressing the direct provision of contraceptive services (see Table 1). The emerging consensus and homogeneity in fertility-related population policies adopted over the past 25 years not only represent governments' commitments to internal change but also signal their alliance with the international community concerned with population growth (Barrett and Tsui 1999). How has this shift in normative climate concerning population issues and policy been manifested in the structure and content of population programs?

The record of population programs as family planning programs

A population program is the enactment of nationally defined policies or organized strategies to affect demographic trends and patterns. It can encompass legislative, regulatory, and programmatic mechanisms that directly influence the size, distribution, composition, and growth of a population. Thus it can address mortality, migration, and fertility rates or behaviors at both the macro and micro levels. The modification of fertility levels has been the predominant demographic rationale for the design and implementation of population programs.

Governments in the poorer regions of the world, once having identified the management of population change as a necessary public good, have tended to legislate national population policies with specific expectations regarding the future course of fertility. This recognition arrives either as a result of internal deliberations or in response to external incentives, such as overseas development assistance. These policy mechanisms often identify voluntary family-limitation behaviors as the outcomes to be encouraged and national family planning programs as the means through which to filter that encouragement.

Family planning programs have been described as "organized efforts to assure that couples who want to limit their family size and space their children have access to contraceptive information and services and are encouraged to use them as needed" (Simmons 1986: 175). Organized efforts to provide contraceptive information and services can range from the extensive to the nominal, that is, from broad governmental efforts coordinated by a national board, as with the original National Family Planning Coordinating Board in Indonesia, to a specific Ministry of Health division supervising the delivery of maternal and child health and family planning services, or to a private nonprofit organization dependent on external financial contributions and voluntary labor, such as a family planning association. Countries that have all three types of provider groups, as well as an active commercial sector, are perceived as having strong national effort. In other countries where contraceptive imports may be embargoed and local manufacturing is nil, where the public health program does not provide contraceptives, or where only a local family planning affiliate in the capital is operative, the national effort is considered weak. Weak or strong, the nationally organized effort, to a large extent, represents the aggregate output of activities pursued by a diverse array of service organizations and providers.

A quantitative measure of family planning program strength, or "effort," has been devised and employed by Mauldin and Berelson (1978), Lapham and Mauldin (1985), Mauldin and Ross (1991), and Ross and Mauldin (1996). These authors have scored program effort for 93 to 98 developing countries on 30 dimensions for several time points—1972, 1982, 1989, and 1994.[1] These scores have been criticized as expert opinions or reputational rankings biased by a priori knowledge of the outcomes (e.g., Schultz 1993). They have been extensively analyzed and critiqued for their internal construction and construct validity (e.g., by Entwisle 1989; Bulatao 1996). Other researchers, however, have accepted them prima facie and related them to fertility and contraceptive behavioral outcomes (e.g., Cutright 1983; Bongaarts et al. 1990). Validation with objective data has been reported in Mauldin et al. (1995). Although imperfect, these scores are presently the only cross-national time-series data on national family planning program effort.

The scores offer a relatively standardized means for monitoring nationally organized efforts for family planning. Table 2 traces change be-

TABLE 2 Family planning program effort scores as a percent of maximum effort, by method of weighting and region, for 1972, 1982, 1989, and 1994, 77 countries

Weighting/region	1972	1982	1989	1994
Unit weights				
Total	22	32	47	50
East Asia	61	73	76	76
South/Southeast Asia	35	43	53	55
North Africa/Middle East	10	23	38	43
Sub-Saharan Africa	5	15	38	44
Latin America	32	40	54	52
Weights by numbers of females aged 15–49				
Total	53	61	69	70
East Asia	82	83	86	91
South/Southeast Asia	51	60	68	66
North Africa/Middle East	16	27	46	49
Sub-Saharan Africa	5	14	39	44
Latin America	16	47	51	54

SOURCE: Ross and Mauldin 1996: Table 3.

tween 1972 and 1994 among a panel of 77 developing countries, by region and weighted both by unit (country) and population (females aged 15 to 49). The table tracks national program effort, which has risen from 22 percent to 50 percent of maximum overall, with differential trends by region. Least change is seen in East Asia, which began at 61 percent and rose to 76 percent, as compared to sub-Saharan African countries which showed only 5 percent effort in 1972, climbing to 44 percent by 1994. Still, the 1994 scores for sub-Saharan African countries, along with those of the other regions, were below those that East Asia received more than two decades earlier. Overall, the time trends in Table 2 signal quite clearly, whether weighted by country units or female population of reproductive age, an expanded delivery of contraceptive information and services over this 22-year period.

Table 3 shows change between 1982 and 1994 in the categories of program activities.[2] The category "Method availability" might be viewed as the service provision output of the other components of program effort;

TABLE 3 Family planning program effort scores (percent of maximum) by component and region: 1982 and 1994

Component and year	All	East Asia	South/ South-east Asia	Sub-Saharan Africa	Middle East/ North Africa	Latin America
Program effort						
1982	29	63	42	15	20	40
1994	48	67	54	44	41	50
Change	19	4	12	29	21	10
Policy and stage setting						
1982	34	66	45	25	26	39
1994	53	64	61	55	45	48
Change	19	–2	16	30	19	9
Service and service-related						
1982	25	58	38	12	16	34
1994	44	60	50	41	36	43
Change	19	2	12	29	20	9
Record keeping						
1982	29	57	43	13	21	42
1994	52	72	53	47	39	60
Change	23	15	10	34	18	18
Method availability						
1982	31	76	45	10	21	53
1994	50	83	53	35	46	62
Change	19	7	8	25	25	9

NOTE: Percentages calculated using unit, not population, weights.
SOURCE: Ross and Frankenberg 1993: Table 2; Ross and Mauldin 1996: Table 1.

its score rose from 31 percent to 50 percent or by 19 percentage points overall and at a greater magnitude in the African regions and much smaller magnitude in the Asian and Latin American regions. Policy and stage-setting activities also rose on average by 19 percentage points, with the largest gain found in sub-Saharan Africa (30 points). Marginal change in both Policy and Service-related activities occurred in Latin America and virtually no change, if not a retrogression, occurred in East Asia. Gains in the Record-keeping score were the highest, rising from 29 to 52 percent, with an especially substantial gain in sub-Saharan Africa (a 34-point increase). While the absence of objective measurements of program activity over time is unfortunate, the picture indicated by these summary scores is of a remarkable strengthening of national family planning programs.

The record linking family planning programs and contraceptive practice in developing countries

The practice of contraception plays a key and obvious role in the regulation of fertility. The substantial change in fertility limitation in developing countries that has transpired over nearly a quarter of a century can be viewed in the trend data on contraceptive practice, shown in Figure 1. Con-

FIGURE 1 Contraceptive prevalence in the developing world, by region

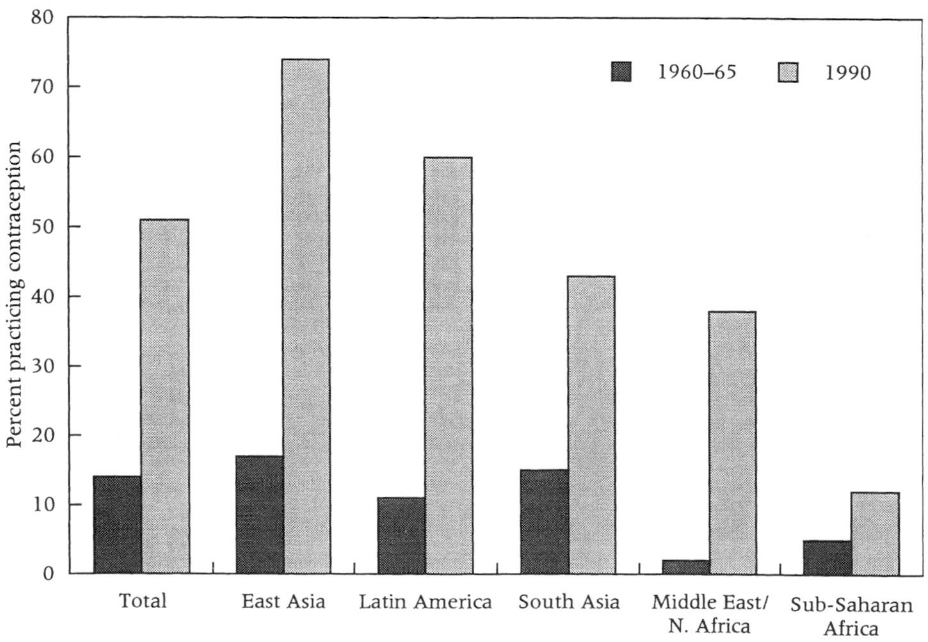

SOURCE: Ross and Frankenberg 1993: Figure 1.

traceptive prevalence rose from 14 percent among couples of childbearing age in developing regions in 1960–65 to 50 percent in 1990. The latest United Nations (2000) estimate is 56 percent of women in union. Regional variation was fairly narrow in the earlier period, ranging between 2 and 17 percent. In 1990, it ranged from 12 percent in sub-Saharan African to 74 percent in East Asian countries. In numerical terms this translates into nearly a ninefold increase in the number of reproductive-aged females currently practicing some form of pregnancy avoidance, from an estimated 54 million couples in 1960 to 504 million in 2000, using United Nations population figures.

The effectiveness of contraceptive use in lowering fertility levels is seen in Figure 2, which relates national and subnational estimates of contraceptive prevalence with total fertility rates in the developing world. This close relationship is represented in the regression line or equation, TFR = 7.29 – .07 CPR, and suggests that for each 15 percentage point change in CPR (contraceptive prevalence rate), the TFR increases (or decreases) by one child. The conversion equation implies that substantial fertility reduction should have taken place, based on the observed increases in contraceptive use.

More than 90 percent of current users rely on modern forms of contraception. National profiles of contraceptive experience in selected countries reveal dynamic shifts over a two-decade period in contraceptive method choice, reflecting changes in both consumer preferences and program sup-

FIGURE 2 Relationship between total fertility rate and contraceptive prevalence in developing countries

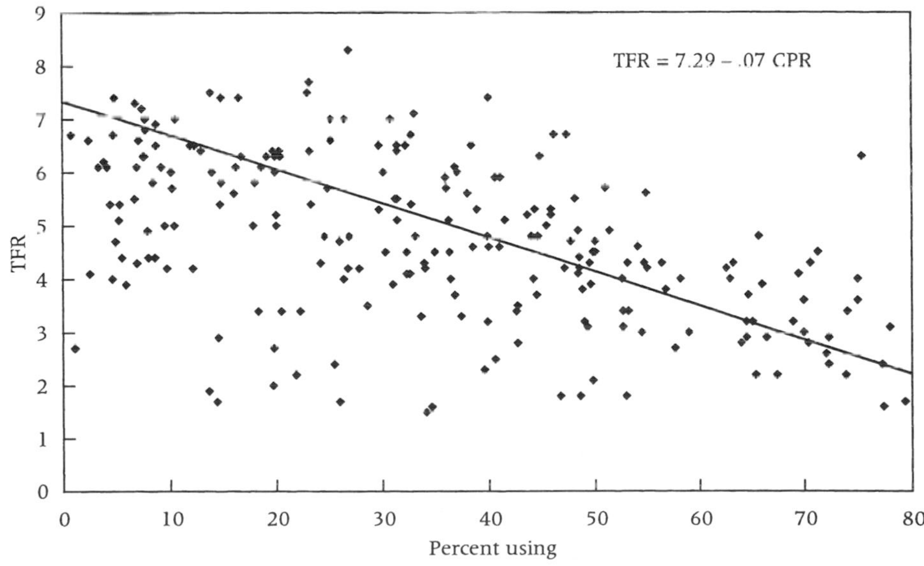

SOURCE: Population Council Databank.

ply. In a study summarizing the contraceptive method-specific experience for 57 developing countries (United Nations 1996: Table 15), 58 percent of married women of reproductive age were practicing some form of contraception, and nearly all (93 percent) of the use is with modern methods. Sterilization, oral contraceptives, and IUDs figure as the most frequently used methods. These data suggest that perhaps a billion individuals have used modern contraception at some time and roughly 390–400 million married women of reproductive age currently modify their sexual and reproductive behaviors by practicing artificial means of contraception.

The data indicate that public programs sponsoring clinical and nonclinical contraceptive services have played an important role in increasing the accessibility of methods. In Demographic and Health Surveys conducted in countries of sub-Saharan Africa and Asia, the overwhelming majority of clinical method users (such as users of surgical contraception, intrauterine devices, or implants) obtain their services from public sources (government hospitals and clinics). In Latin American and Caribbean countries, public and private sources tend to serve contraceptive users equally, except in Colombia where the large nongovernmental organization, Profamilia, serves more than three-fifths of clinical method users. Nonclinical method users (users of the pill, condoms, or injectables, for example) resort to the private sector more frequently than clinical method users; however, private-sector providers, predominantly pharmacists, are often participants in social marketing programs, in which governments and international donors heavily subsidize the sale of contraceptives through private retailers. It thus appears that a significant volume of public resources has been allocated to expanding contraceptive access through a range of service sites and across program networks. Although family-limitation behavior might have increased without modern contraception and the services of public programs (as indeed occurred in Western Europe), such behaviors would likely neither have been as effective as afforded by safe contraceptive technologies nor have gained widespread use as quickly.

One should not overemphasize the role of supply-oriented policies and programs in recent fertility declines and disregard the forces that raise demand for those public goods and services. Demeny (1993) has suggested that the ideology of development planning can result in a disproportionate effort to account for tangibles, such as commodity distribution data, imbuing supply-side programs with a greater sense of value than warranted. National family planning programs, however, for better or worse, have become the modality for population programs in recent decades, and such programs have emphasized family planning service delivery. The trend data for developing countries indicate rising national program efforts, increased public recognition of modern contraceptive methods and knowledge of service sites, and expanded delivery and use of services and methods. Are these trends indicative of effective organized efforts to deliver family planning services nationally, or do supply-side programs yield a larger-than-life view of their impact? In the next section we discuss the range of evidence from recent reviews and present results of a cross-national time-series analysis that can help assess the extent to which population or family planning program strength has accelerated fertility transitions in developing countries.

Cross-national analysis of social, economic, and programmatic change

What would fertility levels in the developing world have been in the absence of family planning programs? Assessing the effect of national population programs on fertility transitions reduces to this counterfactual question. Some analysts question whether such programs have risen independently as instruments of international and national policy, suggesting that they may be endogenous to development planning concerns (Pritchett 1994; Schultz 1994). At one level we can address this issue with a cross-national time-series database of development indicators for 80 developing countries for 1972, 1982, 1989, and 1994, years for which the family planning effort index has been calculated. The database contains social, economic, and demographic indicators of development that are typically used in studies of the determinants of fertility change (e.g., Schultz 1994; Bongaarts et al. 1990), including the total fertility rate, average years of schooling for females, percent of population urban, percent of the labor force in agriculture, average kilocalories consumed daily, and per capita gross domestic product (in constant dollars). In addition, we have data on the percent of the population in the main religions (Catholic, Protestant, Islam).[3]

We use a slightly modified version of family planning program effort score to measure organizational input by netting out scores for six items that measure access to contraceptive methods and abortion.[4] The 24-item score is also lagged to indicate the estimated effort two years earlier (i.e., 1970, 1980, 1987, and 1992). To address potential bias from the perceived subjectivity of the program effort score, we also include a donor-agency per capita population assistance measure.[5]

Table 4, which gives the results of the regression analysis,[6] shows a reasonably strong fit between the data and the model, which controls for the periodicity of the years and the fixed levels of religious composition. The results of the individual predictors are in the expected direction, with male schooling raising fertility and female schooling lowering fertility significantly. Urbanization and (log) per capita gross domestic product are not statistically significant influences on fertility levels, while a larger nonagricultural labor force and more adequate food availability do lower them. Family planning program effort (lagged) has a net negative but statistically

TABLE 4 Regression results for total fertility rate on indicators of social and economic development and family planning program effort for 1972–94 in 78 developing countries[a]

Variable	Coefficient	Standard error	t	Significance level
Constant	4.849	1.143	4.242	0.000
Average years of schooling for males	0.245	0.078	3.129	0.002
Average years of schooling for females	–0.372	0.087	–4.300	0.000
Proportion of population in urban areas	0.001	0.008	0.122	0.903
Percent of labor force in agriculture	0.035	0.010	3.669	0.000
(Log) GDP per capita	0.008	0.113	0.072	0.943
Lagged family planning effort score[b]	–0.004	0.003	–1.409	0.160
Per capita population expenditures by USAID	–1.062	0.367	–2.897	0.004
Average kilocalories consumed annually	–0.463	0.227	–2.037	0.043
Year = 1982	–0.228	0.174	–1.314	0.190
Year = 1989	–0.371	0.238	–1.562	0.120
Year = 1994	–0.446	0.288	–1.551	0.123
R^2 within	0.682			
R^2 between	0.596			
R^2 overall	0.617			
F(11,188)	36.65			
Significance level	0.000			

[a]Fixed-effects estimator; model also controls for proportion Catholic, Muslim, and Protestant in countries.
[b]Total score for 24 nonmethod access items, lagged 2 years.

insignificant effect on fertility. Per capita donor population assistance, which may be correlated with unobserved national government expenditures on family planning, is associated with appreciable fertility reduction. A per capita spending level of US$1 in population assistance is associated with a 1.06 reduction in the TFR.

An easier way to interpret the regression model results is to simulate what the TFRs would have been in the absence of any family planning program effort (lagged FPE). Table 5 gives the average TFRs for the four time points, as well as the predicted TFRs in 1994 if FPE had been absent and if there had also been no US population assistance throughout, for each major region and all countries combined. Overall, if no family planning effort was experienced, the models suggests that the 1994 TFR would

TABLE 5 Total fertility rates circa 1972, 1982, 1989, and 1994 for 75 developing countries and simulated for 1994 with no family planning effort (FPE) and no donor spending, by region

Region	No. of countries	TFR 1972	TFR 1982	TFR 1989	TFR 1994	Predicted 1994 TFR if: No FPE	Predicted 1994 TFR if: No FPE and no aid	Predicted effect of FPE and aid on 1994 TFR
Total	75	5.93	5.32	4.87	4.33	4.61	4.83	–0.50
Africa	28	6.42	6.48	6.20	5.93	5.72	5.82	+0.11
Asia	16	5.14	4.13	3.54	3.21	4.49	4.57	–1.36
Latin America	20	5.19	4.14	3.56	3.29	3.34	3.70	–0.41
Near East	11	6.27	5.47	4.78	4.28	4.49	4.64	–0.36

NOTE: TFRs are averages with countries equally weighted. Predicted 1994 TFR counterfactuals are simulated using regression model in Table 4.

have been 4.61; and if also there was no US population assistance, then the average TFR would have been 4.83, or 0.5 births higher than the observed 1994 average of 4.33.[7] By region, we see that the average difference between the 1994 TFR and the TFR under the assumption of no family planning program effort and no US assistance ranges from negligible (but in the "wrong" direction) for the African countries in the dataset to a substantial –1.36 for the Asian countries.[8] We interpret these differences as evidence of the effect of population programs in accelerating the fertility transitions.[9]

Other similar cross-national impact analyses of family planning effort on fertility have used unwanted fertility rather than total fertility rates as outcomes (Bongaarts 1995) or desired fertility as a predictor of overall fertility (Pritchett 1994). Bongaarts notes that his and Pritchett's estimates of the fertility impact of a 50-point increase in family planning effort in the 1980s, reductions of 1.4 and 1.0 respectively in the TFR, do not differ substantially, are in the range of that estimated in Bongaarts et al. (1990), and average 1.2 fewer births. He suggests, more optimistically than the results shown in Table 5, that organized family planning programs have accounted for about half of the fertility decline occurring since the 1950s. Ahlburg and Diamond (1996) critique the Bongaarts model results for the quality of data and statistical techniques used, suggesting that Schultz's studies (1993, 1994) offer more rigorous approaches. We have attempted to replicate Schultz's cross-national analysis in Table 4 and to supplement it with improved population expenditure information, lagged and adjusted family planning effort scores, and a longer observation period.

The aggregate effect of national family planning program effort on global fertility and population growth levels may be considerable given the proportionate distribution of the developing world's population in Asia.

Consistent with the demographic transition model's arguments at the macro-societal level, the results of our analysis are based on a long time series of cross-national data, follow structural specifications others have used, and apply appropriate estimation procedures. Not all researchers, however, are willing to accept cross-national empirical evidence. Some place more credence on micro-level, country-specific evidence, and others are more interested in broader political and economic influences on the performance of population programs (e.g., Lee et al. 1998).

Determining program effects from micro-level studies presents its own challenges. Hermalin and Khadr's review of studies assessing the effect of family planning programs on fertility (1996) notes the range of study designs and time periods involved and, consequently, the varying magnitudes of effects found. Using 14 national surveys conducted between 1988 and 1995 in 11 developing countries, Angeles et al. (1998) have conducted a comparative analysis of the effects of community-level family planning service access and quality on individual use of modern contraceptives. They find that the net effect of the absence of universal service access independently lowers modern use from 25 percent to 16 percent. On the other hand, they find no significant effect of service quality on use, nor do they find that community-level access and quality measures strongly influence a woman's recent fertility. Ahlburg and Diamond's review of such within-country analyses of family planning program impact on fertility, however, more confidently concludes that "family planning programs contribute to fertility decline, often substantially" (1996: 319). Mauldin and Sinding agree, summarizing:

> At times there has been controversy as to whether socioeconomic development or family planning is more important. The authors believe that this has become a largely academic question as research has repeatedly shown that both contribute to declining fertility and that the more each of them is present, the faster fertility will decline.... No matter how rapid socioeconomic development is, the transition from high to lower fertility will be greatly aided by well-organized family planning programs, as the past decade has clearly demonstrated. (1996: 102)

Likewise, Phillips and Ross (1992) were persuaded that the weight of the evidence affirms program effects on fertility.

The issue of the impact of family planning programs remains primarily relevant for those countries still at the early stages of fertility transition. Most of the demographically significant countries have completed the transition or experienced most of it. Already 22 of the 80 countries analyzed here, considered developing in 1972, have 1994 TFRs below 3.0 and another eight have TFRs between 3.0 and 3.5. The majority of the countries with nascent transitions are poor, or in sub-Saharan Africa, or both. For these countries, the essential question is how the organized delivery of contraceptive information and services can be made more efficient and effective.

Bulatao (1993), Ahlburg and Diamond (1996), Guilkey (1998), and others have identified elements of family planning programs that contribute to their effectiveness in raising contraceptive use. Bulatao suggests programs be organized to provide high-quality services, with a strong client focus, strategic management, effective promotion, and participation by the private sector. Community-based outreach and information-education-communication (IEC) programs show particularly strong effects in the studies Guilkey reviewed. Ahlburg and Diamond list a number of components as key to successful family planning programs: social and cultural acceptability, service accessibility and quality, commitment to meeting client needs, IEC, a supportive political and administrative system, and operations research. Evidence of the selective importance of these structural characteristics, specialized functions, and contextual factors of family planning programs reinforces Phillips and Ross's recommendation (1992) to focus future research on the components of the supply side.

Furthering the understanding of organizations and programs

Researchers of micro-level demography have primarily been interested in the explanatory roles of personal, familial, and household attributes vis-à-vis fertility preferences and outcomes. On occasion their perspective has shifted one step up the social hierarchy to the level of the community. Beyond the community, however, is the seat of national and civic governance, the level at which national policy and public-sector programs are defined, designed, and financed. A mix of institutions operates at this level, including ministries, nonprofit nongovernmental organizations, individual health care providers, and commercial outlets. It is the institutional mix at multiple levels, however, that is relevant for studying the causal pathways by which a national-level, centralized decision may or may not influence the family-formation behaviors of individuals residing in communities.[10] Warwick's study (1986) of Indonesia's National Family Planning Coordinating Board reminds us that at the regional, provincial, and village levels, officials face competing pressures to implement centrally directed development programs (whether for agriculture, health and family planning, public works, or education). The administrative hierarchy does not always facilitate a smooth flow of resources and operations leading to the distribution of benefits to individuals in communities and households as originally intended by national policymakers and program managers.

As organizations mature, they pass through stages of development. Goodman et al. (1997) apply "stage theory" (Lewin 1951) to explain how organizations innovate in goals, programs, technologies, and ideas. Progression through stages requires organizational awareness to innovation, attitude formation, and decisions to implement and carry out the innovation. Institutionalization must occur in the last stage to sustain change. Goodman et al. (1997: 290) propose that "beyond institutionalization is renewal, a stage during which well-established programs evolve to meet changing demands."

Population and family planning programs provide examples of this renewal where single-focus organizations evolve and merge with others sharing similar missions. For example, the Korean Institute for Family Planning (1971–80) became the Korean Institute for Population and Health (1981–89), following a merger with the Korean Health Development Institute; and in 1990, to recognize the transfer and incorporation of a new social welfare research function, KIPH became the current Korea Institute for Health and Social Affairs. During this period the Korean government sharply reduced its population and family planning budgets. Similarly in Malaysia the National Family Planning Board, a ministerial coordinating unit, evolved to become the National Population and Development Board. The Taiwan Institute of Family Planning targets high-quality family planning services to adolescents, the physically and mentally disabled, and economically disadvantaged populations; it has a special program for infertile couples (Freedman 1999). Rapid fertility transitions in Asia have hastened the organizational maturity of national family planning programs, prompting the host organizations themselves and external funding agencies to question their original raison d'être and forcing institutional renewal through redefined missions.

Another pattern of institutional behavior is decentralization. In many modern states, there is pressure from both external and central sources to devolve responsibility for financing and organizing human welfare services to lower operating units, usually province, district, or municipal authorities. Decentralization may diffuse organizational purpose, but it simultaneously allows maximal responsiveness to heterogeneous client demands (Aldrich 1981). It is a change process worth formal study. Applied to family planning programs, decentralization implies shifts in resource flows. There may be more flexibility and responsiveness to local client demands. Program functions may see more duplication and overlap, which can potentially strengthen the overall system's reliability. A centrally oriented flow of benefits may be redirected with more resources going to lower units, and specialized tasks may be increasingly defined, such as the integration of screening and counseling for sexually transmitted diseases with family planning services in high-risk areas.

These patterns of organizational behaviors have implications for the nationally organized delivery of contraceptive information and services that in turn can influence individual family-limitation behaviors. Formal organizations are complex, and their dynamic processes constitute the "black box" of family planning programs, the effects of which are often measured crudely and the particulars of which are rarely studied systematically.

Family planning programs in the future

Population policies and programs, even if reoriented toward reproductive health, aging, migration, or environmental issues, will benefit from new kinds of studies of effectiveness. "Second-generation studies" will focus primarily on factors influencing the efficiency of program performance (see, e.g., Bulatao 1996), program response to clients' service preferences, and the effects of integrating other reproductive health services with contraceptive services. "Third-generation studies" will largely address equity issues, looking at the allocation of public resources to population groups with economic need and to competing social-sector programs. To what extent has public subsidization of health and family planning services benefited those in greatest economic need? Have the free or mostly free services, particularly from family planning clinics in urban public hospitals and clinics, been disproportionately used by individuals able to finance their own care? Mature family planning programs and their service systems will be scrutinized more carefully in the future for evidence of cost efficiency and benefit incidence to maximize returns on the investment of public funds. These types of studies will require the engagement of those with expertise in health economics and the administrative and organizational sciences.

Future needs for governmental and international support of family planning programs are likely to be greatest in the poverty-ridden areas of the developing world, particularly in sub-Saharan Africa and South Asia and in selected Latin American countries. Rising contraceptive prevalence will also add new demands to resources presently allocated to programs in the demographically significant developing countries, although the expansion of private-sector services will provide substantial relief to public financing. There are encouraging signs that individual motivations for contraceptive practice are being established earlier in the reproductive life cycle. Blanc and Way (1998) report current modern contraceptive use among sexually active and unmarried women aged 15 to 19 to be higher than for those currently married in most sub-Saharan African countries surveyed. (The reverse was true for Latin American and Caribbean countries surveyed in the early 1990s.) Overall, modern contraceptives are being used by more and by younger women in developing countries than ever before (see also McDevitt 1996).

The risk of STD transmission is requiring family planning programs to update the skills of clinic and outreach personnel to counsel and provide services to clients when opportunities for screening, diagnosis, and treatment present themselves. The persistent health risks to sexually active men and women will prompt family planning services to shift their focus to reproductive well-being. This, in turn, imbues population programs with a prominent health as well as demographic rationale and agenda for their claim on public resources. The diversification of national population programs to meet additional socially desirable goals need not be limited to reproductive health; it has already accommodated links with environmental quality (e.g., United Nations 1997), aging (e.g., Martin and Preston 1994), and immigration (e.g., Smith and Edmonston 1998).

Many developing countries have recently experienced fertility transitions of historically unprecendented speed and now face new concerns about the social and economic consequences of rapidly aging populations. Differential improvement in individual well-being and greater ease of movement between regions and countries have increased the perceived attractiveness and accessibility of nearby labor markets and residential locations, leading to higher rates of international and internal migration. As a result the face of national population policies will change and diversify. The role and influence of national fertility policy interventions and programs have been established and accepted sufficiently in most regions to inform and shape initiatives along new directions. The challenge will be to adapt research perspectives and data collection to these new varieties of social action to reveal more clearly the pathways of institutional influence on the course of human demographic outcomes.

Notes

1 The activities and design elements of a national family planning program are classified into four categories: policy and stage-setting, service and service-related, record keeping and evaluation, and availability of and access to fertility-control methods. The activities identified range from the legal and regulatory (e.g., laws permitting contraceptive imports, in-country manufacturing, and mass-media advertising) to program management and monitoring (e.g., training, supervision, administrative structure and staff, and record keeping/evaluation), to implementation and service outreach (e.g., contraceptive commodity logistics and transport, home visits by family planning workers, and postpartum family planning programs), and to method access. National effort is determined by a Delphi scoring method, wherein for each round an average of three key informants familiar with each country complete a detailed questionnaire on the family planning program situation. The data are reduced to the 30 items, each scored from 0 to 4 and summed. The summed score is represented as a percent of the maximum value of 120.

2 The figures differ from those in Table 2 because the latter is for a panel of 77 countries, while Table 3 is based on the full complement of 97 countries surveyed in 1982 and 94 in 1994.

3 The data are compiled from various years of the Penn World Tables, the World Bank's *World Development Report*, UN statistical yearbooks, *World Christian Encyclopedia*, and the U.S. Census Bureau's international demographic database.

4 Eliminated from the total score is the subtotal for availability of and access to male

and female sterilization, oral contraceptives or injectables, condoms or other barrier methods, IUDs, and abortion.

5 These data are compiled from US congressional reports of bilateral population assistance over time by the US Agency for International Development (see Barrett and Tsui 1999 for details) and capitated with current national population estimates. As such the data function as a proxy for international donor spending since similar data are not available for other bilateral and multilateral agencies during this 22-year period. They also underestimate total USAID funding since population funding from the technical bureaus is not included. The data are not lagged; per capita spending tends to show only small year-to-year change.

6 We have used a fixed-effects time-series regression model to estimate the influence of the observed change in these variables on change in the TFR over the time points. We have also estimated the model including family planning effort score (FPE) as an instrumental variable, i.e., where it is specified to be a function of other identifying variables (per capita expenditures on population by international donor organizations, population growth, and population size). The two-stage instrumental variable approach showed predicted values of FPE to be statistically significant in the fixed-effects model. Given the similar results, we report only the non-instrumental variable specification model here.

7 Countries are equally weighted in these averages.

8 We have not attempted to replicate this regression analysis with changes in contraceptive practice as the outcome variable, largely because the countries with such trend data are much fewer and selectively biased away from the smaller sub-Saharan African countries. To test the hypothesis directly with fertility outcomes is in fact a more stringent test as it controls for the effects of other proximate fertility determinants.

9 If the average TFR for all 75 countries declined from 5.93 to 4.33, or by 1.60 births in 22 years, the average annual decline was .073 births. The estimated effect of family planning effort was –0.50 births, suggesting that the fertility transition to this point was shortened by 7 years (0.50/.073) on average. Analogous calculations give a shortening by 15 years in Asia and 5 years in Latin America.

10 Here hierarchical linear models offer important statistical estimation advantages.

References

Ahlburg, Dennis A. and Ian Diamond. 1996. "Evaluating the impact of family planning programs," in Dennis A. Ahlburg, Allen C. Kelley, and Karen Oppenheim Mason (eds.), *The Impact of Population Growth on Well-being in Developing Countries*. Berlin: Springer, pp. 299–336.

Aldrich, Howard. 1981. "Centralization versus decentralization in the design of human service delivery systems: A response to Gouldner's lament," in Oscar Grusky and George A. Miller (eds.), *The Sociology of Organizations: Basic Studies*. New York: Free Press, pp. 370–394.

Allison, Chris. 1993. "Population programmes: Assessment of needs," in *Proceedings of the United Nations Expert Group Meeting on Population Policies and Programmes*. Cairo, Egypt, 12–16 April 1992. ST/ESA/SER.R/128. New York: United Nations, pp. 115–120.

Angeles, Gustavo, Jason Dietrich, David Guilkey, Dominic Mancini, Thomas Mroz, Amy Tsui, and Fengyu Zhang. 1998. "The impact of family planning programs on fertility preferences, contraceptive method choice and fertility: Estimation of reduced form models." The EVALUATION Project, Carolina Population Center, University of North Carolina at Chapel Hill.

Angeles, Gustavo, David Guilkey, and Thomas Mroz. 1998. "Purposive program placement and the estimation of family planning program effects in Tanzania," *Journal of the Statistical Association of America* 93: 884–899.

Barrett, Deborah and Amy Ong Tsui. 1999. "Policy as symbolic statement: International response to national population policies," *Social Forces* 78(1): 213–234.

Blanc, Ann K. and Ann A. Way. 1998. "Sexual behavior and contraceptive knowledge and use among adolescents in developing countries," *Studies in Family Planning* 29(2): 106–116.

Bongaarts, John. 1982. "The fertility-inhibiting effects of the intermediate fertility variables," *Studies in Family Planning* 13(6/7): 179–189.

———. 1995. "The role of family planning programs in contemporary fertility transitions," paper presented at the Annual Meeting of the Population Association of America, San Francisco, 6–8 April.

Bongaarts, John, W. Parker Mauldin, and James F. Phillips. 1990. "The demographic impact of family planning programs," *Studies in Family Planning* 21(6): 299–310.

Brennan, Ellen. 1997. "The United Nations Population Inquiries," paper presented at the IUSSP/EVALUATION Project Seminar on Methods for the Evaluation of Family Planning Program Impact, Costa Rica, 14–16 May.

Bulatao, Rodolfo. 1993. *Effective Family Planning Programs.* Washington, DC: The World Bank.

———. 1996. *Evolving Dimensions of Family Planning Effort from 1982 to 1994.* Report prepared for The Futures Group International, Inc., Glastonbury, CT.

Coleman, James S. 1974. *Power and the Structure of Society.* New York: W. W. Norton.

Cutright, Phillips. 1983. "The ingredients of recent fertility decline in developing countries," *International Family Planning Perspectives* 9(4): 101–109.

DeGraff, Deborah S., Richard E. Bilsborrow, and David K. Guilkey. 1997. "Community-level determinants of contraceptive use in the Philippines: A structural analysis," *Demography* 34(3): 385–398.

Demeny, Paul. 1993. "Policies seeking a reduction of high fertility: A case for the demand side," in *Proceedings of the United Nations Expert Group Meeting on Population Policies and Programmes.* Cairo, Egypt, 12–16 April 1992. ST/ESA/SER.R/128. New York: United Nations, pp. 247–254.

Druckman, Daniel, Jerome Singer, and Harold Van Cott (eds.). 1997. *Enhancing Organizational Performance.* Washington, DC: National Academy Press.

Entwisle, Barbara. 1989. "Measuring components of family planning program effort," *Demography* 26(1): 53–76.

Finkle, Jason L. and C. Alison McIntosh (eds.). 1994. *The New Politics of Population: Conflict and Consensus in Family Planning.* Supplement to *Population Development Review* 20. New York: Population Council.

Freedman, Ronald. 1997. "Do family planning programs affect fertility preferences? A literature review," *Studies in Family Planning* 28(1): 1–13.

———. 1999. "Observing Taiwan's demographic transition: A memoir," paper prepared for the IUSSP Seminar on Family Planning Programs in the 21st Century. Bangladesh, 16–19 January 2000.

Goodman, Robert M., Allan B. Steckler, and Michelle Kegler. 1997. "Mobilizing organizations for health enhancement: Theories of organizational change," in K. Glanz, F. Lewis, and B. Rimer (eds.), *Health Behavior and Health Education.* San Francisco: Jossey-Bass Publishers, pp. 287–312.

Guilkey, David K. 1998. "The impact of family planning programs on contraceptive use: A review of the literature." The EVALUATION Project, Carolina Population Center, University of North Carolina at Chapel Hill.

Guilkey, David K. and Susan Jayne. 1997. "Fertility transition in Zimbabwe: Determinants of contraceptive use and method choice," *Population Studies* 51(2): 173–189.

Hage, J. T. 1999. "Organizational innovation and organizational change," *Annual Review of Sociology* 23: 597–622.

Hannan, Michael and John Freeman. 1989. *Organizational Ecology.* Cambridge, MA: Harvard University Press.

Hermalin, Albert and Zeinab Khadr. 1996. "The impact of family planning programs on fertility: A selective assessment of the evidence." The EVALUATION Project, Carolina Population Center, University of North Carolina at Chapel Hill.

Lapham, Robert J. and W. Parker Mauldin. 1985. "Contraceptive prevalence: The influence of organized family planning programs," *Studies in Family Planning* 16(3): 117–137.

Lee, K., L. Lush, G. Walt, and J. Cleland. 1998. "Family planning policies and programs in eight low-income countries: A comparative policy analysis," *Social Science and Medicine* 47(7): 949–959.

Lewin, Kurt. 1951. *Field Theory in Social Science*. New York: Harper & Row.

Martin, Linda G. and Samuel H. Preston (eds.). 1994. *Demography of Aging*. Washington, DC: National Academy Press.

Mauldin, W. Parker and Bernard Berelson. 1978. "Conditions of fertility decline in developing countries, 1967–75," *Studies in Family Planning* 9(5): 89–147.

Mauldin, W. Parker and John A. Ross. 1991. "Family planning programs: Efforts and results, 1982–89," *Studies in Family Planning* 22(6): 350–367.

Mauldin, W. Parker, John A. Ross, John Kekovole, Barkat-e-Khuda, and Abul Barkat. 1995. "Direct and judgmental measures of family planning program inputs," *Studies in Family Planning* 26(5): 287–295.

Mauldin, W. Parker and Steven Sinding. 1996. "Review of existing family planning policies and programmes: Lessons learned," in *Proceedings of the United Nations Expert Group Meeting on Family Planning, Health and Family Well-Being*. Bangalore, India, 26–30 October 1992. ST/ESA/SER.R/131. New York: United Nations, pp. 61–101.

McDevitt, Thomas. 1996. "Trends in adolescent fertility and contraceptive use in the developing world," U.S. Bureau of the Census, Report IPC/95-1. Washington, DC: Economics and Statistics Administration, U.S. Department of Commerce.

Moss, Nancy. 1983. "An organization-environment framework for assessing program implementation," *Evaluation and Program Planning* 6: 153–164.

Ness, Gayl D. and Hirofumi Ando. 1984. *The Land Is Shrinking: Population Planning in Asia*. Baltimore, MD: Johns Hopkins University Press.

Nortman, Dorothy L. 1985. *Population and Family Planning Programs. A Compendium of Data Through 1983*. 12th edition. New York: Population Council.

Phillips, J. F. and J. A. Ross. 1992. *Family Planning Programmes and Fertility*. Oxford: Clarendon Press.

Piotrow, Phyllis, D. Lawrence Kincaid, Jose G. Rimon, and Ward Rinehart. 1997. *Family Planning Communication: Lessons for Public Health*. Westport, CT: Praeger Press.

Porras, J. I. and P. J. Robertson. 1987 "Organization development theory: A typology and evaluation," in R. W. Woodman and W. A. Pasmore (eds.), *Research in Organization Change and Development*, Vol. 1. Greenwich, CT: JAI Press.

Pritchett, Lant H. 1994. "Desired fertility and the impact of population policies," *Population and Development Review* 20(1): 1–55.

Rogers, Everett M., Peter W. Vaughan, Ramadhan M.A. Swalehe, Nagesh Rao, Peer Svenkerud, and Suruchi Sood. 1999. "Effects of an entertainment-education radio soap opera on family planning behavior in Tanzania," *Studies in Family Planning* 30(3): 193–211.

Ross, John A. and Elizabeth Frankenberg. 1993. *Findings from Two Decades of Family Planning Research*. New York: Population Council.

Ross, John A. and W. Parker Mauldin. 1996. "Family planning programs: Efforts and results, 1972–94," *Studies in Family Planning* 27(3): 137–147.

Rutenberg, Naomi and Susan Cotts Watkins. 1997. "The buzz outside the clinics: Conversations and contraception in Nyanza Province, Kenya," *Studies in Family Planning* 28(4): 290–307.

Schultz, T. Paul. 1993. "Sources of fertility decline in modern economic growth: Is aggregate evidence on the demographic transition credible?" in M. R. Rosenzweig and O. Stark (eds.), *Handbook of Population and Family Economics*. Amsterdam: North Holland.

———. 1994. "Human capital, family planning and their effects on population growth," *American Economic Association Papers and Proceedings* 84(2): 255–260.

Sen, Amartya. 1995. "Population policy: Authoritarianism versus cooperation," International Lecture Series on Population Issues. 17 August. Chicago, IL: John D. and Catherine T. MacArthur Foundation.

Simmons, George. 1986. "Family planning programs," in Jane Menken (ed.), *World Population and U.S. Policy: The Choices Ahead.* New York: W. W. Norton, pp. 175–206.

Smith, James P. and Barry Edmonston (eds.). 1998. *The Immigration Debate: Studies on the Economic, Demographic, and Fiscal Effects of Immigration.* Washington, DC: National Academy Press.

Smith, Janet and Vijay Rao. 1996. "Market-based services: Strategic role in family planning service expansion," *Proceedings of the United Nations Expert Group Meeting on Family Planning, Health and Family Well-Being,* Bangalore, India, 26–30 October 1992. ST/ESA/SER.R/131. New York: United Nations, pp. 449–458.

Steele, Fiona, Ian Diamond, and D. Wang. 1996. "The determinants of the duration of contraceptive use in China: A multilevel multinomial discrete-time hazards modeling approach," *Demography* 33: 12–23.

Tsui, Amy O. and Luis H. Ochoa. 1992. "Service proximity as a determinant of contraceptive behavior: Evidence from cross-national studies of survey data," in J. F. Phillips and J. A. Ross (eds.), *Family Planning Programmes and Fertility.* Oxford: Clarendon Press, pp. 222–256.

United Nations. 1993. *Proceedings of the United Nations Expert Group Meeting on Population Policies and Programmes.* Cairo, Egypt, 12–16 April 1992. ST/ESA/SER.R/128. New York: United Nations.

———. 1996. *Levels and Trends of Contraceptive Use as Assessed in 1994.* ST/ESA/SER.A/146. New York: United Nations.

———. 1997. *Government Views on the Relationships between Population and Environment.* ST/ESA/SER.R/147. New York: United Nations.

———. 1998a. *National Population Policies.* ST/ESA./SER. A/171. New York: United Nations.

———. 1998b. *World Population Monitoring 1996: Selected Aspects of Reproductive Rights and Reproductive Health.* New York: United Nations.

———. 2000. *World Population Monitoring 1998. Health and Mortality: Selected Aspects.* New York: United Nations.

U.S. Census Bureau. 1998. *World Population Profile: 1998.* Report W.P./98. Washington, DC: U.S. Government Printing Office.

Warwick, Donald P. 1986. "The Indonesian family planning program: Government influence and client choice," *Population and Development Review* 12(3): 453–490.

Westoff, Charles F. and Germán Rodríguez. 1995. "The mass media and family planning in Kenya," *International Family Planning Perspectives* 21(1): 26–31, 36.

Yoder, P. Stanley, Robert Hornick, and Ben C. Chirwa. 1996. "Evaluating the program effects of a radio drama about AIDS in Zambia," *Studies in Family Planning* 27(4): 188–203.

Comment: Population Programs and Fertility

LUIS ROSERO-BIXBY

THIS COMMENT ADDRESSES two key aspects of family planning programs: their rationale and their indirect impact on fertility.

Program rationale

Understanding the rationale and sources of support for population programs is crucial for assessing their impact and chances of survival. One of the most notable features of population agencies and programs is that not long ago—in the 1950s—they were unthinkable. "To govern is to populate" was the unquestioned principle of good government attributed to Juan Bautista Alberdi, the nineteenth-century statesman and philosopher from Argentina. How did governments come to abandon this principle and establish birth control programs (later called euphemistically "family planning" and "reproductive health" programs)? The answer "rapid population growth" or "high demographic density" may seem obvious to demographers but it is not so obvious for politicians, especially considering the opposition to birth control by religious authorities and other powerful interest groups and the nationalist pride associated with large populations.

One may distinguish two rationales behind the adoption and implementation of family planning programs: the macro-level, or Malthusian rationale and the micro-level thinking represented by activism of the kind associated with Margaret Sanger. High-level government officials are more likely to be moved by macro-level consideration of the problems associated with rapid population growth, particularly the drag on economic development and the burden that demographic (that is, capital-widening) investments represent for public services. In turn, those directly involved in the provision of services support family planning because of micro-level concern with the benefits for health and well-being that it brings, especially to women. Economists and men tend to support family planning because of macro considerations, whereas women, health practitioners, and social workers tend to support it because of its micro effects. I have observed this gender division in focus groups with ordinary people discussing the causes of fertility transition in Costa Rica: men cite socioeconomic considerations, while women explain the adoption of birth control in terms of health, sexuality, their bodies, and the availability of information and services (Rosero-Bixby and Casterline 1995).

A reason to revisit the matter of the rationale behind family planning programs is the dramatic shift that took place in 1994 at the International Conference on Population and Development, held in Cairo. The Program of Action approved by consensus at this conference moved away from demographic rationales and justified population programs in terms of reproductive health and reproductive rights. Given this shift, we may ask whether the rationale of family planning agencies has implications for their political and public support, their funding, their effectiveness, and their chances of survival. If politicians and taxpayers were willing to support population activities only because they thought these were good investments to promote development and to prevent social unrest, environmental degradation, migration to cities, and the like, then the Cairo shift to a reproductive health rationale might be the beginning of the end of population programs. This shift could also be, however, a clever *aggiornamento* that will increase the chances of survival of these programs in times when social engineering is discredited, the "laissez-faire, laissez-passer" is glorified, and the perception spreads that the population bomb has been defused.

Indirect effects and nonlinearities

The fertility theory most commonly used to frame the debate on program impact is that of Easterlin and the US National Academy of Sciences (Bulatao and Lee 1983). This is the demand–supply paradigm that distinguishes the motivational forces favoring small families—that is, the demand for family planning—from the costs or barriers to contraception as determined by the supply of family planning services and information. Theoretical work on ideational change and social interaction (e.g., Cleland and Wilson 1986; Bongaarts and Watkins 1996) identifies innovation diffusion as a third force driving the fertility decline. This third causal pathway opens the possibility of indirect or multiplicative effects of program impact, which are more difficult to observe and measure, and it may imply nonlinear effects, which are difficult to capture in conventional quantitative analyses.

Figure 1 simulates a fertility transition with a simple mathematical model that helps to clarify the meaning and potential role of the three sets of factors in fertility decline: diffusion, supply of birth control methods, and demand for such methods (Rosero-Bixby and Casterline 1993). The figure shows the evolution over time of the total fertility rate and "unmet

FIGURE 1 Simulation of a fertility transition with and without interaction effects

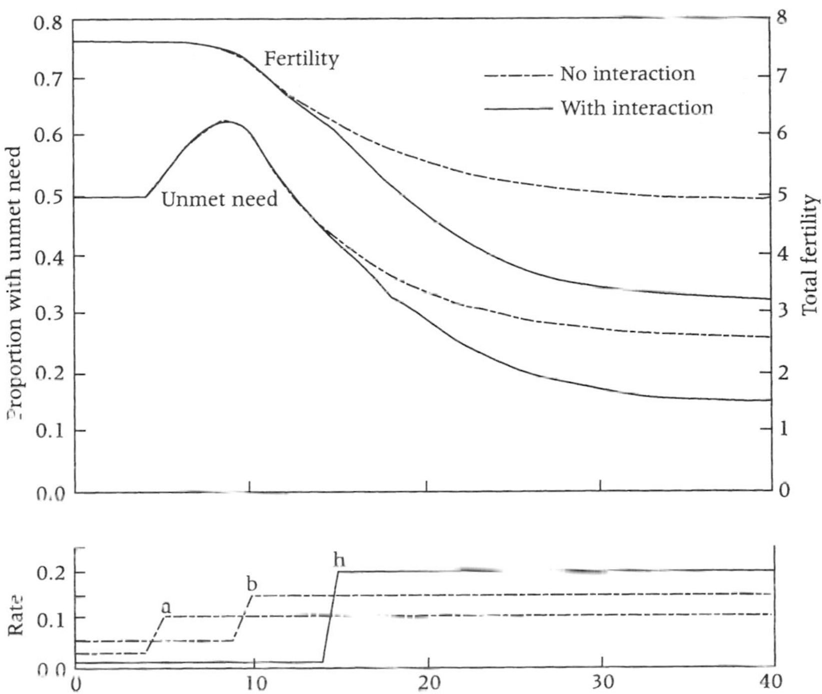

need" (the proportion of couples who are not using contraception among those motivated to control their fertility). Dashed lines represent outputs from a simulation with no diffusion effects. The difference between dashed and solid lines represents the diffusion effect on fertility transition. The inputs of the model are "rates" of demand (or motivation) for and supply (or costs) of birth control, as well as a rate of ideational diffusion due to interaction. These rates denote the proportion of a population that becomes birth controllers in a year due to the respective factor (details in the original article). The impact of programs is usually taken as working through shifts in the supply, although it can also occur through induced changes in demand and the multiplier effect of diffusion.

The simulation in the figure starts from an equilibrium situation with very low rates of demand, supply, and interaction. Then, it is fueled with increases in demand (point *a* in the chart) in year 5, supply (point *b*) in year 10, and interaction (point *h*) in year 15. In response to the increase in demand in year 5, there is a surge in unmet need, but there is no noticeable effect on fertility because of the low level of supply. When supply increases in year 10, a substantial decline in both unmet need and fertility starts. This development provides the first lesson for the assessment of program impact. Demand and supply effects are very difficult to separate. In this case one might be tempted to attribute the entire fertility decline that starts in year 10 to the increase in supply that year. In truth, however, such an effect was possible only because there was an increase in motivation 5 years earlier. What one actually has, therefore, is a synergistic or concurrent effect of supply and demand.

In the final stage a substantial increase in the rate of interaction (and, consequently, of spread of information and diffusion of ideas and *mentalités*) is introduced into the simulation in year 15, which results in acceleration of the fertility decline. The difference between the curves with and without interaction suggests a potentially large independent effect of diffusion in both the pace of fertility decline and the post-transition level of equilibrium. In this simulation, diffusion accounts for a reduction in the total fertility rate of almost two births at the new equilibrium level. But, again, in this situation one can argue that this diffusion effect is actually dependent on the earlier demand and supply improvements.

Another feature of this simulation model is that in order to simulate a pretransition equilibrium at high fertility levels, one must also assume that diffusion was nil in the past. In other words, the diffusion hypothesis is not compatible with the coexistence of high fertility and pockets of forerunners with reduced fertility. Why did the birth control movement not spread from the pockets of the upper classes in Latin America that started using contraception in the 1920s and 1930s? The model suggests that the diffusion hypothesis requires additional assumptions of a change in the interaction rate. That change could be, for example, that family planning and sexual matters stopped being taboo topics, people started talking about them, and ideational diffusion took place. It can also be that a critical mass is needed for the innovation to take off. A report explaining the recent drop in crime in New York City (Gladwell 2000) graphically illustrates nonlinear effects with what one could call the "ketchup effect," as stated in the ditty:

> Tomato ketchup in a bottle—
> None will come and then the lot'll.

The point is that family planning programs can be the key factor in opening up taboo areas, or creating a critical mass, which makes possible the diffusion process, and that this kind of nonlinearity is quite difficult to capture in conventional quantitative analyses and regression models.

References

Bongaarts, John and Susan Cotts Watkins. 1996. "Social interactions and contemporary fertility transitions," *Population and Development Review* 22(4): 639–682.

Bulatao, Rodolfo A. and Ronald D. Lee. 1983. "A framework for the study of fertility determinants," in Rodolfo A. Bulatao and Ronald D. Lee (eds.), *Determinants of Fertility in Developing Countries*. Vol. 1, pp. 1–26. New York: Academic Press.

Cleland, John and Christopher Wilson. 1987. "Demand theories of the fertility transition: An iconoclastic view," *Population Studies* 41(1): 5–30.

Gladwell, Malcolm. 2000. *The Tipping Point: How Little Things Can Make a Big Difference*. New York: Little, Brown.

Rosero-Bixby, Luis and John B. Casterline. 1993. "Modelling diffusion effects in fertility transition," *Population Studies* 47(1): 147–167.

———. 1995. "Difusión por interacción social y transición de la fecundidad: evidencia cuantitativa y cualitativa de Costa Rica," *Notas de Población* 61: 29–78.

PART THREE

LOW-FERTILITY REGIMES

Paths to Subreplacement Fertility: The Empirical Evidence

Tomas Frejka
John Ross

In the mid-1990s 44 percent of the world's population lived in countries with fertility at or below the replacement level. This includes practically all of Europe, the overseas English-speaking countries, almost all countries of East Asia (including China and Japan), and Thailand and Cuba. An era of below-replacement fertility is taking hold. Evidence presented in this chapter suggests that in most of these countries fertility is likely to remain very low. A number of other countries are also heading in this direction. Such demographic developments will have profound economic, political, and social consequences.

This study examines the empirical record of the fertility transition in countries that as of the mid-1990s have had subreplacement fertility and investigates effects of three proximate determinants of fertility—marriage, contraception, and abortion—with limited attention to the social frameworks of change. This exploration may shed light on whether other societies are likely to follow similar paths and, if so, what the patterns and time frames of fertility change might be.

Our findings are for 54 countries: all European countries; the successor states of the Soviet Union except for those of central Asia; the United States, Canada, Australia, New Zealand; and Japan as well as other Asian countries that have recently reached subreplacement fertility, namely the People's Republic of China, the Republic of Korea (South Korea), the Republic of China (Taiwan), Hong Kong, Singapore, and Thailand.[1] We refer to these as the low-fertility countries.

We have relied on secondary data sets from both vital statistics and surveys to obtain long time series. The sources include United Nations publications, Council of Europe 1997, and many other publications listed in the References. Decisions on how far back in time to go were arbitrary; the interesting period for East Asia was clearly after World War II, but the other regions experienced substantial fertility reductions, often to subreplacement, much earlier. We therefore chose to include the period before the war, using time series that for the most part started in the late nineteenth century, but with emphasis on the period after 1960.

A specific methodological note is apropos. Three measures can be used to depict long-term fertility change: the period total fertility rate (PTFR), the completed cohort fertility rate (CCFR), and the net reproduction rate (NRR). Demographers are continually improving knowledge of the advantages and shortcomings of each of these. Most recently Bongaarts and Feeney (1998) and Lesthaeghe and Willems (1999) have refined our knowledge of how period total fertility rates can be affected by cohorts' postponing or advancing births. However, analysis of this relationship is possible only in countries that have detailed data sets of fertility by birth order and corresponding age at birth. For our analysis, which is focused on global long-term change, we rely primarily on the three aforementioned measures.

The era of subreplacement fertility

The global fertility transition has been underway for a little over a century. There were countries and regions where fertility was relatively low or had been declining for extended periods in the eighteenth and nineteenth centuries, as in France and the United States; however, only a very small proportion of the world population was involved, and the declines were gradual. Toward the end of the nineteenth century notable and rapid fertility declines started in a number of countries (Chesnais 1992). Although fundamental economic and social changes that tend to generate fertility declines had been in progress for several decades, the decisive changes in reproductive behavior did not commence on a widespread basis until the last quarter of the nineteenth century.

Not only did fertility decline rapidly in many Western and Central European countries during the first quarter of the twentieth century, but the descent was so steep that by the 1920s more than half of Europe's population was reproducing at below-replacement level. In the early 1930s, Austria, Germany, Estonia, and Sweden had net reproduction rates (NRRs) significantly below 0.8 (Kirk 1946). Almost all of the other Western and Central European countries had NRRs below unity: England and Wales (.81), Latvia (.82), Switzerland (.86), Norway (.89), Belgium (.91), France (.93), Czechoslovakia (.95), Denmark (.96), and Scotland (.98).[2] Figure 1 depicts trends in Germany, Hungary, and what is at present the Czech Republic. The NRR fell below replacement in the Czech Republic in 1925 and bottomed out at 0.66 in the mid-1930s. We do not have a time series of NRRs for Germany; however, during the 1920s and early 1930s its PTFR was consistently lower than that in the Czech Republic, implying that its

FIGURE 1 Total fertility rates and net reproduction rates, Czech Republic, Germany, and Hungary, 1880–1940

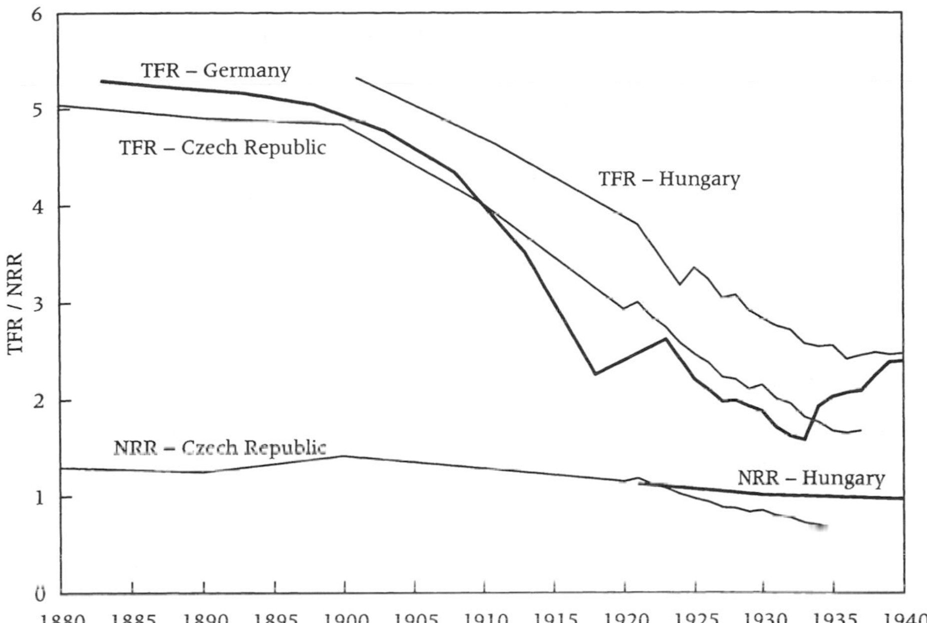

NRR was significantly below replacement. This was confirmed by Kirk (1946), who gave the NRR figure of .70 for Germany in 1933. Although Hungary was a "medium"-fertility country in the European context between the world wars, its reproduction rate was hovering around replacement.

Throughout Europe, as in the overseas English-speaking countries, a secular fertility decline was underway. By the late 1930s, fertility was around replacement in Canada, the United States, and Australia, where the average PTFRs in the period 1936–40 were 2.7, 2.2, and 2.2 children per woman (Chesnais 1992). The latter two were below the replacement level given mortality levels of that time.

Following World War II, the late 1940s and the 1950s were marked by increased fertility—the "baby boom"—in most Western and North European countries, and particularly in the overseas English-speaking countries. In the late 1950s the average PTFR for the latter countries was 3.7 children per woman; for the former it was 2.7. In the socialist countries of Eastern Europe and in the Soviet Union, fertility also increased after the war; however, the long-term decline resumed in the 1950s. In many other developed countries the secular decline reappeared in the 1960s. At about that time, the fertility transition started in many developing countries of Latin America and Asia, especially in East Asia, and it picked up speed in the 1970s and 1980s.

We now turn to a more detailed description of trends in the low-fertility countries. First we explore indicators that measure various aspects of fertility. Then we describe the principal trends in the main proximate determinants of fertility. Finally, we offer a rough assessment of the roles of population-related policies. In the tables and discussion, Eastern countries are all the formerly socialist countries of Central and Eastern Europe; Western countries are all the remaining developed countries; and the rapidly developing Asian countries are the People's Republic of China, Hong Kong, the Republic of Korea, Singapore, Taiwan, and Thailand.

Period total fertility rates

A major shift in fertility as reflected in PTFRs occurred between 1960 and the mid-1990s (see Table 1). In 1960, only four countries had a total fertility rate below 2.1: the Czech Republic, Hungary, Japan, and Latvia. In contrast, 53 countries in Table 1 had PTFRs below 2.1 in the mid-1990s. The one exception in Europe is Albania with a PTFR estimate of 2.70, a somewhat suspect estimate. Among the countries with the lowest PTFRs in the mid-1990s were the Czech Republic (1.17, 1997), Spain (1.15, 1997), Latvia (1.11, 1997), Bulgaria (1.09, 1997), and the former East Germany (0.95, 1996).

On average in 1960, fertility was higher in the Western compared to the Eastern countries; this persisted as of the mid-1990s. A few countries in the East had high fertility around 1960 (Albania, Armenia, and Azer-

TABLE 1 Distribution of low-fertility countries by total fertility rates, 1960–97

	1960				1997 or latest available year			
Total fertility rate	**Total**	**West**	**East**	**Asia**	**Total**	**West**	**East**	**Asia**
Below 1.20	—	—	—	—	5	1	4	—
1.20–1.49	—	—	—	—	18	7	10	1
1.50–1.79	1	—	1	—	18	10	5	3
1.80–2.09	3	1	2	—	12	7	3	2
2.10–2.39	12	5	7	—	—	—	—	—
2.40–2.69	9	5	4	—	—	—	—	—
2.70–2.99	7	5	2	—	1	—	1	—
3.00–4.99	15	9	5	1	—	—	—	—
5.00 +	7	—	2	5	—	—	—	—
Total	54	25	23	6	54	25	23	6
Median	2.75	2.72	2.49	5.50	1.57	1.71	1.40	1.77

NOTE: Eastern countries are all the formerly socialist countries of Central and Eastern Europe; Western countries are all the remaining developed countries; and the rapidly developing Asian countries are the People's Republic of China, Hong Kong, the Republic of Korea, Singapore, Taiwan, and Thailand.

baijan), but the majority of countries had already experienced a significant fertility decline in the 1950s. In contrast, many of the Western countries were still around the peak of their postwar fertility in 1960. At this time, the Asian developing countries were beginning their fertility transition from a median PTFR of 5.5.

By the mid-1990s practically all low-fertility countries were below the replacement level. The Asian developing countries had a median PTFR of 1.8. The median PTFR of the Western countries was 1.7; that of the Eastern countries was lower at 1.4 children per woman. As will be demonstrated below, the Eastern countries experienced a rapid fertility decline during the 1990s.

In the mid-1990s the range of the PTFR for all low-fertility countries was quite narrow; all had a value below replacement, with the possible exception of Albania for which reliable data are not available. This range was narrowing steadily from around 1960 when the developing countries of Asia had PTFRs around 5–6 and a number of other countries had high fertility: for instance, Albania 6.9, Iceland 4.2, Canada 3.9, New Zealand 3.9, the United States 3.5, Australia 3.3, Netherlands 3.1, and Slovakia 3.1.

Recent analyses by Bongaarts and Feeney (1998) and Lesthaeghe and Willems (1999) suggest that in a number of countries the period total fertility rates of the mid-1990s are distorted downward as a result of the postponement of births. However, in a number of countries below-replacement fertility has lasted for over two decades, which implies that in these countries the postponement effect has largely run its course. This is particularly so for the Western countries. In the mid-1990s over 80 percent of these countries had PTFRs below 1.8. Even if their PTFRs were adjusted, it is unlikely that they would be at or above replacement. As will be demonstrated below, this is confirmed by the trends in completed cohort fertility.

A clear regional pattern emerges for when countries reached subreplacement fertility. There are exceptions to the rule, but rather few.

During the 1950s and 1960s, the socialist countries of Central and Eastern Europe, as well as the countries of Northern Europe, experienced fertility declines leading to subreplacement (see Table 2). The countries of Western Europe entered the path of sharp fertility descent in the 1960s; however, they reached subreplacement fertility in the 1970s. The overseas English-speaking countries experienced even faster downward trends than did Western Europe, and they too reached subreplacement fertility in the 1970s. This decade was also notable because the first developing country/city-state, Singapore, reached such low fertility. The 1980s was the "South European decade," when Greece, Portugal, and Spain reached subreplacement fertility. It was also the decade when certain rapidly developing countries did so: Hong Kong, the Republic of Korea, and Taiwan. Finally, in the 1990s, the Transcaucasian countries reached replacement-level fertility, al-

TABLE 2 Period when low-fertility countries reached replacement-level fertility, 1960s–90s

Period	Country	Number of countries
Before 1960	Czech Republic, Hungary, Japan, Latvia	4
1960–69	Bulgaria, Croatia, Denmark, Finland, Romania, Russian Federation, Slovenia, Sweden, Ukraine	9
1970–79	Australia, Austria, Belarus, Belgium, Canada, Cyprus, Estonia, Federal Republic of Germany, France, German Democratic Republic, Italy, Lithuania, Luxembourg, Malta, Netherlands, New Zealand, Norway, Singapore, Switzerland, United Kingdom, United States	21
1980–89	Bosnia and Herzegovina, Greece, Hong Kong, Iceland, Ireland, Poland, Portugal, Republic of Korea, Slovakia, Spain, Taiwan, Yugoslav Federal Republic	12
1990–96	Albania, Armenia, Azerbaijan, Georgia, Moldova, People's Republic of China, Thailand, Former Yugoslav Republic of Macedonia	8

though Azerbaijan by some estimates might still have been above replacement in the mid-1990s.

We now analyze the regional patterns of fertility change in greater detail. First we will look at the Western, Eastern, and the Asian rapidly developing countries separately, and then analyze smaller groupings of countries.

The median fertility decline in all the low-fertility countries in the period 1960–97 was 47 percent (see Table 3). If one compares the period 1960–80 to 1980–97, the decline averaged 26 percent in both periods. This was, however, a consequence of differential decline in the East and in the West. In most of the Western countries the fertility decline was rapid during 1960–80, but relatively slow during 1980–97. In the Eastern countries most of the fertility decline was concentrated in the 1990s. In the Asian rapidly developing countries the average decline was rapid in both periods.

During 1960–97 distinct regional patterns of fertility change were evident in smaller country groupings. West European countries experienced a moderate fertility increase following World War II to a range around a PTFR of 2.5–3.0 that peaked in the mid-1960s (see Figure 2A).[3] Then during the late 1960s and most of the 1970s these countries fell to below replacement, each country stabilizing within a relatively narrow range during the 1980s and 1990s.

Scandinavian countries experienced PTFR trends not very different from the West European countries, albeit with some fluctuations, particularly in Sweden before and after the decline of the late 1960s/early 1970s (Figure 2B).

TABLE 3 Distribution of low-fertility countries by percent change in total fertility rate, 1960–97 (or latest available year)

Fertility change (percent)	1960–80				1980–97 (or latest available year)				1960–97 (or latest available year)			
	Total	West	East	Asia	Total	West	East	Asia	Total	West	East	Asia
Increase	2	—	2	—	6	5	—	1	—	—	—	—
Decline												
0.0– 9.9	6	2	4	—	10	10	—	—	—	—	—	—
10.0–19.9	8	2	6	—	7	5	2	—	1	1	—	—
20.0–29.9	11	4	6	1	8	1	6	1	4	3	1	—
30.0–39.9	11	10	1	—	13	1	9	3	12	7	5	—
40.0–49.9	10	6	3	1	8	3	5	—	18	9	8	1
50.0–59.9	5	1	1	3	2	—	1	1	10	5	5	—
60.0–69.9	1	—	—	1	—	—	—	—	6	—	4	2
70.0 +	—	—	—	—	—	—	—	—	3	—	—	3
Total number of countries	54	25	23	6	54	25	23	6	54	25	23	6
Median decline in percent[a]	26	29	14	47	26	8	33	34	47	41	49	70

[a]The median rate of decline is calculated from individual country data. The rate for the 20-year period 1960–80 is controlled for period length, i.e., the data are prorated to be comparable to the 17-year period 1980–97.

Total fertility rates around 2.5–3.0 lasted into the mid- to late-1970s in South European countries (Figure 2C). The notable fertility decline in these countries occurred about ten years later than in the West European countries. By the mid-1990s the PTFRs in South European countries were lower than in the West European and Scandinavian countries. This was apparently due to a considerable tempo effect as shown by the comparison of calculations for Italy and Belgium in Lesthaeghe and Willems (1999). PTFRs in Southern Europe may increase once the postponement of births runs its course; however, since the PTFRs in this region are between 1.2 and 1.5 the elimination of the tempo effect would not raise them to replacement level.

Many of the formerly socialist countries of Central and Eastern Europe experienced a fertility decline during the 1950s, and by 1960 their PTFRs were close to replacement (Figures 2D and 2E). Throughout the 1960s, 1970s, and 1980s their PTFRs fluctuated around the replacement level. To a significant extent these swings were influenced by various pronatalist measures or by policies modifying abortion legislation and the availability of modern contraceptives (David 1970, 1999; Frejka 1980, 1983, 1993; Stloukal 1995). Most prominent among these measures was the total ban on induced abortions in Romania in 1965, where the population relied heavily on abortion for fertility regulation; the PTFR increased from under 2 to above 3.5 from one year to the next. A slow fertility decline in

FIGURE 2 Period total fertility rates, selected low-fertility countries, 1960–97

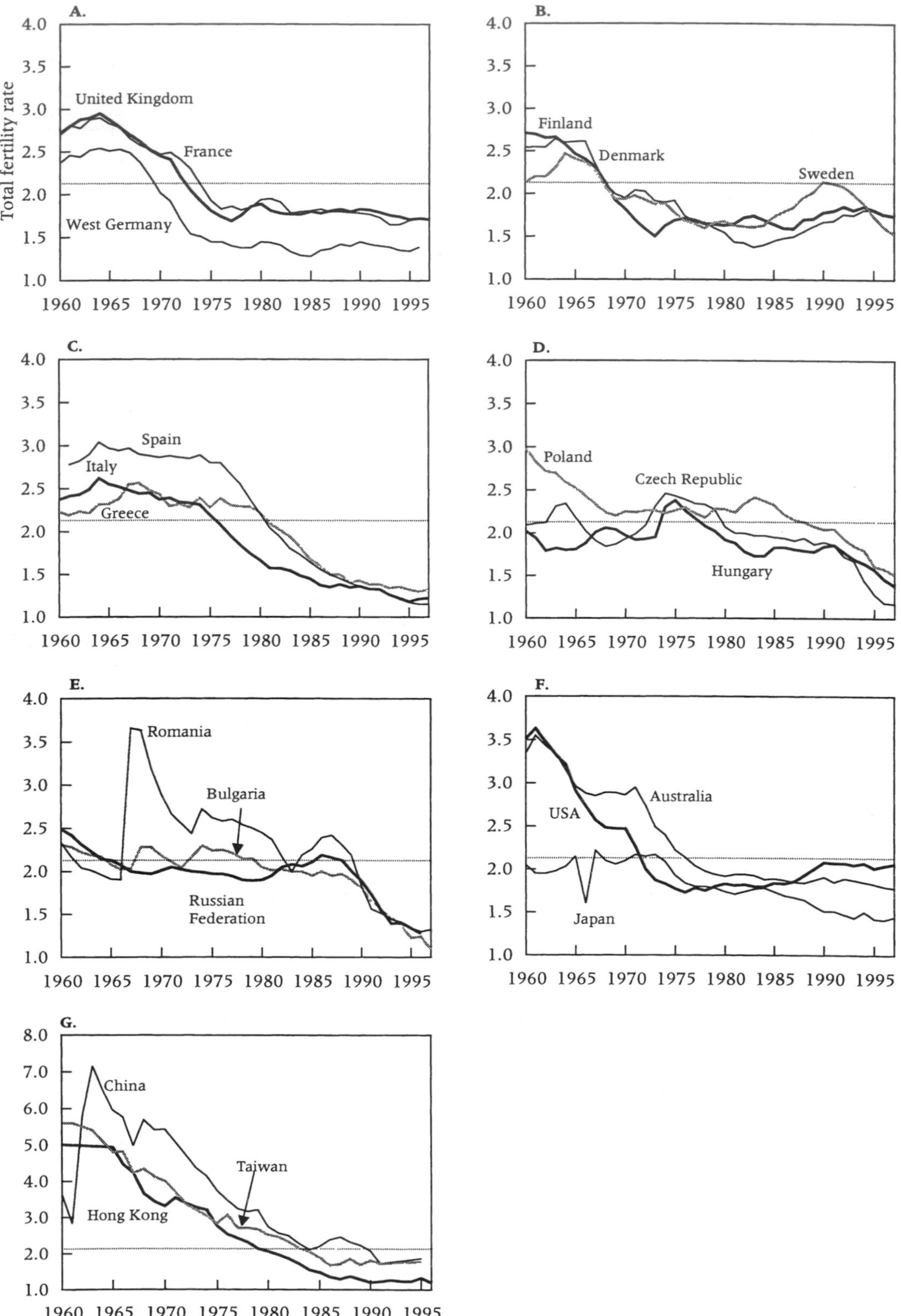

most of these countries started in the late 1980s and accelerated following the disintegration of the socialist regimes throughout Central and Eastern Europe around 1990. In the Czech Republic the PTFR declined from 1.89 in 1990 to 1.17 in 1997; in Romania from 2.42 in 1987 to 1.83 in 1990 and to 1.32 in 1997. In practically all these countries the fertility decline was still in progress in the mid-1990s.

The postwar fertility increase was more pronounced in the non-European developed countries, rising to a PTFR as of 1960 around 3.5 (Figure 2F). The fertility decline in these countries started in the early 1960s and lasted longer than in Europe, through the late 1970s. Period fertility then stabilized slightly below replacement in a quite narrow range. Bongaarts and Feeney (1998) argue that the postponement of childbearing has caused a distortion of the period TFR. The PTFR adjusted for the tempo effect was still only around 2 children per woman throughout the period from the early 1970s through the mid-1990s.

Japan experienced its rapid fertility decline in the late 1940s and the 1950s (Frejka 1960). The total fertility rate declined from its postwar high of 4.5 births per woman in 1947 to 2.0 in 1957, a decline of 56 percent in ten years. During the 1960s its PTFR hovered around the replacement level (Figure 2F) and has since been slowly declining, to a level of around 1.5 or less during the 1990s.

In the rapidly developing Asian countries the PTFR was 5–7 prior to sustained fertility decline in the 1960s to 1980s (Figure 2G). In the mid-1990s these countries were within a PTFR range of 1.3 in Hong Kong to 1.9 in China. Bongaarts and Feeney (1998) demonstrated that in the case of Taiwan the tempo effect in the late 1980s and early 1990s was considerable and the adjusted PTFR would have been around the replacement level.

Net reproduction rates

In 1970, the majority of low-fertility countries still had net reproduction rates above 1.0 (see Table 4). Only ten countries had a net reproduction rate below unity, and only two of those (Croatia and Finland) had a NRR below 0.9.

In the mid-1990s all but four of the low-fertility countries had NRRs clearly below unity. The data for three out of the four countries listed with a NRR of 1.0 or above in the mid-1990s were outdated; they refer to 1990 (Albania, Azerbaijan, and Georgia). Their NRRs have probably declined since then. The one remaining country, Cyprus, had a NRR of 1.00 in 1996.

At least seven countries had NRRs below 0.6 in the mid-1990s: Belarus 0.59, Estonia 0.59, the Czech Republic 0.57, Spain 0.56, Bulgaria 0.52, Latvia 0.52, and the former German Democratic Republic 0.45. But it is possible that as many as ten countries had such low fertility, because the latest fig-

TABLE 4 Distribution of low-fertility countries by net reproduction rates, 1970 and 1997 (or latest available year)

	1970				1997 or latest available			
Net reproduction rate	Total	West	East	Asia	Total	West	East	Asia
Below 0.60	—	—	—	—	7	1	6	—
0.60–0.79	—	—	—	—	23	11	11	1
0.80–0.99	10	4	6	—	20	12	3	5
1.00–1.19	24	14	10	—	2	1	1	—
1.20–1.39	10	6	4	—	2	—	2	—
1.40–1.99	7	1	2	4	—	—	—	—
2.00 +	3	—	1	2	—	—	—	—
Total	54	25	23	6	54	25	23	6

ures for Georgia (1.04) and Bosnia and Herzegovina (0.81) were for 1990; for Italy (0.64) for 1993; and for Russia (0.60) for 1996.

Fertility by age of women

In gross terms, fertility has become more concentrated in the middle of the reproductive period. Large reductions have certainly occurred at the older ages. It is difficult to generalize about the younger ages because of variance by region and country; nevertheless, the considerable concentration of fertility into a span of 15 years has occurred in almost all countries.

Fertility of women above age 40 declined faster than the PTFR in all countries studied (see Table 5).[4] The same was true at ages 35–39 in the majority of countries in the East and in Asia; however in the West there were about as many countries where fertility declined more slowly than the PTFR in this age group as there were with equal or faster declines.

For the other age groups, clear patterns emerge in the smaller regional groupings of countries.

—In the West and North European countries fertility declined considerably faster than the PTFR not only in the ages above 40, but also under 25. The one exception was Great Britain where the fertility decline of the 15–19 age group was relatively slow. In the middle of the reproductive ages (25–39), and particularly at ages 30–34, fertility in these countries declined considerably more slowly than the PTFR.

—In the South European countries the age-specific decline was more evenly distributed. For ages 20–39 the fertility trend was not very different from the PTFR decline. In Greece and Spain fertility declined very slowly among women under age 20.

—In the formerly socialist countries of Central Europe fertility declined rapidly in the age groups above 34 and below 25. These trends were most

TABLE 5 Distribution of low-fertility countries by changes in age-specific fertility rates, 1960–96 (or latest available year)

Change in relation to total fertility rate	15–19	20–24	25–29	30–34	35–39	40–44	45–49
West: 25 countries							
Decline larger than TFR decline	16	19	1	—	8	25	25
Decline equal to TFR decline (within 10 percent)	—	6	10	2	7	—	—
Decline smaller than TFR decline or increase	9	—	14	23	10	—	—
East: 23 countries							
Decline larger than TFR decline	8	3	6	15	22	23	23
Decline equal to TFR decline (within 10 percent)	—	6	7	4	1	—	—
Decline smaller than TFR decline or increase	15	14	10	4	—	—	—
Asia: 5 countries							
Decline larger than TFR decline	2	1	—	1	3	5	5
Decline equal to TFR decline (within 10 percent)	2	3	2	1	2	—	—
Decline smaller than TFR decline or increase	1	1	3	3	—	—	—

pronounced in Hungary. In Poland on the other hand, especially up to age 34, age-specific fertility declined quite closely in line with the overall decline.

—In the formerly socialist countries of Eastern Europe there was a rapid fertility decline at all ages above 30, whereas fertility declined slowly among young women, especially in the Russian Federation.

—In the overseas developed countries, as in other Western countries, a rapid fertility decline occurred among women in their early 20s, but not in the 15–19 age group. As elsewhere, a rapid fertility decline emerged among women over age 40.

—In the Asian developing countries age-specific fertility rates fell quite evenly. The declines were large but fairly uniform across all age groups, although they were slightly faster in the age groups over 40. There was one outstanding exception, in Thailand, where fertility at the young ages declined very slowly.

Shifts in the age concentration of fertility appear also in the peak age-specific fertility rate. In almost all countries in Northern Europe and half of those in Central Europe, the peak shifted from ages 20–24 to ages 25–29. This was also the case in all the overseas English-speaking countries. In the Asian countries, the peak age-specific fertility rate was in the 25–29 age group for the entire period, except in Thailand, where there was a move to the younger ages. In the former Soviet Union and former Yugoslavia, about half of the countries had their peak fertility in the 20–24 age group around 1960, whereas by the mid-1990s almost all had shifted their peak up to ages 25–29.

Live births by order

The change to smaller families is essentially universal. Between the early 1960s and the mid-1990s, in almost all countries the proportion of births that were first- and second-order increased.[5] Around 1960, the median proportion of first- plus second-order births was 64 percent. By the mid-1990s, the median had risen to over 84 percent.

At the other extreme, the proportion of fourth- and higher-order births declined almost everywhere. Around 1960, there were only six countries in which fourth- and higher-order births made up less than 10 percent of the total. By the mid-1990s, 42 countries were below that mark. Those countries above 10 percent were so by only a few points; the highest proportion, 14 percent, was in Ireland.

The proportions of third-order births also declined in most countries. Only 11 of 51 countries had increases (by 1–3 percentage points) in third-order births.

Mean age of women giving birth

On balance, the mean age at childbearing in the mid-1990s was considerably higher than it was 25 years earlier. In over half (24) of the countries with available data, the mean age was above 28 years compared to only nine countries at that level around 1970.

In Western countries there was a tendency toward a declining age at childbearing in the 1960s and early 1970s (see Figure 3A); however, to a significant extent this was the result of the changing weights in birth orders, that is, the proportion of first- and second-order births was increasing at the expense of higher-order births. This lowered the mean age at childbearing even though the age at each order may not have changed much. (The United States case is illustrated in Bongaarts and Feeney 1998.) Subsequently, despite the continuous shift to higher proportions of lower-order births, the mean age at childbearing increased considerably, implying a strong shift toward a pattern of later childbearing. By the mid-1990s most Western countries had a mean age at childbearing around 29 years.

In Central and Eastern European countries childbearing has historically occurred on average at younger ages than in Western Europe. In addition, the social policies of the formerly socialist countries were conducive to early childbearing (David 1970, 1999; Frejka 1980; Stloukal 1995)

FIGURE 3A Mean age at childbearing, selected Western countries, 1960–96

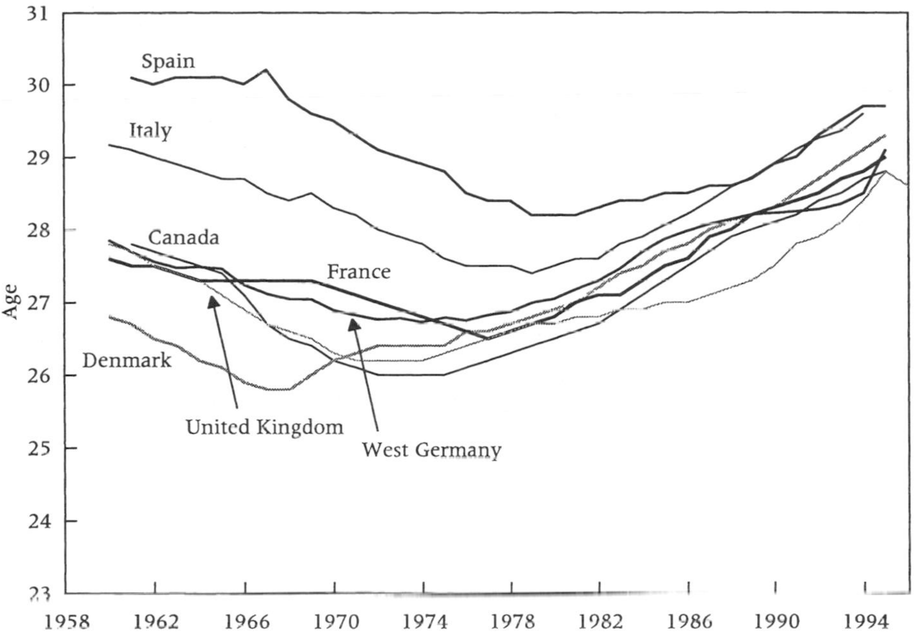

FIGURE 3B Mean age at childbearing, selected Central and Eastern European countries, 1958–96

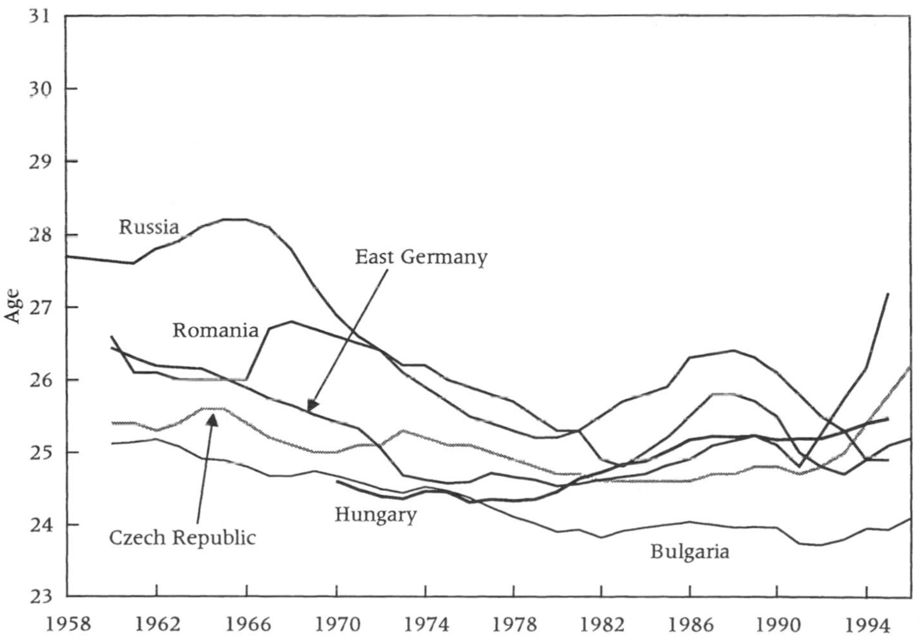

so that between 1960 and 1990 the mean age at childbearing was around 24 to 26 (see Figure 3B). In the 1990s the age at childbearing has increased. In former East Germany and in the Czech Republic the increase was very steep, reflecting the precipitous decline of fertility at young ages. In spite of this, the mean age was still in the range of 25–27 years in most Eastern countries, much lower than in the Western countries. In an interesting contrast to the Central European formerly socialist countries, the mean age at childbearing has been declining in nearly all the successor states of the Soviet Union, reflecting relatively high fertility at young ages (as well as a rise in the proportions of lower-order births). The trend in the Russian Federation is a case in point.

The other outstanding exceptions are China and South Korea. There the dynamics are very different owing to the sharp decline of childbearing among older women, whereas the decline among younger women has been more modest. Furthermore, the increase in the relative weight of lower-order births has been rapid.

Completed cohort fertility rates

"Real" fertility levels and trends are probably best reflected in completed cohort fertility rates (CCFRs). By definition, these are available only after women have reached the end of their childbearing years, that is, with a considerable time delay. To partially mitigate this shortcoming, one can quite reliably estimate CCFRs for cohorts that have nearly completed their fertility, when only trivial additions remain. In the majority of developed low-fertility countries this certainly includes women in their 40s, and often even those who are in their late 30s. Such data are available for over 30 countries.[6]

Data in Table 6 show declines in completed cohort fertility rates. In all countries for which data for the 1930 birth cohort were available, the CCFR was above 2.1 children per woman. Among the birth cohorts of 1950—those that had reached age 45 by the mid-1990s—over two-thirds had CCFRs below 2.1. With the exception of Yugoslavia and Ireland, all birth cohorts of the 1960s in Europe and North America will apparently have CCFRs below 2.1. In two-thirds of these countries cohort fertility will likely be below 1.9 children per woman.

The lowest estimated CCFRs among the birth cohorts of the 1960s (below 1.7) are in the German-speaking countries, in Italy and Spain, and in Russia. Already about 20 birth cohorts have experienced CCFRs below 1.9 in former East and West Germany and in Switzerland; in Austria the first birth cohort with such low fertility was that of 1949 (see Figure 4A). The estimated CCFR is 1.47 for the 1965 cohort in the former East Germany and in the former West Germany it is 1.55 for the 1961 cohort.

TABLE 6 Distribution of low-fertility countries by completed cohort fertility rate, birth cohorts 1930–65

Completed cohort fertility rate	Birth cohort 1930	1950	1965 or latest cohort (at least 1960)[a]
Below 1.70	—	1	7
1.70–1.89	—	12	15
1.90–2.09	—	10	9
2.10–2.29	10	6	1
2.30 +	13	4	1
Total	23	33	33

[a]Estimate for cohorts younger than 50 years at the time of observation equals actual observed fertility plus estimated fertility for remaining years.

In Italy and Spain the first birth cohorts to experience CCFRs below 1.9 were those of 1950 and 1956, respectively (see Figure 4B). In both countries there appears to be a distinct decline in the CCFR from one birth cohort to the next. This is more pronounced in Spain than in Italy; their respective estimated CCFRs are 1.66 and 1.59 for the birth cohorts of 1961. In Russia, all birth cohorts starting with that of 1941 have had CCFRs below 1.9. The estimate for the 1965 birth cohort is 1.65.

A general decline in CCFRs is present in almost all other countries (see Figure 4C). The estimated CCFR of the 1960 cohort is the highest in Ireland at 2.40; however, the decline from cohort to cohort was steep. In contrast, the CCFR in the Czech Republic fluctuated within a narrow band of 2.15 to 2.02 from the 1930 to the 1960 birth cohort, but then the estimate for the 1965 cohort falls to a value of 1.89. A very different pattern is observed in Slovakia, with a relatively steady decline from 2.86 for the 1930 cohort to 2.02 for the 1965 cohort. The Netherlands experienced a smooth decline from the 1930 cohort to the cohorts of the late 1940s, a leveling off for about ten years, and then a slow decline for the cohorts born in the late 1950s and early 1960s. Finland exemplifies a steady decline among the cohorts of the 1930s followed by stabilization and even a modest increase among the cohorts of the 1950s. Similar trends occurred (not shown) in Denmark and Norway.

In the United States and Canada CCFRs declined rapidly from the birth cohorts of the early 1930s through the cohorts of the late 1940s (see Figure 4D). In Canada the declining trend continued among the cohorts of the 1950s, and the 1960 birth cohort will probably have a CCFR of about 1.72. In the United States it appears that the completed fertility of the cohorts of the 1950s and 1960s will be around 2.0. US data permit decomposition by race (see Figure 4E). Data for whites and non-whites are pub-

FIGURE 4 Completed cohort fertility rate, selected countries, birth cohorts 1930–65

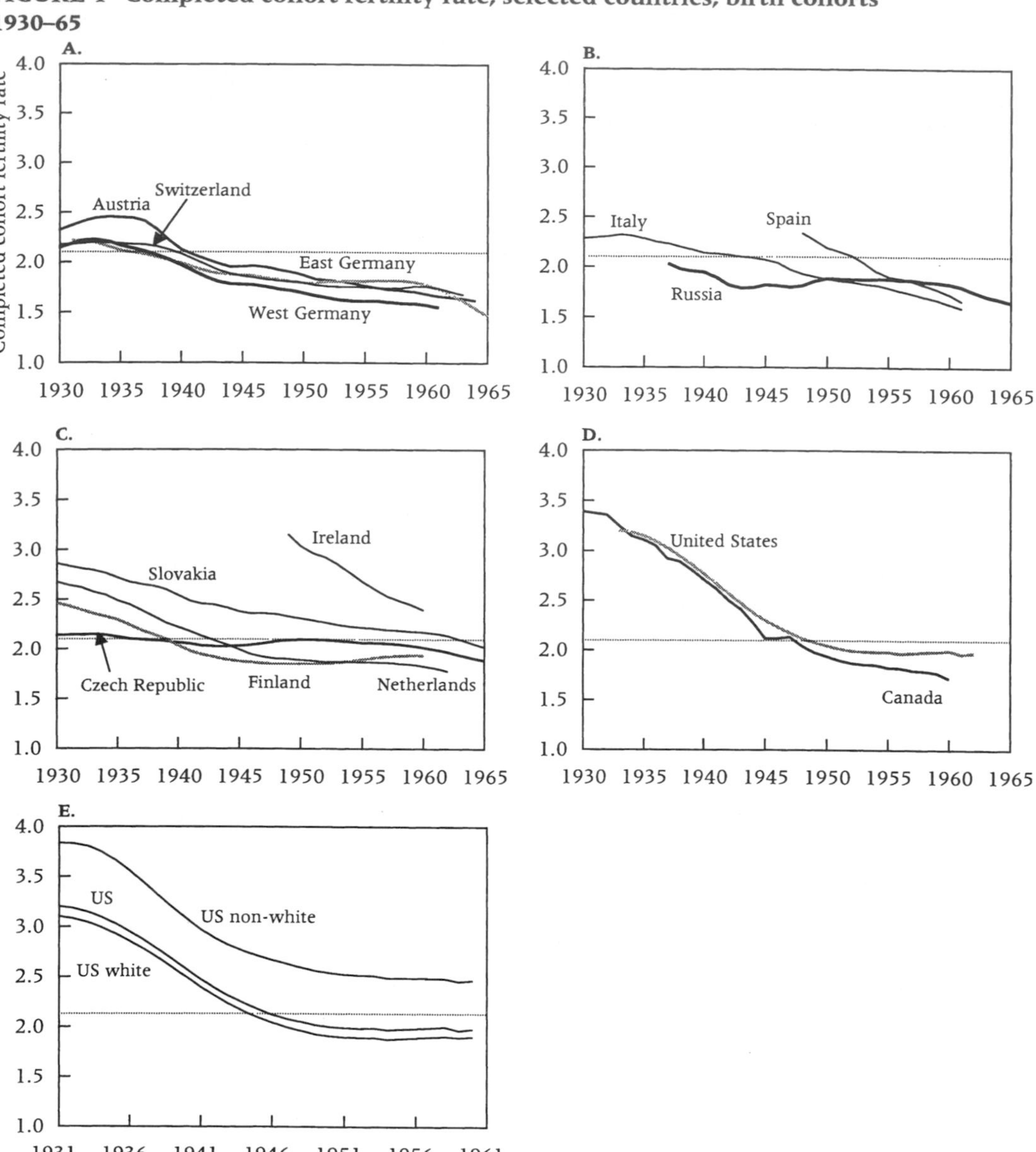

lished separately. These two groups followed similar trends during the period under consideration, with a steady differential of about 0.5–0.6 children. The white birth cohorts of the mid-1940s reached replacement and the cohorts of the 1950s appear to be stabilizing with CCFRs of about 1.9. CCFRs for the 1950s cohorts for non-whites, which undoubtedly conceal other differentials by race, have stabilized at close to 2.5 children per woman.

The main conclusion from these data is that significant shifts are taking place in completed cohort fertility, not just in period fluctuations. Completed cohort fertility is below the replacement level for the birth cohorts of the 1950s and the early 1960s in almost all European and North American countries, and with very few exceptions the trend among the most recent cohorts is one of decline.

Parity

Data on completed fertility by parity of birth cohorts of women are analytically valuable but rarely available. Table 7 presents such data for Germany, Hungary, and Russia.

A drop in family size is clear: the proportions of higher-order parities in the more recent birth cohorts are significantly smaller than in earlier cohorts. In the three countries the proportions at 3+ parity in the 1955, 1960, and 1950–54 birth cohorts were 18–20 percent compared to higher percentages in earlier cohorts.

More tellingly, from the perspective of replacement fertility, in all three countries the combined proportion of parities zero and one is larger than the proportions of 3+ parities. With a generous allowance for the fraction at 4+, the overall result is clear; it confirms that completed cohort fertility is below replacement. In Russia the combined proportion of parity 0 and 1 in the 1955 birth cohort was 34 percent and for parity 3+ only 18 percent; the respective proportion for the 1960 German cohort was 45 percent compared to 18 percent; in Hungary these proportions were 28 percent compared to 20 percent in the 1950–54 birth cohort. These data are in logical consonance with the estimated completed cohort fertility rates for the respective birth cohorts. These are 1.88 births per woman for the 1955 Russian birth cohort, 1.56 for the 1960 German cohort, and 1.94 for the 1950–54 Hungarian birth cohort.

TABLE 7 Distributions of completed fertility by parity, Federal Republic of Germany, Hungary, and Russian Federation, selected birth cohorts 1905–60 (in percent)

	Federal Republic of Germany		Hungary		Russian Federation	
Parity	1940	1960	1926–30	1950–54	1905	1955
0	10	23	12	8	11	7
1	24	22	25	20	14	27
2	39	37	36	52	16	48
3	27	18	15	15	15	13
4+			12	5	44	5
Total	100	100	100	100	100	100

Proximate determinants of fertility

Among the proximate determinants of fertility, we concentrate on cohabitation, contraceptive use, and induced abortion. Ideally one would want to measure the relative effect of each determinant through decomposition. Because data permit such an exercise only on a country level, we identify the basic direction of impact of the respective determinants in various country groupings.

Cohabitation

Major changes in cohabitation patterns occurred in all countries we have studied. Until the 1960s, it was common to get married during the childbearing years in all low-fertility countries. Few men and women did not enter into marriage. Total first marriage rates[7] (TFMRs) for women were close to unity in the early 1960s in all countries with available data. Thirteen of these are illustrated in Figures 5A and 5B.

In several Western countries the female TFMRs started to decline in the mid-1960s and reached a value of near 0.6 in all of them by the mid-1980s (Figure 5A), implying that only 60 percent would ever marry. But the data presented in this section are period rates, subject to timing effects. The long-term cohort marriage behavior may differ.

In the Scandinavian countries this process occurred earlier than elsewhere, as illustrated by the data for Denmark. In Southern Europe this trend did not start until the mid-1970s, but the decline was faster and steeper than elsewhere, as depicted by the trend in Spain. A significant proportion of the decline in formal marriage in the Western countries is offset by increases in consensual unions; however, this compensation is only partial.

As with all general indicators, TFMRs are indicative only of main trends and can conceal structural changes. For example, although age-specific first marriage rates have been declining among women in their teens and early 20s, in more recent years among women in their late 20s and early 30s they have either been relatively stable or have even increased in many Western countries.

In the Central and Eastern European countries the female TFMRs were near unity until around 1980 (Figure 5B). A moderate decline is discernible during the 1980s followed by a universally steep decline in the 1990s. Age-specific marriage rates (not shown) followed similar paths. In the Czech Republic, for instance, the declines in the young age groups were so abrupt that between 1960 and 1996 the proportions currently married plummeted to historic lows, from 8 percent to 2 percent at ages 15–19 and from 62 percent to 38 percent at ages 20–24.

TFMRs were not available for the Asian countries; however, age-specific proportions married provide evidence of distinct changes in family for-

FIGURE 5A Total first marriage rates for women, selected Western countries, 1960–96

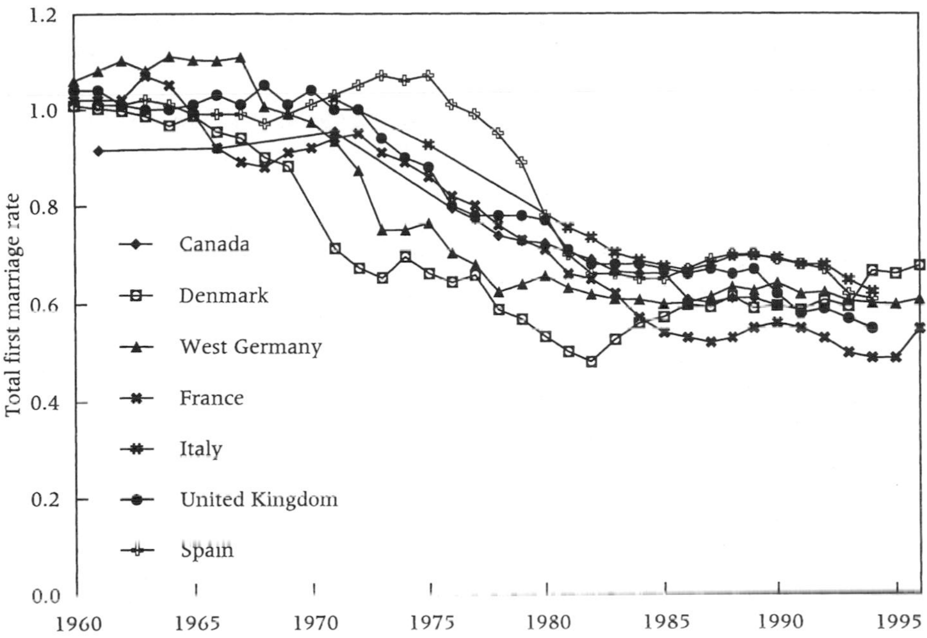

FIGURE 5B Total first marriage rates for women, selected Central and Eastern European countries, 1960–96

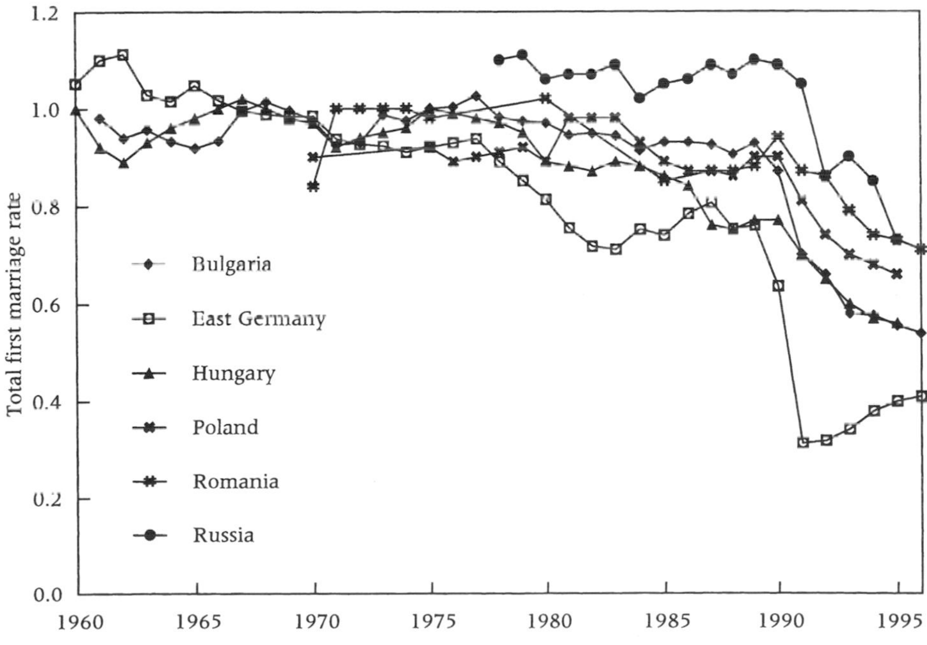

NOTE: See endnote 7 for definition of total first marriage rates.

mation (see Figure 6A). Among women aged 20–24 in Taiwan, 70 percent were married in the mid-1950s but only 20 percent by the mid-1990s. Japan and Korea experienced similar declines at ages 20–24 and also at higher ages; the proportions married in the late 20s and early 30s also fell in Japan, Korea, and Taiwan, but commencing after a delay of several years. The proportions of women married in their 40s have not changed.

In some countries patterns of family formation were modified by exceptional demographic structures created by manmade cataclysms. The low proportion of women married in Russia in the late 1950s was in part the consequence of unbalanced sex ratios arising from extremely high male mortality during World War II and possibly also from the incarceration of millions of men in the Gulag. As sex ratios became more balanced, the proportions of women married at ages 20–24 increased after 1950 but fell off again around 1990 (see Figure 6B). In China, marriage patterns were modified by demographic imbalances emerging from high famine-induced mortality and a temporary collapse of fertility around 1960, as well as by comparatively strict policy measures that in some periods restricted entry into marriage to relatively high ages.

The proportions of women cohabiting, either in formal marriages or in informal unions, are considerably smaller in the mid-1990s in the low-fertility countries than ever before. The 1901 to 1961 female birth cohorts

FIGURE 6A Proportions of women married at ages 20–24, Japan, Republic of Korea, and Taiwan, 1950–96

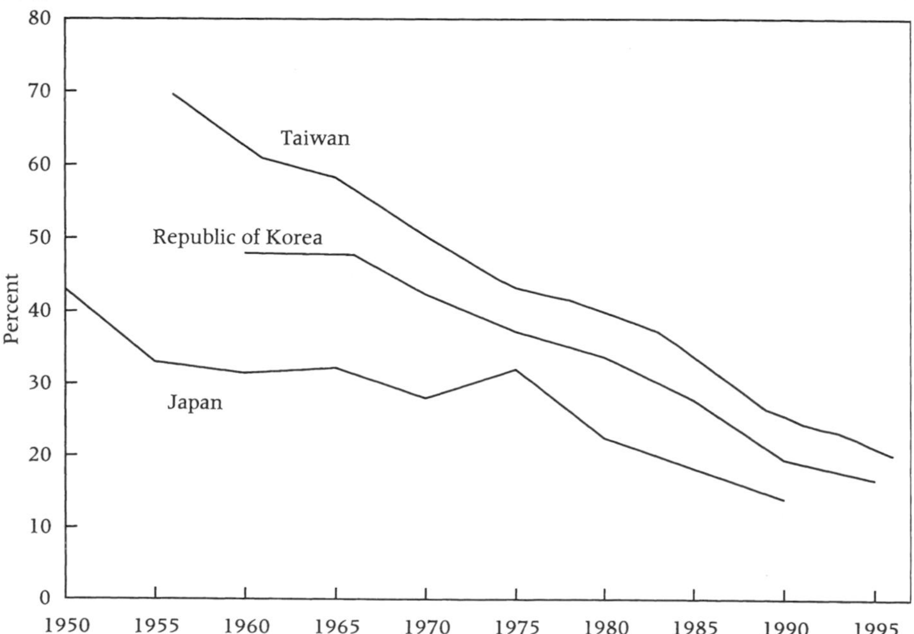

FIGURE 6B Proportions of women married at ages 20–24, Czech Republic, Hungary, and Russia, 1950–96

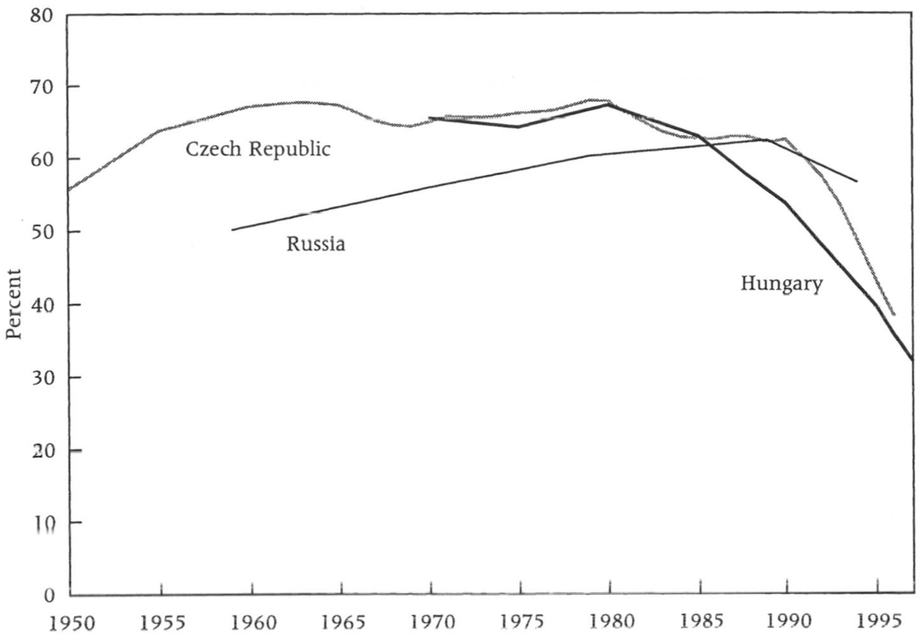

in Spain are illustrative (see Figure 7). For the cohorts born in the 1940s and earlier, at least 80 percent of women were ever married. Since then these proportions have been declining rapidly with only 68 percent of the 1961 birth cohort ever married. With some variation in timing, similar trends have probably been taking place in all low-fertility countries. This is a significant factor in lowering the probabilities of conceiving, even though sexual activity also occurs outside the bounds of cohabitation.

Contraceptive use

Profound changes have taken place in the use of contraception during the last four decades of the twentieth century, both in total use and in reliance on modern methods.

The increase in use was remarkably fast in the rapidly developing Asian countries (see Figure 8). Between the mid-1960s and the mid-1980s the proportions of women in union using contraception rose from 20 percent to 80 percent in Taiwan and in the Republic of Korea. Without doubt a similar process transpired in China, but the early years were not documented.

In the developed countries contraceptive use was commonplace earlier, yet even there some growth took place in the latter part of the century (Figure 8). Data for Hungary, the Netherlands, and the United States

FIGURE 7 Proportions ever married, Spain, female birth cohorts 1901–61

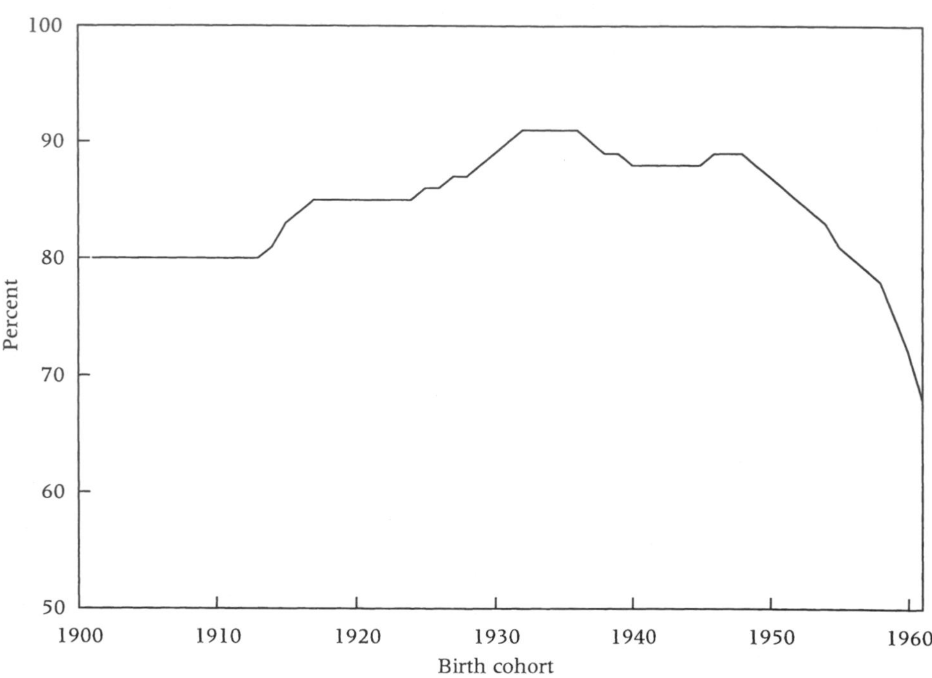

indicate that from the 1950s to the mid-1990s contraceptive use increased from around 60 percent to roughly 75 percent.

The other major development in contraceptive use was the rapid and widespread proliferation of modern methods. Early forms of the intrauterine device had been known (and sparsely used) since the 1920s, but a number of new versions were developed. Hormonal methods were invented and gradually refined, in particular oral contraceptives. Methods of surgical contraception were substantially improved. The quality of condoms was also improved. All of these contraceptives became accessible to, and were progressively used by, large segments of populations in developed and developing countries, essentially because of their effectiveness and convenience of use. Also, their prices were reasonable in comparison to other needs, or prices were subsidized for those who would otherwise not have had the means to purchase them.

In the West the contraceptive revolution got underway in the late 1950s and early 1960s. In 1955, for instance, in the United States 84 percent of users were relying on traditional contraceptives, including condoms (see Figure 9A). In less than two decades this number declined to 31 percent and it remained at that level through the 1980s. While 70 percent of users have been relying on modern contraceptives since the early 1970s, structural changes have occurred. The oral contraceptive was preferred by

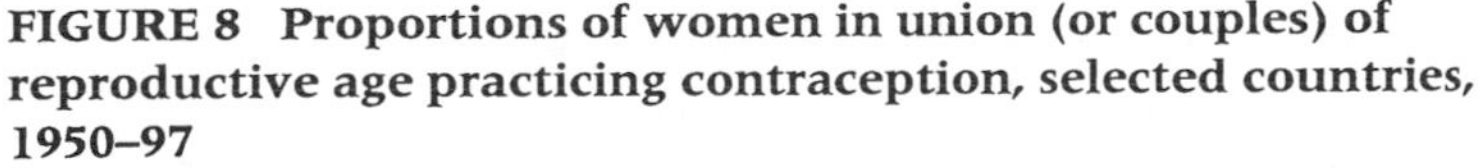

FIGURE 8 Proportions of women in union (or couples) of reproductive age practicing contraception, selected countries, 1950–97

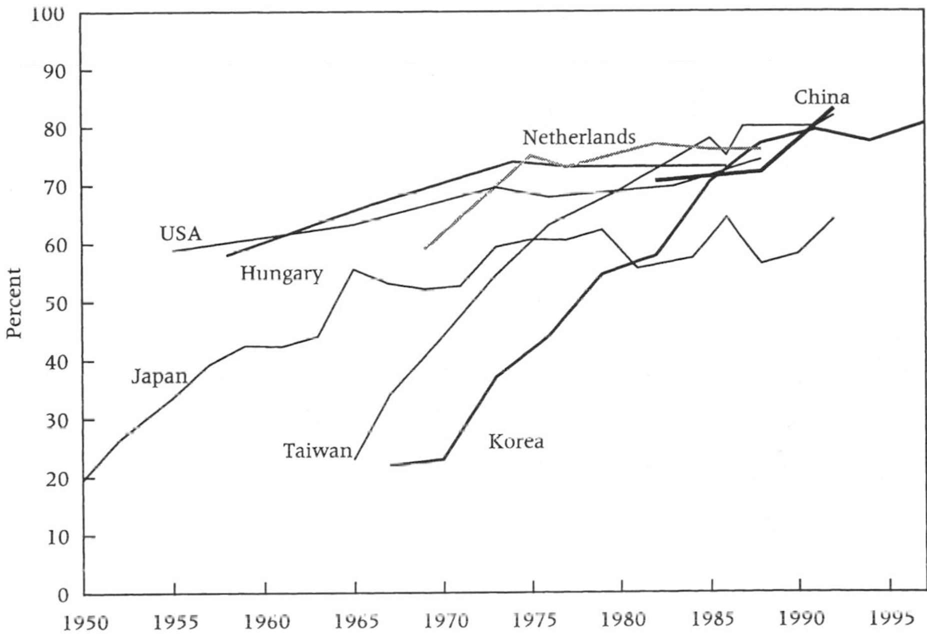

over one-third of users in the 1970s; this declined to one-fifth by the late 1980s. Use of the IUD increased to almost 10 percent by 1973, but fell to only 2 percent by the late 1980s. There has been a steady increase in the adoption of male and female sterilization; in 1988 one-half of all birth control users living in unions were sterilized. In sum, among the majority of users modern methods have replaced traditional ones. With many variations in composition and timing this has occurred in most Western countries.

In the formerly socialist countries of Central and Eastern Europe, the transformation from traditional to modern contraception has been much slower than in the West and has taken a different path. Most governments blocked the use of oral and surgical contraception. Hungary was an exception. Its relatively permissive government, which came into power in the late 1960s and gradually introduced social and economic reforms, supported the use of oral contraception and the IUD. As a result, modern contraceptive use rose from zero in 1966 to 62 percent in 1977 (see Figure 9B).

The spread in the use of the IUD (mostly the older versions) and especially of oral contraception was slow, with large differences between countries. In the Czech Republic in 1991, for instance, 22 percent of users were employing IUDs and less than 10 percent oral contraceptives; 70 percent of users were still relying on traditional methods.

FIGURE 9A Contraceptive use by method, United States, 1955–88

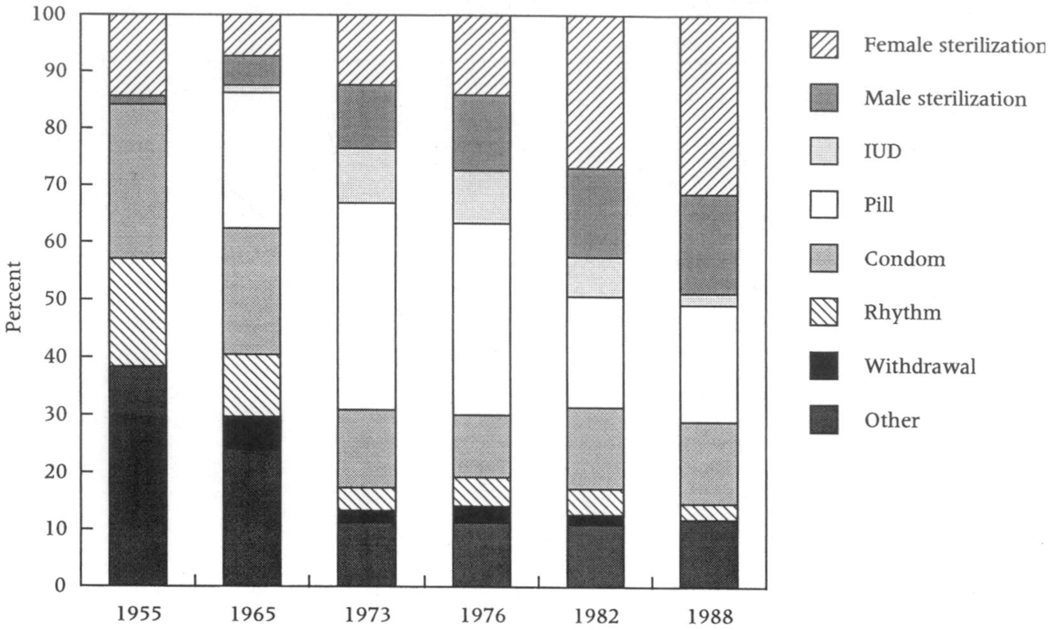

FIGURE 9B Contraceptive use by method, Hungary, 1958–93

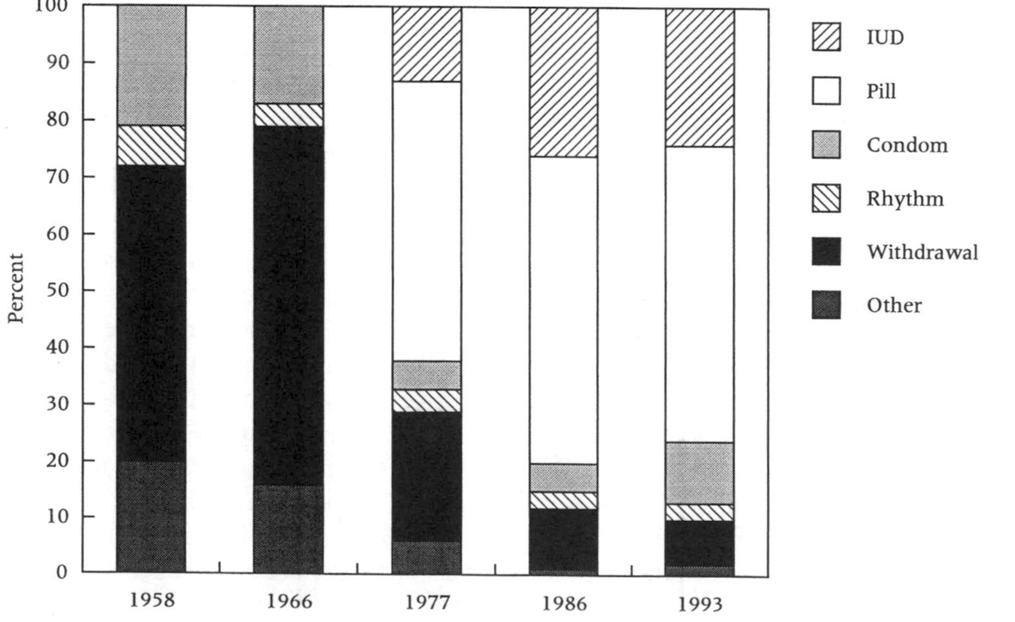

Changes in the use of contraception were very different in the developing countries. Traditional method use had always been trivial, so the spread of contraception was directly tied to modern contraceptives. Moreover, modern contraceptives were at first supplied and promoted mostly by public family planning programs with the assistance of international organizations. Even in the mid-1960s when only about 20 percent of women living in union were using contraception in Taiwan and Korea, 83 and 77 percent of these women, respectively, relied on modern contraception (see Figures 9C and 9D).[8] These proportions remained quite stable over the next several decades, and as the numbers of users increased rapidly so did the numbers relying on modern contraception.

At the same time, there were significant changes in method mix. In the 1960s, IUDs were in the forefront. Their use later diminished, more so in South Korea than in Taiwan where an earlier version of the IUD, the Ota ring, had been in use. The proportion using oral contraceptives was around 20 percent in South Korea in the early 1970s; that has decreased steadily to almost zero in 1997. In Taiwan pill use rose into the mid-1970s; thereafter a slow decline set in. The use of the condom has been increasing since the early 1980s with around 20 percent of users relying on it in both countries in the 1990s. Resort to sterilization has been quite important in Taiwan; since the mid-1980s one-third of users rely on it. In the Republic of Korea by 1979 almost 40 percent and by 1988 62 percent of users were sterilized. Although this proportion has since been declining it was still at 46 percent in 1997.

Even though modern contraceptives now dominate, the method mix differs from one country to another (see Figure 10). In China, South Korea, Canada, and the United States around 50 percent or more of users are sterilized. But in Hungary over 50 percent rely on oral contraceptives and an additional 24 percent on IUDs. In Japan 65 percent of couples using a method employ the condom. In Taiwan 33 percent of users are sterilized and almost 30 percent use IUDs. In the Czech Republic in the early 1990s over 30 percent of users were relying on withdrawal, and almost 30 percent the condom; less than 40 percent employed modern contraceptives. There, as in practically all other Central and Eastern European countries, induced abortion is an important means of fertility regulation.

Induced abortion

Induced abortion has played a significant role in the fertility transition of all low-fertility countries. During the first half of the twentieth century when numerous European countries were approaching replacement-level fertility, induced abortions were legally restricted everywhere (except for the Soviet Union[9]). Understandably, there is no official information on the

FIGURE 9C Contraceptive use by method, Taiwan, 1965–92

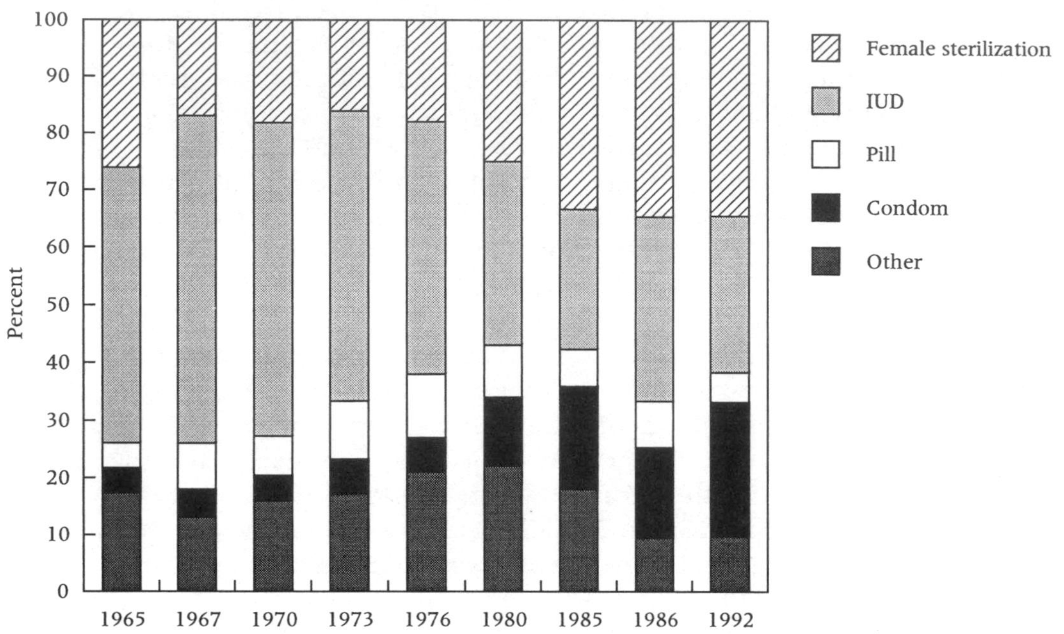

FIGURE 9D Contraceptive use by method, Republic of Korea, 1967–97

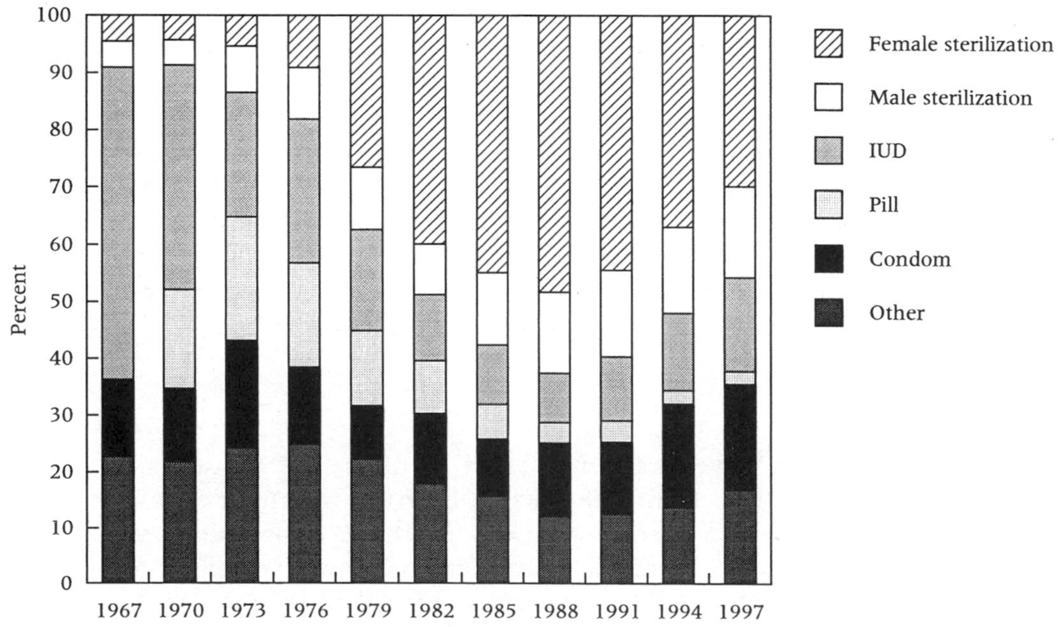

FIGURE 10 Contraceptive use by method, selected countries, 1988–97

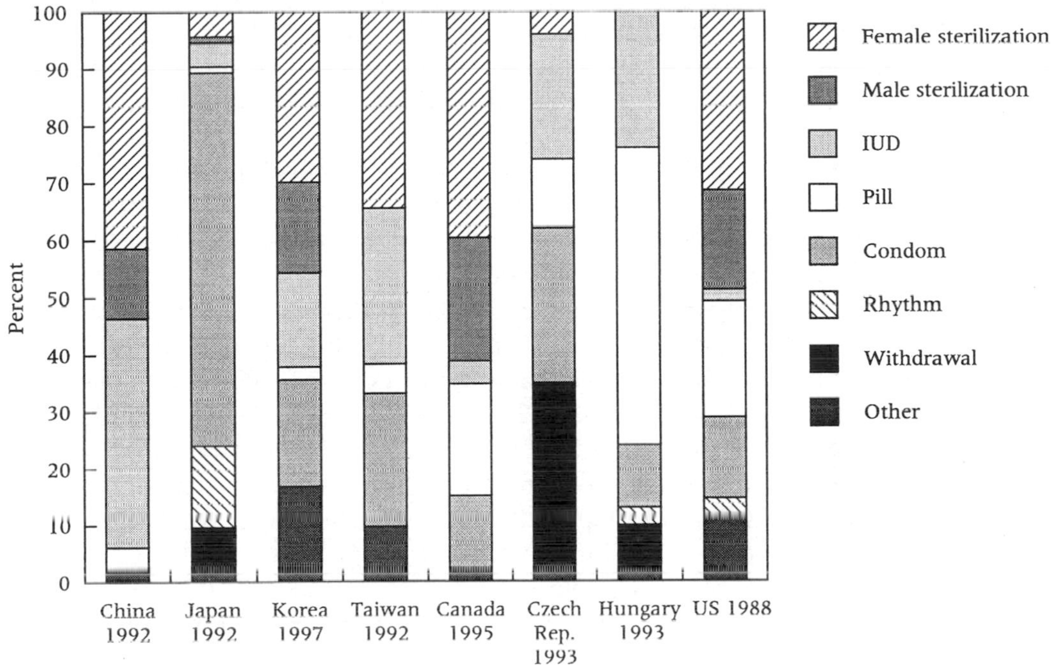

incidence of abortion for those years;[10] however contemporary observers believed the incidence to be high, especially in the worst years of the Depression in the 1930s (Carr-Saunders 1936; UN 1954; Glass 1940, reprinted in 1967, McLaren 1990).

During the second half of the century, legalization of induced abortion occurred in many countries (Tietze 1983; Rahman, Katzive, and Henshaw 1998). The effects tend to be multiple. The absolute number of abortions may or may not increase much; many legal abortions simply replace illegal ones. The liberalization of abortion laws lowers the health and mortality risks associated with induced abortion, because most of the abortions that would have been performed by unqualified personnel under unsanitary conditions can be and usually are performed by physicians in appropriate facilities. Liberal legislation has also enabled more or less complete registration of abortions, thus providing reasonable information on actual incidence and, frequently, on certain personal characteristics.

The fertility effect of liberalized legislation depends very much on the extent to which contraception is practiced. Wherever a large proportion of the population is already practicing contraception, the fertility effect tends to be small, since relatively few unwanted pregnancies occur, and birth intervals are in any case long on average. On the other hand, if contraception is not widely practiced, the fertility effect can be large (Tietze and Bongaarts 1976). During the modernization process, when desired family size is falling, legalization can reinforce the growing use of abortion, which can even serve as a primary method of birth limitation. Moreover, some contraception may be replaced by induced abortion. Overall abortion incidence in such cases tends to increase considerably, reaching and remaining at high levels (Frejka 1983). In the Asian rapidly developing countries similar processes took place; however, the prevalence of contraception, mostly modern, was increasing alongside the rise in abortion and has gradually replaced it, leading to declines in abortion incidence.

Around 1950 only a few countries had legislation that gave women easy access to induced abortion. In the mid-1930s three Nordic countries—Iceland (1935), Sweden (1937), and Denmark (1938)—liberalized their abortion laws. In 1948 the Eugenic Protection Law was promulgated in Japan; it permitted the termination of pregnancy for a woman "whose health may be affected seriously by continuation of pregnancy or by delivery from the physical or economic viewpoint." During the 1950s abortion laws were liberalized in the Soviet Union, in most countries of Central and Eastern Europe, and in China. Some Western countries followed during the 1960s as did Singapore, but the main wave of liberalization of abortion laws in the West did not take place until the late 1970s (Tietze 1983). In Korea practice has generally been more liberal than legislation. It was so before some liberalization occurred in 1973 and continued to be more liberal even afterward. In Hong Kong liberalization occurred a year earlier, in 1972.

The development and widespread use of new procedures for performing induced abortions is another characteristic of recent decades. This certainly contributed to lowered morbidity and mortality and may well have influenced incidence. The main improvements consisted in substituting dilation and curettage with suction (machine and manual), and the development of nonsurgical medical abortion. Moreover, on average abortions are performed earlier in pregnancy than before. The concepts of "menstrual regulation" in many developing countries, and "mini-abortions," as in the former Soviet Union, have become commonplace.

Although some mode of registration is in place in practically all low-fertility countries, there is a great difference in its completeness from one country to another. Caution in interpreting available abortion data is called for; however, crude comparisons in space and time make sense, especially if the relative reliability of the respective data is known (Henshaw, Singh, and Haas 1999).

In the second half of the twentieth century induced abortions were employed as a means of fertility regulation especially in countries of Central and Eastern Europe and in the former Soviet Union. Experts differ on estimates of the incidence of induced abortion in the former Soviet Union. Some estimate that in addition to registered abortions,[11] which for decades indicated a total abortion rate (TAR) on the order of 2.5 to 3.0 abortions per woman (see Table 8 and Figure 11), there were at least as many un-

TABLE 8 Estimated legal total abortion rates (TAR), selected countries, 1950–96

Region and country	1950 or year as shown	1960 or year as shown	1970 or year as shown	1980 or year as shown	1990 or year as shown	1996 or year as shown
Central and Eastern European countries						
Albania[a]	—	—	—	0.1	0.2	0.8
Bulgaria	0.02(1953)	0.9	1.9	2.3	2.2	1.6
Czechoslovakia	0.03(1954)	1.0	1.0	0.9	1.4	—
Czech Republic	—	—	0.8(1975)	1.0	1.5	0.6
Slovakia	—	—	0.7(1975)	0.9	1.2	0.6
East Germany	0.2	0.01	0.2	0.7	0.6(1989)	0.3
Hungary	0.02	2.3	2.5	1.1	1.2	1.1
Poland[a]	0.01	0.7	0.6	0.5	0.2	0.0
Romania[a]	—	5.6	1.9	2.7	5.5	2.3
Soviet Union[a]	0.4(1955)	3.4	3.3(1971)	3.1	2.6	—
Russian Federation[a]	—	—	—	—	4.1(1989)	2.9(1995)
Yugoslavia[a]	—	0.5	1.3	1.8	2.7	1.6(1993)
Other European countries						
Denmark	0.2(1954)	0.1	0.3	0.6	0.5	0.5(1995)
England and Wales	—	0.1(1968)	0.2	0.4	0.5	0.5
Finland	0.1(1951)	0.2(1961)	0.4	0.4	0.3	0.3
France[a]	—	—	0.4(1976)	0.5	0.4	0.4
Italy[a]	—	—	—	0.6	0.4	0.3
Netherlands	—	—	0.2(1973)	0.2	0.2	0.2
Norway	—	0.1(1964)	0.3	0.5	0.5	0.5
Sweden	0.1(1954)	0.1	0.3	0.6	0.6	0.6
West Germany[a]	0.0	0.01(1968)	0.0	0.3	0.2	0.2
Selected countries outside Europe						
Canada	—	—	0.1	0.3	0.4	—
China	—	—	0.7(1971)	1.3	1.2(1991)	0.8(1995)
Cuba	—	—	1.2	1.4	2.6	2.3
Israel[a]	—	—	—	0.5	0.5	0.4(1995)
Japan[a]	1.2(1952)	1.3(1962)	0.8	0.7	0.5	0.4
Korea (South)[a]	—	—	1.9(1975)	1.9	1.1	0.6
New Zealand	—	—	0.2(1976)	0.3	0.4	0.5(1995)
Singapore	—	—	0.7(1975)	0.9	0.7	0.5
United States	—	0.003(1963)	0.5(1973)	0.9	0.8	0.7

[a]Reporting incomplete or completeness unknown.
SOURCES: Frejka 1983; Henshaw, Singh, and Haas 1999; Barkalov and Ivanov 1997 (for Russian Federation).

FIGURE 11 Total abortion rates, selected countries, 1950–96

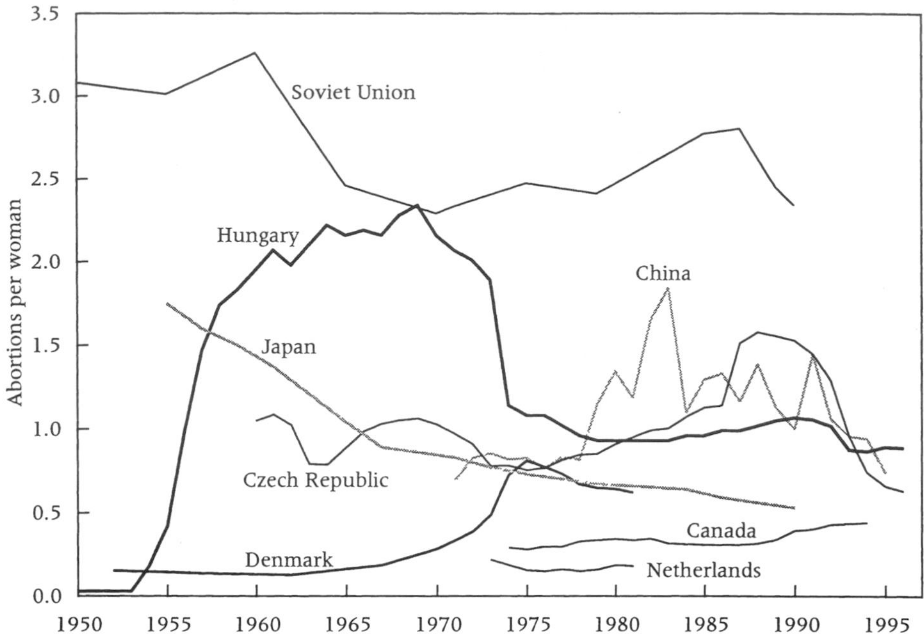

registered ones, which would imply annual TARs above 5.0, and two to three times more abortions than births (Popov et al. 1993). In Romania, which had a reliable registration system, the TAR was between 6.0 and 7.5 in the period 1961 to 1966 (Tietze 1983) and subsequently, in 1990, it again increased to 5.5 (Henshaw, Singh, and Haas 1999)—these are to our knowledge the highest rates ever reasonably reliably recorded. Throughout the 1960s the TAR in Hungary was above 2.0. Bulgaria and Yugoslavia also experienced years when the TAR was above 2.0. In Czechoslovakia the TAR fluctuated around 1.0; in East Germany and Poland it was even lower, but Poland's data were never complete.

In East Asia induced abortions were also an important factor in the fertility transition. Frejka (1993) estimated that in the late 1980s induced abortions compared to contraception accounted for about one-quarter of the fertility decline in East Asia. It was in Japan that induced abortions were first widely employed as a method of birth control in the late 1940s. Official statistics are grossly incomplete but experts estimate total abortion rates for the 1950s and 1960s between 3 and 4 abortions per woman (Muramatsu 1973). In the other countries of East Asia the incidence of induced abortion was lower, as it accompanied the intensive introduction of modern contraception. Nevertheless, in China, for instance, throughout the 1980s the TAR was between 1.0 and 1.9. In Korea TARs for married women, as distinct from all women in Table 8, fluctuated from 2.1 to 2.9 between 1973 and 1985, declining thereafter, though still at 1.4 in 1994 (Cho 1997). In Taiwan, from 1985 through 1991, a third of married women reported ever having had an abortion.[12]

In the West the incidence of induced abortion tends to be relatively low, with TARs of around 0.5 or less, because of the widespread use of modern contraception.

In the remainder of the low-fertility countries in Asia, in the countries of the former Soviet Union, and in Central and Eastern Europe the resort to induced abortion has declined in recent years. In the countries of East Asia this trend has been in progress for possibly two decades, as documented in Korea and Japan. In the states of the former Soviet Union and in Central and Eastern Europe the decline is mainly a feature of the 1990s. According to one estimate the TAR in Russia declined from 4.1 to 2.9 between 1989 and 1995 (Barkalov and Ivanov 1997). Access to modern contraception has become easier than under the previous socialist regimes; however, it will likely be some time before induced abortion is employed primarily as a backup to contraception.

Policy measures

Policy measures can have direct and immediate effects on reproductive behavior. Indeed, they have had an important impact in the Asian low-fertility countries and at times in the formerly socialist countries.

The fertility transition in the Asian low-fertility countries has occurred at a much faster pace than that in the industrialized countries. Within two to three decades fertility declined from TFRs of about 6 to replacement. Without national family programs, the principal policy measure in the developing countries, this decline might have taken significantly longer. In Taiwan, for example, "the family planning services provided by the program were the immediate proximate cause of the fertility decline" (Freedman, Chang, and Sun 1994: 327). The authors continue by noting that "as late as 1985, just after reaching replacement-level fertility, 73 percent of all current users had obtained their contraceptive services from the family planning program" (ibid.). Also, organized efforts to provide access to family planning services to many population strata commenced in some countries even before any significant or widespread economic development took place. In China this was as early as the mid-1950s and in Korea in the early to mid-1960s. Still, early fertility declines assisted by family planning programs materialized because of existing latent demand for family limitation. In 1964, on the basis of the experience of designing and implementing one of the first large-scale family planning programs, Berelson and Freedman (1964: 29) concluded that "people do not need to be motivated. They want to plan their families, but they need to know how. Teaching them how—implementing a family planning program—has proved to be feasible."

In almost all low-fertility countries in Asia—in Hong Kong, the Republic of Korea, Singapore, Taiwan, and Thailand—family planning programs while vigorous were essentially noncoercive. They employed large staffs, operated with adequate material resources provided by local funds and international aid, and carried out effective information, education, and communication projects. In general they relied heavily upon a substantial existing interest in contraceptive use in the population.

In China the approach was different. The government provided similar services, but specific policies were authoritarian, backed by strong and strict enforcement. Initially, the national program was based on the *wan xi shao* approach—later (marriage), longer (birth intervals), fewer (births)—promulgated in 1971. As this policy was perceived not to be sufficiently effective, in 1979 the one-child principle was adopted. That policy, with certain modifications, including a partial relaxation in 1984 regarding minorities and rural couples whose first child was a daughter, has since formed the national approach. Fertility decline in China has possibly been faster than in any of the other countries. Feeney and Wang (1993: 95), who conducted a detailed analysis of China's fertility decline, concluded: "It is likely that over half of this decline may be attributed to government intervention specifically aimed at reducing fertility."

In Korea, Taiwan, Singapore, and Hong Kong, by the late 1980s or early 1990s, fertility declines had made family planning programs largely superfluous and they have been largely dismantled. Individuals themselves decide and finance their means of fertility control. The programs have turned their attention to special issues; in Korea for instance the focus is on adolescents and single persons, with more attention to reproductive health and such issues as home health care and private medical insurance (Cho, Seo, and Tan 1990). Furthermore, some governments, for instance in Singapore and Taiwan, have become concerned with low fertility and have initiated efforts to raise fertility and stabilize it around replacement level.

A unique "population policy" decision in 1948 turned out to have a major effect in Japan during the 1950s and later. The government in an atmosphere of postwar rapid population growth—a baby boom, a sharp mortality decline, and the repatriation of more than 5 million persons from various Asian countries—together with major economic and political problems, adopted the Eugenic Protection Law. The interpretation of this law by the medical profession and by government authorities made abortion available on request (Tietze 1983). By 1955 the annual number of recorded induced abortions was 1.2 million compared to 1.7 million births, and the annual number of sterilizations (also permitted by the Eugenic Protection Law) had increased to 44,000 (Terao 1959). It can be argued whether the Eugenic Protection Law concerned population policy, but there is no question that it provided Japanese couples with an effective means of fertility control, and it hastened the secular fertility decline to below replacement. As discussed above, the total fertility rate declined from its postwar high of 4.5 births per woman in 1947 to 2.0 in 1957.

In the formerly socialist countries of Central and Eastern Europe and in the former Soviet Union a wide variety of population-related policy measures were taken in the four decades following World War II. The pronatalist orientation of these policies was rooted in Marxist ideology, reinforced by the simplistic notion that since fertility is declining in capitalist societies it must increase, or at least remain "high," in socialist ones. Thus, many of the adopted policies, including a range of social welfare measures, were intended to stimulate fertility. Other policies of a broader economic nature (such as giving priority to large-scale labor-intensive investments) were implemented for different reasons but had fertility consequences, usually quickening the declines. Measures to legalize induced abortion were adopted to prevent the deleterious consequences of poorly performed illegal abortions; in the process women's rights were enhanced although this was rarely a primary consideration. Occasional decisions to restrict the use of abortion were made to lessen its perceived excessive use by certain strata of the population and to reduce its impact on fertility decline. Other measures were taken to bar or limit the introduction of modern contraceptives. These were justified on ideological grounds (modern contraceptives were developed in the capitalist West, especially in the imperialist United States), or by concerns about health side effects, or by the state's need to raise fertility.

The deliberate measures to raise fertility included liberal maternity leave, financial support for mothers staying at home with young children, family and child care allowances, birth grants, subsidized prices for child clothing and free textbooks, subsidized public child care, loans to newlyweds, and rents and pensions tied partially to family size (Frejka 1980; Klinger 1984; Centre for Demography and Human Ecology 1997). At times their effect was ambiguous, but, particularly when several measures were introduced simultaneously and when they were materially attractive, the fertility effects were discernible. This happened in Czechoslovakia in the period 1968–73, in Hungary in 1973, in East Germany in 1976, and to some extent in the former Soviet Union in the early 1980s. Czechoslovakia, for instance, experienced an increase in age-specific fertility rates and the total fertility rate, an increase in first marriage rates, an increase in second and third births, and increases in parity progression ratios for cohorts that were entering their prime childbearing years in the early 1970s. Thus the completed fertility of these cohorts was also affected. Invariably the fertility effect was limited to the cohorts in their prime childbearing years at the time the measures were adopted. After a few years they were taken for granted and had little or no effect on subsequent cohorts.

In addition to the social policy measures directly aimed at increasing fertility, many features of the social infrastructure motivated young people to have children and to have them earlier rather than later. This included preferential allocation of housing, which was in short supply in the tightly regulated state-controlled systems (Frejka 1980; Klinger 1984; Centre for Demography and Human Ecology 1997; David 1999). Also, there was a lack of sex education, lack of knowledge about contraception, and a general preference for getting married to accommodate a first, early and unintended pregnancy rather than to interrupt it (David 1999). There was also a wide belief that first pregnancies of young women should not be terminated because this might impede later childbearing. Large and increasing proportions of first births occurred less than eight months after weddings (Centre for Demography and Human Ecology 1997). Induced abortions were practiced mainly by married women, usually in their late 20s or older, who had already achieved their desired family size (Tietze 1983).

While numerous countervailing forces were present, some depressing rather than stimulating the desire for children, in the 1970s and 1980s fertility was higher than it would have been without the socialist system of centralized economic management and social welfare policies.[13] This conclusion appears to be supported by period TFRs in the formerly socialist countries that were on average higher by about 20 percent compared to Western European ones.[14] Subsequently, by the mid-1990s—after the dissolution of the authoritarian governments in Central and Eastern Europe and in the former Soviet Union, and after the value of the social welfare measures had eroded (Rychtaříková 1996)—period rates declined rapidly to values on average lower than in the West. In the Czech Republic, for instance, fertility declined especially among women under 25 years of age; age-specific first marriage rates for women under 25 declined by more than 50 percent within six years; the mean age at childbirth increased from 24.7 in 1991 to 26.2 in 1996. Obviously it is too early to assess longer-term effects, but there are indications, including evidence provided above, that cohort fertility is also generally on the decline.

Our arguments appear to contradict what others in the profession have concluded, namely that "the effects [of pronatalist policies] are nil or negligible" (Demeny 1986: 350). However, the policy relevance now seems limited, since the fertility-enhancing effect of such policies in the formerly socialist countries was achieved under circumstances that are not likely to be replicated in any country in the foreseeable future.

Conversely, the experience with the implementation and functioning of family planning programs in the East Asian countries has had and continues to have a great deal of policy relevance. For instance, Freedman (1998), in an article evaluating social science and operations research, writes: "Taiwan's program, because it was an early success, was visited by thousands of people concerned with programs in developing countries" (p. 39).

And further: "In retrospect, Taiwan's family planning history has significant value...for other countries in the early stages of their demographic transitions" (p. 43).

Conclusions

Never before in history have there been such enormous changes in fertility behavior in so many societies as took place in the twentieth century. This phenomenon clearly reflects the profound changes in technology, labor productivity, urban occupations and living arrangements, and social infrastructure and lifestyles—in short a consequence of major changes in social and economic frameworks. The fertility responses have not mirrored these changes mechanically and uniformly, but have frequently been modified also by political structures and by national cultures. At the beginning of the century total fertility rates around the world were on the order of 5 to 7 children per woman. In contrast, in the mid-1990s 44 percent of the world's population lived in countries where total fertility rates were at or below 2.1, the replacement level for low-mortality populations.

Is subreplacement fertility likely to prevail in these countries for at least two to three decades or is it a temporary phenomenon? The evidence presented here points to the former scenario.

Completed cohort fertility for the majority of these countries is and apparently will remain below replacement. Large proportions of women remain childless or have only one child. Only small proportions of women have more than three children. The proportions of women married and cohabiting are at historically low levels and declining further. People have access to and are using effective means of fertility regulation—pills, IUDs, condoms, sterilization, and induced abortion. Key social changes in the status of women, in the place of the family, and in Western cultures unite to undermine childbearing. In the developing countries population policies have been effective in assisting people to limit their family size, whereas population policies inducing people to raise their fertility, which showed some results in the formerly socialist countries, usually have only temporary effects. All things considered, it appears that an era of subreplacement fertility has taken hold and will endure.

Notes

We owe substantial debts to numerous individuals who helped to advance this study. Erik Klijzing of the UN Economic Commission for Europe greatly expedited our access to much European information, and Gérard Calot and Alain Confesson of the Observatoire Démographique Européen provided numerous data sets in electronic form. Additional data were provided by Aminur R. Khan, Bhakta Gubhaju, Sergei Ivanov, and Mary Beth Weinberger of the United Nations Population Division. Griffith Feeney was constantly helpful with counsel on parity progression rates and available data sets. We also thank the Advisory Group of the Fertility and Family Surveys (FFS) program of comparative research for its permission, granted under identification number 24, to use FFS data. We owe special debts to other individuals who provided documents or data. Alphabetically by country they are Douglas Norris for Canada, Jitka Rychtaříková for the Czech Republic, Charlotte Höhn and Jürgen Dorbritz for Germany, Peter Józan for Hungary, Chai Bin Park and Nam Hoon Cho for Korea, Sergei Zakharov, Elena Ivanova, Ward Kingkade, and Ludmila Pashina for Russia, Joaquin Arango for Spain, and T. H. Sun and M. C. Chang for Taiwan. We especially thank Laura Heaton and Robert McKinnon for assistance with data processing, and Cathy Johnson, chief of the production unit of the Futures Group International.

1 For the purpose of this analysis:

a. As a rule, countries are considered legal entities as they existed on 1 January 1998. Each of the successor states of the former Soviet Union, Yugoslavia, and Czechoslovakia are units of analysis. The one exception is Germany. The preunification Federal Republic of Germany and the former German Democratic Republic are each treated as a unit.

b. Only low-fertility countries with more than 250,000 inhabitants on 1 January 1998 were included. The full list of the 54 countries appears in Table 2.

2 In a detailed analysis of the demography of Europe in which some 600 small political divisions were surveyed, even lower net reproduction rates were observed. In numerous cities across the continent, fertility was extremely low. In the early 1930s, the NRR stood as low as 0.25 in Vienna, 0.36 in Oslo, 0.37 in Berlin, 0.40 in Stockholm, 0.47 in Riga, 0.48 in Hamburg, and 0.61 in Copenhagen (Kirk 1946). The NRR was well below replacement in London, Paris, Prague, Budapest, Belgrade, and Warsaw.

3 In Figures 2A through 2F a "replacement fertility" straight line is drawn with the value of 2.1. This is strictly for illustrative purposes. In the 1990s replacement-level fertility is close to 2.1 in almost all countries shown; however, in earlier decades in a number of countries, particularly in the Asian developing countries, replacement fertility was much higher owing to higher mortality.

4 Only 53 countries are included in this analysis, because no data on age-specific fertility rates are available for the People's Republic of China.

5 Data for Malta, the Republic of Korea, and Thailand were not available.

6 Estimates for cohorts younger than age 50 years at the time of observation equal actual observed fertility plus estimated fertility for remaining years. For each year of age above the observed age, the respective age-specific fertility rate of the most recent cohort for which an observation was possible is applied. For instance, if fertility for the 1960 birth cohort was observed through 1995, when it completed age 35, the observed age-specific fertility rate at age 36 for the 1959 birth cohort plus the observed age-specific fertility rate at age 37 for the 1958 birth cohort were added. The methodology applied was developed by Gérard Calot of the Observatoire Démographique Européen. The data for the European countries were provided by this institution. Canadian data were provided by François Nault. Detailed tables of US cohort fertility were provided by Stephanie Ventura of the National Center for Health Statistics, Centers for Disease Control and Prevention and the estimates were completed by the authors (calculations of the US completed cohort fertility rates are based on 5-year moving averages; in the table and figures these are centered on the respective year as indicated).

The proportions of the completed cohort fertility rates that are estimated provide evidence of the degree of accuracy. In the CCFRs for the US cohorts of the early 1950s, about 0.7 percent of the total was estimated; for those of the late 1950s about 5.5 percent was estimated; and for the cohorts of 1961 and 1962 about 15 percent of the CCFR was estimated. Thus the estimates of the 1950s cohorts were clearly close to what they will actually turn out to be, and there is some room for error in the birth cohorts of 1961 and 1962, although even here the margin of error is not likely to be large. The proportions of the CCFRs that are estimated are similar in the other countries.

Countries included in this analysis for which at least short time series of completed cohort fertility rates were available are the following: Austria, Belarus, Belgium, Bosnia-Herzegovina, Bulgaria, Canada, Croatia, Czech Republic, Denmark, Estonia, Federal Republic of Germany (former), Finland, Former Yugoslav Republic of Macedonia, France, Georgia, German Democratic Republic (former), Greece, Hungary, Ireland, Italy, Luxembourg, Malta, Netherlands, Norway, Poland, Portugal, Romania, Russian Federation, Slovakia, Slovenia, Spain, Sweden, Switzerland, United Kingdom, United States, and Yugoslavia.

7 The total first marriage rate is calculated as the probability of first marriage for a person if she or he were to pass through her/his lifetime conforming to age-specific first marriage rates of a given year. Although one person cannot have more than one first marriage, the value of the measure can exceed unity, if there is a burst of first marriages in several age cohorts in the single reference year.

8 In the developing countries condoms are included in the category of modern contraception, because they were part of national and international introduction efforts.

9 Legislation pertaining to abortion was liberalized in the Soviet Union in 1920, but in 1935 and 1936 severe limitations were reinstated (David 1970).

10 Data are available for some parts of the Soviet Union. Reasonably reliable data from Moscow, for instance, document a rise in the use of abortion during the 1920s: from about 20 per 100 births in 1921–24, rising to 56 per 100 in 1926 and to 75 in 1927 (Stloukal 1995). This rate continued to increase thereafter and, according to Soviet medical statistics, in Moscow there were 271 and 221 abortions per 100 births in 1934 and 1935, respectively.

11 The records were confidential and were not open to the public until the 1990s.

12 Sex-selective abortions are employed throughout East Asia to ensure a male birth at parity two and above. In Korea in 1988, for example, there were almost 200 male births per 100 female births at parity four (Cho, Seo, and Tan 1990).

13 Some demographers have voiced similar conclusions, albeit less forcefully. For instance, Andorka (1996: 28), in a chapter summarizing population developments in Hungary since 1960, concluded that "in the absence of family benefits, the level of fertility would be much lower than it is now."

14 The average (unweighted) TFR during 1971–90 for the Czech Republic, German Democratic Republic, Hungary, and Russia was 1.95; for Denmark, the Federal Republic of Germany, and Italy it was 1.62. The TFR was 21 percent higher in the former group compared to the latter.

References

Andorka, R. 1996. "Demographic changes and their main characteristics from 1960 to our days," in P. P. Tóth and E. Valkovics (eds.), *Demography of Contemporary Hungarian Society*. Highland Lakes, NJ: Atlantic Research and Publications.

Arango, J. 1998. Unpublished data, personal communication, Instituto Universitario Ortega y Gasset, Madrid.

Avdeev, A. 1994. "Contraception and abortion: Trends and prospects for the 1990s," in W. Lutz et al. (eds.), *Demographic Trends and Patterns in the Soviet Union Before 1991*. London, New York, and Laxenburg: Routledge and IIASA.

Barclay, G. 1954. *Colonial Development and Population in Taiwan*. Princeton, NJ: Princeton University Press.

Barkalov, N. and S. Ivanov, 1997. "Contraception and induced abortion in Russia: A review," unpublished manuscript.

Berelson, B. and R. Freedman. 1964. "A study in fertility control," *Scientific American* 21(5): 29–37.

Blum, A. and S. Zakharov. 1997. "The demographic history of the USSR and Russia in the mirror of cohorts," *Population and Society*, No. 17, Centre for Demography and Human Ecology, Moscow.

Bongaarts, J. and G. Feeney. 1998. "On the quantum and tempo of fertility," *Population and Development Review* 24(2): 271–291.

Breslin, M. 1997. "Japanese women want more children than their total fertility rate suggests," *Family Planning Perspectives* 29(6): 291–292.

Calot, G. 1998. Unpublished data, personal communication, Observatoire Démographique Européen, Paris.

Carr-Saunders, A. N. 1936. *World Population: Past Growth and Present Trends.* Oxford: Clarendon Press.

Centre for Demography and Human Ecology. 1996. *The Population of Russia 1995.* Moscow.

———. 1997. *The Population of Russia 1996.* Moscow.

Chang, M. C. 1993. "Sex preference and sex ratio at birth: The case of Taiwan," presented at the Annual Meeting of the Population Association of China, Taipei, 5–6 February.

Chang, M. C., R. Freedman, and T. H. Sun. 1981. "Trends in fertility, family size preferences, and family planning practice: Taiwan, 1961–80," *Studies in Family Planning* 12(5): 211–228.

———. 1987. "Trends in fertility, family size preferences, and family planning practice: Taiwan, 1961–85," *Studies in Family Planning* 18(6): 320–337.

Chen, C. H. C. et al. 1997. "Contraceptive prevalence in China: Findings from the 1992 National Family Planning Survey," in *1992 National Fertility and Family Planning Survey, China.* Beijing: State Family Planning Commission.

Chen, S. 1997. "Demographic change from 1982 to 1992," in *1992 National Fertility and Family Planning Survey, China.* Beijing: State Family Planning Commission.

Chesnais, J-C. 1990. "Demographic transition patterns and their impact on the age structure," *Population and Development Review* 16(2): 327–336.

———. 1992. *The Demographic Transition.* Oxford: Clarendon Press.

Cho, N. H. 1996. *Achievements and Challenges of the Population Policy Development in Korea.* Seoul: Korea Institute for Health and Social Affairs.

———. 1997. Unpublished data, personal communication.

Cho, N. H., M. H. Seo, and B. A. Tan. 1990. "Recent changes in the population control policy and its future direction in Korea," *Journal of Population, Health and Social Welfare* 10(2): 152–173.

Coale, A. J. 1981. "A further note on Chinese population statistics," *Population and Development Review* 7(3): 512–518.

Council of Europe. 1997. *Recent Demographic Developments in Europe 1997.* Strasbourg: Council of Europe Publishing.

Czech Statistical Office; Factum non Fabula; WHO Collaborating Center for Perinatal Medicine/Institute for the Care of Mother and Child, Prague; and Centers for Disease Control and Prevention, USA. 1995. *1993 Czech Republic Reproductive Health Survey: Final Report.* Prague.

Darsky, L. E. 1994. "Quantum and timing of births in the USSR," in W. Lutz et al. (eds.), *Demographic Trends and Patterns in the Soviet Union Before 1991.* London, New York, and Laxenburg: Routledge and IIASA.

David, H. P. (ed.). 1970. *Family Planning and Abortion in the Socialist Countries of Central and Eastern Europe.* New York: Population Council.

——— (ed.). 1999. *From Abortion to Contraception: A Resource to Public Policies and Reproductive Behavior in Central and Eastern Europe from 1917 to Present.* Westport, CT: Greenwood Press.

Davis, K., M. S. Bernstam, and R. Ricardo-Campbell (eds.). 1986. *Below-Replacement Fertility in Industrial Societies: Causes, Consequences, Policies,* Supplement to *Population and Development Review* (12).

Delgado, M. 1992. "Spain," in H-P. Blossfeld (ed.), *The New Role of Women.* Boulder: Westview Press.

Delgado, M. and M. Livi-Bacci. 1992. "Fertility in Italy and Spain: The lowest in the world," *Family Planning Perspectives* 24(4): 162–171.

Demeny, Paul. 1986. "Pronatalist policies in low-fertility countries: Patterns, performance, and prospects," *Population and Development Review* 12 (Supp): 335–358.

Dorbritz, J. and C. Höhn. 1998. "The future of the family and future fertility trends in Germany," manuscript, provided as a personal communication to authors.

Feeney, G. 1991. "Fertility decline in Taiwan: A study using parity progression ratios," *Demography* 28(3): 467–479.

———. 1994. "Fertility decline in East Asia," *Science* 266(5190): 1518–1523.

———. 1996. "Fertility in China: Past, present, prospects," in W. Lutz (ed.), *The Future Population of the World: What Can We Assume Today?* London: Earthscan Publications.

Feeney, G. and F. Wang. 1993. "Parity progression and birth intervals in China: The influence of policy in hastening fertility decline," *Population and Development Review* 19(1): 61–101.

Feeney, G. and J. Yu. 1987. "Period parity progression measures of fertility in China," *Population Studies* 41: 77–102.

Fernandez, C. J. A. 1986. "Analysis longitudinal de le fecundidad en Espana," in Ministerio de Economia y Hacienda, *Tendencias demograficas y planificacion economica*, Madrid.

Freedman, R. 1986. "Policy options after the demographic transition: The case of Taiwan," *Population and Development Review* 12(1): 77–100.

———. 1998. "Operations and other types of research in Taiwan's family planning history," in J. R. Foreit and T. Frejka (eds.), *Family Planning Operations Research: A Book of Readings*. New York: Population Council.

Freedman, R., M. C. Chang, and T. H. Sun. 1994. "Taiwan's transition from high fertility to below-replacement levels," *Studies in Family Planning* 25(6): 317–331.

Frejka, T. 1960. "The development and present state of the population in Japan" (in Czech), *Demografie* 2(2): 250–256.

———. 1980. "Fertility trends and policies: Czechoslovakia in the 1970s," *Population and Development Review* 6(1): 65–93.

———. 1983. "Induced abortion and fertility: A quarter century of experience in Eastern Europe," *Population and Development Review* 9(3): 494–520.

———. 1993. "The role of induced abortion in contemporary fertility regulation," in IUSSP, *International Population Conference*, vol. 1. 209–213, Montreal.

Frejka, T. and E. Frejka. 1965. "Women in the labor force" (in Czech), *Planovane Hospodarstvi* 18(7–8): 169–176.

Glass, D. V. 1940, reprinted 1967. *Population Policies and Movements in Europe*. London: Cass.

Henshaw, S. K., S. Singh, and T. Haas. 1999. "The incidence of abortion worldwide," *International Family Planning Perspectives* 25 (Supp): S30–S38.

Höhn, C. 1991. "From one to two to one Germany," in J. L. Rallu and A. Blum, *European Population, I. Country analyses*, Paris: EAPS, IUSSP, INED, pp. 83–112.

———. 1996. "Fertility and family policy in Germany: Experiences from one to two to one Germany," manuscript, provided as a personal communication to authors.

Hongsheng, H. and G. Ling. 1997. "Sex preference and its effects on fertility in China," in *1992 National Fertility and Family Planning Survey, China*. Beijing: State Family Planning Commission.

Ilyina, I. 1994. "Marital status composition of the Soviet population," in W. Lutz et al. (eds.), *Demographic Trends and Patterns in the Soviet Union Before 1991*. London, New York, and Laxenburg: Routledge and IIASA.

Instituto Nacional de Estadistica. 1997. Unpublished data, personal communication, Madrid.

Ivanova, E. 1996. "Female nuptiality in Russia," *Population and Society*, No. 12, Centre for Demography and Human Ecology, Moscow.

Józan, P. 1997. Unpublished data, personal communication, Hungarian Central Statistical Office, Budapest.

Kamarás, F. 1994. *Reproductive Behavior in Hungary*. Hungarian Central Statistical Office.

———. 1995. "The impacts of the population-related policies on fertility in Hungary," *European Population Conference*, Milan, 4–8 September.

———. 1996. "Birth rates and fertility in Hungary," in P. P. Tóth, and E. Valkovics (eds.), *Demography of Contemporary Hungarian Society*. Highland Lakes, NJ: Atlantic Research and Publications.

———. 1997. "Birth control practice in Hungary," Hungarian Central Statistical Office.

Kerr, G. H. 1945. "Formosa: Island frontier," *Far Eastern Survey* 14(7): 80–85.

Kim, T. I., J. A. Ross, and G. C. Worth. 1972. *The Korean National Family Planning Program: Population Control and Fertility Decline*. New York: Population Council.

Kirk, D. 1946. *Europe's Population in the Interwar Years*. League of Nations, Princeton University Press.

Klinger, A. 1984. *The Impact of Policy Measures, Other Than Family Planning Programmes, on Fertility*. Budapest: Demographic Research Institute.

Lee, H. T. and N. H. Cho. 1992. "Consequences of fertility decline: Social, economic and cultural implications in Korea," in *Impact of Fertility Decline on Population Policies and Programme Strategies*. Seoul: Korea Institute for Health and Social Affairs.

Lesthaeghe, R. and P. Willems. 1999. "Is low fertility a temporary phenomenon in the European Union?" *Population and Development Review* 25(2): 211–218.

Lyle, K. C. and J. S. Aird. 1982. "China," in *International Encyclopedia of Population*. New York: Free Press,.

Mauldin, W. P. and J. A. Ross. 1989. "Historical perspectives on the introduction of contraceptive technology," in S. J. Segal, A. O. Tsui, and S. M. Rogers (eds.), *Demographic and Programmatic Consequences of Contraceptive Innovations*. New York: Plenum Press,

McLaren, A. 1990. *A History of Contraception: From Antiquity to the Present Day*. Oxford: Basil Blackwell.

Monnier, A. 1998. "The demographic situation of Europe and the developed countries overseas: An annual report," *Population: An English Selection* 10(2): 447–473.

Mundigo, A. I. 1992. "The determinants of impact and utilization of fertility research on public policy: China and Mexico," in J. F. Phillips and J. A. Ross (eds.), *Family Planning Programmes and Fertility*. Oxford: Clarendon Press.

Muramatsu, M. 1973. "An analysis of factors in fertility control in Japan—An updated and revised version," *Bulletin of the Institute of Public Health* 22(4): 228–236.

Norris, D. 1998. Unpublished data, personal communication, Statistics Canada, Ottawa.

Ogawa, N. and R. D. Retherford. 1993. "The resumption of fertility decline in Japan: 1973–92," *Population and Development Review* 19(4): 703–741.

Park, C. B 1992. "Family building in the Republic of Korea: Recent trends," in *Impact of Fertility Decline on Population Policies and Programme Strategies*. Seoul: Korea Institute for Health and Social Affairs.

———. 1995. "Transition of family formation in South Korea: Cohort perspectives," unpublished manuscript.

Pavlík, Z. 1964. *An Outline of the World Population Development* (in Czech). Prague: Czechoslovak Academy of Sciences.

Peterson, P. G. 1999. *Gray Dawn: How the Coming Age Wave Will Transform America—and the World*. New York: Times Books.

Popov, A. 1994. "Family planning and induced abortion in the post Soviet Russia of the early 1990s: The unmet needs in information supply," Centre for Demography and Human Ecology, Moscow, Working Papers, Vol. 16, August.

Popov, A. et al. 1993. "Contraceptive knowledge, attitudes, and practice in Russia during the 1980s," *Studies in Family Planning* 24(4): 227–235.

Quo, S. K. 1950. "The population growth of Formosa," *Human Biology* 22(4): 293–301.

Rahman, A., L. Katzive, and S. K. Henshaw. 1998. "A global review of laws on induced abortion, 1985–1997," *International Family Planning Perspectives* 24(2): 56–64.

Romaniuc, A. 1984. *Fertility in Canada: From Baby-Boom to Baby-Bust*. Ottawa: Statistics Canada.

Ross, J. A. and K. S. Koh. 1975. "Transition to the small family: A comparison of 1964–1973 time trends in Korea and Taiwan," in Y. Chang and P. J. Donaldson (eds.), *Population Change in the Pacific Region*. Vancouver: The Thirteenth Pacific Science Congress.

Russian Centre for Public Opinion Research (VCIOM), Centers for Disease Control and Prevention (CDC), and United States Agency for International Development (USAID).

1997. *1996 Russia Women's Reproductive Health Survey: A Study of Three Cities. Preliminary Report,* January.

Rychtaříková, J. 1996. "Current changes of the reproduction character in the Czech Republic and the international situation," *Demografie* (Czech) 38(2): 72–89.

———. 1998. Unpublished data, personal communication, Charles University, Prague.

Song, K. Y and S. H. Han. 1974. *1973 National Family Planning and Fertility Survey: A Comprehensive Report.* Seoul: Korean Institute for Family Planning.

Srb, V. 1967. *Demographic Handbook.* Svoboda, Prague.

State Committee of the Russian Federation on Statistics (Goskomstat). 1996. *The Demographic Yearbook of Russia.* Moscow.

Statistics Canada, Canadian Centre for Health Information:

Selected Birth and Fertility Statistics, Canada. 1993. *1921–1990.* Pub. March.

Selected Marriage Statistics. 1992. *1921–1990.* Pub. Sept.

Statistics Canada, General Social Survey, 10th round, 1995, special tabulations for contraception data.

Statistics Canada, Health Statistics Division:

Therapeutic Abortions, 1994. 1996. Pub. Sept.

Selected Therapeutic Abortion Statistics, 1970–1991. 1994. Pub. Nov.

Births and Deaths, 1995. 1997. Pub. May.

Marriages, 1995. 1996. Pub. Dec.

Stloukal, L. 1995. "Demographic aspects of abortion in Eastern Europe: A study with special reference to the Czech Republic and Slovakia," Ph.D. thesis, Australian National University, Canberra.

———. 1997. "Abortion," in Z. Pavlík and M. Kucera (eds.), *Population Development in the Czech Republic 1996,* Department of Demography and Geodemography, Charles University, Prague, pp. 35–41.

Taeuber, I. 1944. "Colonial demography: Formosa," *Population Index* 10(3): 147–157.

———. 1946. "The population potential of postwar Korea," *The Far Eastern Quarterly.* New York: Columbia University, May.

———. 1958. *The Population of Japan.* Princeton, NJ: Princeton University Press.

Taeuber, I. B. and G. W. Barclay. 1950. "Korea and the Koreans in the northeast Asia region," *Population Index* 16(4): 278–297.

Terao, Takuma. 1959. *Outline of Birth Control Movement.* Tokyo.

Thornton, A. and H. S. Lin (eds.). 1994. *Social Change and the Family in Taiwan.* Chicago, IL: University of Chicago Press.

Tietze, Christopher. 1983. *Induced Abortion: A World Review, 1983.* New York: Population Council.

Tietze, Christopher and John Bongaarts. 1976. "The demographic effect of induced abortion," *Obstetrical and Gynecological Survey* 31(10): 699–709.

United Nations. 1954. *Foetal, Infant and Early Childhood Mortality: The Statistics.* ST/SOA/SER.A/13, New York.

———. 1996. *Levels and Trends in Contraceptive Use As Assessed in 1994.* New York.

———. 1999. "Fertility trends among low-fertility countries," *Population Bulletin of the United Nations* Nos. 40/41: 35–125.

United Nations Development Programme. 1996. *Human Development Report 1995: Russian Federation.* New York.

United Nations Population Division. 1992. *Patterns of Fertility in Low-Fertility Settings.* New York.

United Nations Population Fund. 1998. *Population and Reproductive Health in the Russian Federation: Needs Assessment Mission, 12–30 May 1997.* New York.

Van de Kaa, D. 1987. "Europe's second demographic transition," *Population Bulletin* 42(1). Washington, DC: Population Reference Bureau.

Weinstein, M. et al. 1990. "Household composition, extended kinship, and reproduction in Taiwan: 1965–1985," *Population Studies* 44(2): 217–239.

Westoff, C. F. and N. B. Ryder. 1977. *The Contraceptive Revolution*. Princeton, NJ: Princeton University Press.

Zakharov, S. V. 1994. "Changes in spatial variation of demographic indicators in Russia," in W. Lutz et al. (eds.), *Demographic Trends and Patterns in the Soviet Union Before 1991*. London, New York, and Laxenburg: Routledge and IIASA.

———. 1999. "Fertility trends in Russia and the European newly independent states: Crisis or turning point?" in *Population Bulletin of the United Nations* Nos. 40/41: 292–317.

Comment: A March Toward Population Recession

JEAN-CLAUDE CHESNAIS

AT THE DAWN of the twenty-first century, demographers face a phenomenon until recently unanticipated either by insiders (experts in charge of national population policies) or by outsiders (population forecasters affiliated with international bodies like Eurostat, the United Nations, and the World Bank). When the secular fertility decline begins, the trend is commonly rapid, deep, and nonreversible. Contrary to expectations derived from demographic transition theory, the fertility curve does not converge to a level around replacement; nobody knows the lower limit, except of course the theoretical limit of zero. Present population trends (persistent mortality decline, sustained below-replacement fertility, thus extreme aging of the population) are confounding. Among the fathers of demographic transition theory, only one, Adolphe Landry (1934), envisaged a scenario of "permanent disequilibrium."

The post-transitional stage as a new regime of permanent disequilibrium

There are strong arguments in favor of the eventual globalization of the birth deficit. Let us select four:

—In the mid-1990s, according to the stocktaking illustrated in the chapter by Tomas Frejka and John Ross, some 44 percent of the world's population lived in countries having fertility at or below replacement. The corresponding share of the total world population living in such countries by the year 2000—if we include countries with a total fertility rate between 2.1 and 2.5—is approximately 50 percent. What was previously a marginal behavior is becoming predominant and potentially universal.

—The phenomenon of depressed fertility is not new. It was a prevailing feature of twentieth-century populations of Europe. If we take into account early mortality (deaths before childbearing ages), we find that the completed fertility of nearly all European birth cohorts in the twentieth century was below the level required for them to replace themselves. In the past, this shortfall resulted from the combination of high premature mortality and relatively low fertility; now, it is the reflection of very low fertility. In any case, the net reproduction rate of birth cohorts was generally below 1.0 throughout the twentieth century.

—The long-term downward trend seems irreversible. To date, there has been no sign of lasting and spontaneous reversal, even in the cases where the lowest thresholds (total fertility rates of 1.2 children per woman or less) have been reached or crossed. Fertility can remain at much below replacement levels; there is no proof that this is a provisional stage or temporary phenomenon related to, for example, economic cycles or timing effects. As a consequence, we have to revise the textbooks on the theory of demographic transition.

—The long-term effect of the post–World War II baby boom is much milder than usually presented in the current literature. In Europe, the baby boom was a short and limited parenthesis both in space (it occurred only in Western countries) and in time (its duration was two decades or less). Even in France, where the baby boom was more pronounced than elsewhere in Europe, its impact on the age structure has already been offset by the opposite trend, the baby bust: the median age of the population was 35 years in 1946; by 1998 it was 37 years.

Mapping the global fertility transition

At the beginning of the 1960s, the world demographic landscape seemed to be stable, unchanged since World War II; the average total period fertility rate (TPFR) in the more developed countries was 2.7 while in the less developed countries it was 6.0; the gap between the two sets of countries was wide and clearcut. In all industrialized countries, the total period fertility rate was below 4 children per woman, whereas in the third world it was peaking at a very high level, most commonly above an average of 5 or 6 children per woman. The contrast between the Northern and Southern Hemispheres was sharp. Only a few Southern Hemisphere countries, all of European descent (Australia, New Zealand, Argentina, Uruguay), had moderately high fertility, with values of the TPFR from 2.5 to 4; the large majority of countries from Latin America, Africa, and Asia maintained traditional—that is, very high—fertility levels, thus exhibiting a seemingly high degree of homogeneity. At the other extreme, the low-fertility zone—where women on average had fewer than 2.5 children—was limited to Japan and parts of Central, Eastern, and Northern Europe.

By 1990–95, some three decades later, a massive shift had occurred. The change has been worldwide; the low-fertility countries (using the same definition of TFRs below 2.5) included Russia, all of Europe, Northern

America, Australia, New Zealand, Japan, China, Thailand, and Brazil. In Latin America as well as in East and South Asia, fertility has fallen to low or intermediate levels. Only two regions remain with high fertility (above 5.5): sub-Saharan Africa and the Middle East. But even in these two cases, the countries that were formerly characterized by very high fertility (above 6.5) have become a minority mainly limited to Yemen, the Sahel zone, and politically unstable zones of Africa.

A sweeping change thus happened in a relatively short time; fertility decline became global, reaching all continents. But the meaning of "low" fertility became radically new, with unprecedentedly small family sizes characterizing whole countries. From year to year, in countries that are labeled traditional or poor, fertility continues to slump. In a growing number of countries, what was considered unlikely or impossible 10–15 years ago is becoming real: not only are fertility levels below replacement, but under present standards the actual number of children represents only half the number of parents. Thus, a huge potential for population decline will appear in the next decades, with the progressive reversal of the age pyramid; if fertility stabilizes at the present level, the annual rate of population *decrease* could reach 1.5 percent. This picture is common in much of Europe, except in the North.

Given the difficulty of predicting the onset and speed of secular fertility decline, demographers have to be modest; all explanatory frameworks can be shaky when confronted with empirical data. However, what we can reliably do is to try to establish a list of common mechanisms at work in different settings.

In search of common denominators

The first and probably by far the strongest factor behind the fertility decline is the progressive disappearance of mortality at young ages. If couples want to reproduce themselves, they do not need to have large families as in past centuries. The conventional mortality profile by age was a U shape, with high risks at the two extremes of human existence: among children and among the elderly. In traditional societies, half of newborn children could die before adulthood; this left branch of mortality at young ages has virtually disappeared, except in a few impoverished societies. Thus, while the left branch of the curve is falling, the right branch tends to shift outward to older and older ages. Extreme longevity may tend to create a new psychological context that confers a feeling of eternity (people forget they are mortal); this mentality dampens the desire for self-replication and as a consequence exerts a downward pressure on birth rates.

Many other intertwined factors can play a crucial role in the globalization of fertility decline: the clustering or concentration of people; the progress of female literacy; increasing social tolerance of new sexual and family norms, consumerism, and the preference for immediate gratification; the acceleration of social atomization; and finally the diffusion of modern family planning techniques.

Let us consider these various points.

The real meaning of urbanization, especially in big cities, is a radical change of civilization; it is foremost a deruralization, an uprooting, and the end of enclaves; it is also the adoption of new mentalities, strongly constrained by time, money, and space. Paradoxically, world population growth is moving toward increasing concentration of inhabitants with an abandonment of whole territories: hamlets, villages, and small towns have become depopulated. Most people live in human concentrations, strongly interconnected by a host of networks (infrastructure, radio, television, phone, fax, Internet); fashions and innovations can spread faster than at any time in the past.

Aggregate evidence shows a strong correlation between female literacy and the stage of demographic transition. Educational attainment has a deep impact on the main demographic choices, such as marriage (age at union, choice of spouse), fertility (timing and number of children), family arrangement and management (hygiene, health care, food intake and distribution, education of children, role of girls and women, extra-domestic activities, cohabitation with older generations).

Tolerance of formerly atypical and exceptional norms tends to grow among highly urbanized and educated young generations. In Japan, for example, where marriage was nearly universal, female celibacy and thus childlessness are becoming widespread; singlehood has become a socially accepted lifestyle. Similarly, there is a convergence between male and female education (classes are mixed) and even of clothing and hairstyle. The impact of this new unisex style is, of course, not measurable but we can presume that it has a negative influence on the view of sex differentiation and correlatively on marriage and fertility.

The consumer-goods society, strongly supported by advertising, tends to produce a marked preference for the present or the short-term future. In such a context, individuals hesitate to make long-term and irreversible commitments such as to family-building and childbearing. Individual independence and personal freedom become key values: enjoying life *hic et nunc* is the basic rule of consumerism.

Another feature of present structural change is the continuation of the process of individualization or social atomization. Marriages and consensual unions are centered on new objectives that are more egocentric: the pursuit of personal happiness and self-fulfillment are at the top of the agenda. As the functional and external differentiation between males and females diminishes, the preference for sons—at least in Westernized societies—is progressively vanishing. So, the perception of population "replacement" has changed: a couple replaces itself through the birth of a single child.

The last several decades have witnessed an impressive change in the efficiency of birth control techniques: the pill, IUD, safe and legal abortion and sterilization, and many other modern methods have radically transformed the lives of couples; the number and spacing of children, once accepted largely as matters of chance, are now a matter of free choice.

Conclusion

All of the above-mentioned factors contributing to exceptionally low fertility can lead to new types of societies where there is no more self-regulation. If fertility drops much below replacement levels, there is no spontaneous force to reverse the trend. If the present fertility decline persists, the ultimate world population size will not be 10 to 12 billion as was commonly assumed until the beginning of the 1990s. It might be only 8 billion and, after reaching that peak, it could stabilize and then decrease. Another consequence of the combination of longevity and low fertility is a sudden reversal of the age pyramid: excessively aging populations may well become one of the major challenges of the twenty-first century.

If we consider countries with "high" fertility (i.e., with a total fertility rate of at least 5 children per woman), we find that their cumulated population in 2001 has fallen to one-tenth of the total world population. In other words, it has become purely residual. Such a fact tends to reinforce the idea of massive and universal change, leading to a new paradigm dominating the twenty-first century. After the population explosion of the twentieth century, mankind could progressively experience population implosion.

Reference

Landry, Adolphe. 1934. *La révolution démographique: études et essais sur les problèmes de la population*. Paris: Librairie du Recueil Sirey.

Fertility and Reproductive Preferences in Post-Transitional Societies

JOHN BONGAARTS

THE TIMING OF the onset of contemporary fertility transitions and the pace of change during their early phases have been central concerns of researchers and policymakers in recent decades. Demographers and social scientists have studied survey data with detailed information about reproductive behaviors and attitudes of individuals in many countries. This research has provided new insights into the determinants of reproductive behavior and has contributed to the development of increasingly refined and realistic theories of fertility change. Policymakers and program managers in the developing world have been concerned about the contribution of high fertility to rapid population growth and poor reproductive health, and they have focused on implementing effective programs—in practice, mostly family planning programs—to reduce high and unwanted fertility.

Until recently, less attention had been given to determinants and consequences of fertility in post-transitional societies. Conventional demographic theories have little to say about the level at which fertility will stabilize at the end of the transition. However, it is usually assumed that population growth in the long run will be near zero, which implies that fertility will on average be close to the replacement level of about 2.1 births per woman (Demeny 1997; Caldwell 1982; Freedman and Berelson 1974). This assumption is, for example, incorporated in past population projections of the United Nations and the World Bank (medium variants). If fertility in contemporary post-transitional societies had indeed leveled off at or near the replacement level, there would have been limited interest in the subject because this would have been expected. However, fertility has dropped below the replacement level—sometimes by a substantial margin—in virtually every population that has moved through the demographic transition. If future fertility remains at these low levels, populations will decline in size and will age rapidly. These demographic developments in turn are likely to have significant societal consequences (Coale 1986). Concern about these effects has led to a recent surge in scientific, programmatic, and popular interest in this topic.

This chapter examines the relationship between reproductive preferences and observed fertility. Conventional fertility theories have focused on explaining how social and economic development and changing ideas and values determine the desired number of children (see van de Kaa 1998 for a discussion of the determinants of post-transitional preferences). These theories often assume implicitly or explicitly that couples are able to implement their preferences without much difficulty and that observed fertility is not very different from average desired family size. A declining desired family size is indeed one of the principal forces driving fertility transitions, but in reality levels of fertility often deviate substantially from stated preferences.

Examples of such deviation are found in most contemporary developed countries, where desired family size is typically two children while fertility is well below replacement. This divergence between actual fertility and desired family size is a new and unexamined phenomenon. It is of much more than theoretical interest because it raises the possibility that the low fertility observed in contemporary post-transitional societies is depressed because of temporary factors. If that is the case, fertility may be expected to rise to a level closer to the preferred level in the future, and concern over the undesirable demographic implications of prolonged very low fertility in post-transitional societies may be overstated.

In this chapter I examine the causes of this discrepancy between actual and preferred fertility and its implications for future fertility trends. After a brief overview of levels and trends in fertility and reproductive preferences at the end of the transition, I discuss the factors responsible for elevating or reducing fertility relative to desired family size. I conclude with an assessment of future prospects.

Trends in late-transitional fertility

In the developed world, fertility (as measured by the total fertility rate) reached its post–World War II maximum at 2.8 births per woman during the peak of the baby boom in the late 1950s. Steep declines in the 1960s and 1970s left fertility below replacement, reaching 1.7 births per woman in 1990–95. These broad trends have been observed in Europe, North America, and Australia/New Zealand (see Figure 1). In Japan fertility had already reached the replacement level in the late 1950s and it has declined further over the past quarter-century. In the late 1950s regional fertility levels ranged from a high of 3.7 births per woman in North America to a low of 2.1 in Japan, but they converged by 1980 to approximately 1.8 births

FIGURE 1 Trends in total fertility rates in selected populations in the industrialized world, 1950–95

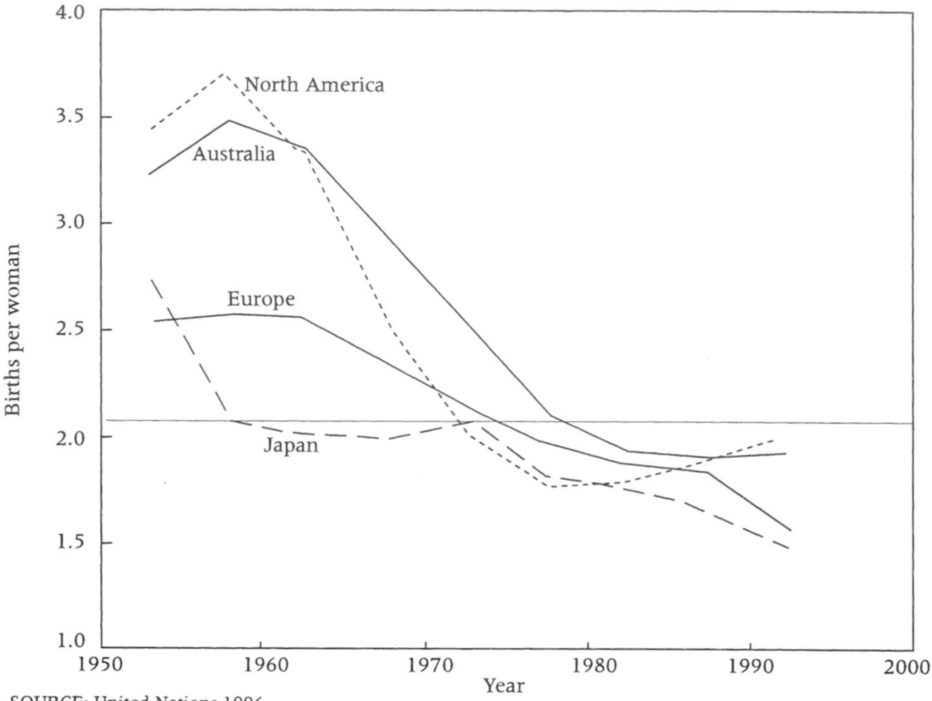

SOURCE: United Nations 1996.

per woman. Since 1980 fertility levels have diverged again, with North America's fertility rising to 2.0 births per woman while Japan and Europe have continued to drop further to about 1.5 births per woman. In the early 1990s fertility was below replacement in nearly all of the 46 countries in the developed world; the only exceptions were New Zealand (2.12), Moldova (2.15), Iceland (2.19), and Albania (2.85) (United Nations 1996).[1]

Variations in fertility among countries within regions can be substantial. For example, within Europe fertility was lowest in the south and east, where sharp declines have occurred since 1975. Italy and Spain, with total fertility rates of 1.24 and 1.27 births per woman, respectively, were competing for the world's record lowest level of fertility. In contrast, fertility in Northern Europe (averaging 1.8 births per woman) was higher than elsewhere in the continent and it has changed relatively little over the past two decades. In a few countries fertility has actually risen since 1975, most notably in Sweden (from 1.65 to 2.01 births per woman).

Below-replacement fertility is now the norm in the developed world, but it is also observed in a small but growing number of populations elsewhere, in particular in those Southeast Asian countries where economic

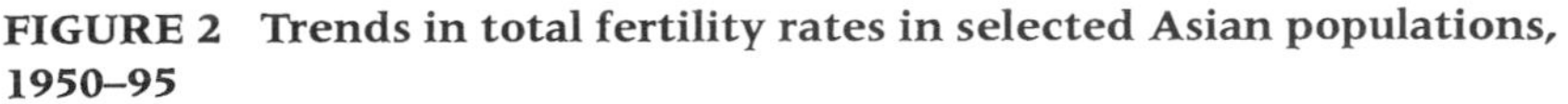

FIGURE 2 Trends in total fertility rates in selected Asian populations, 1950–95

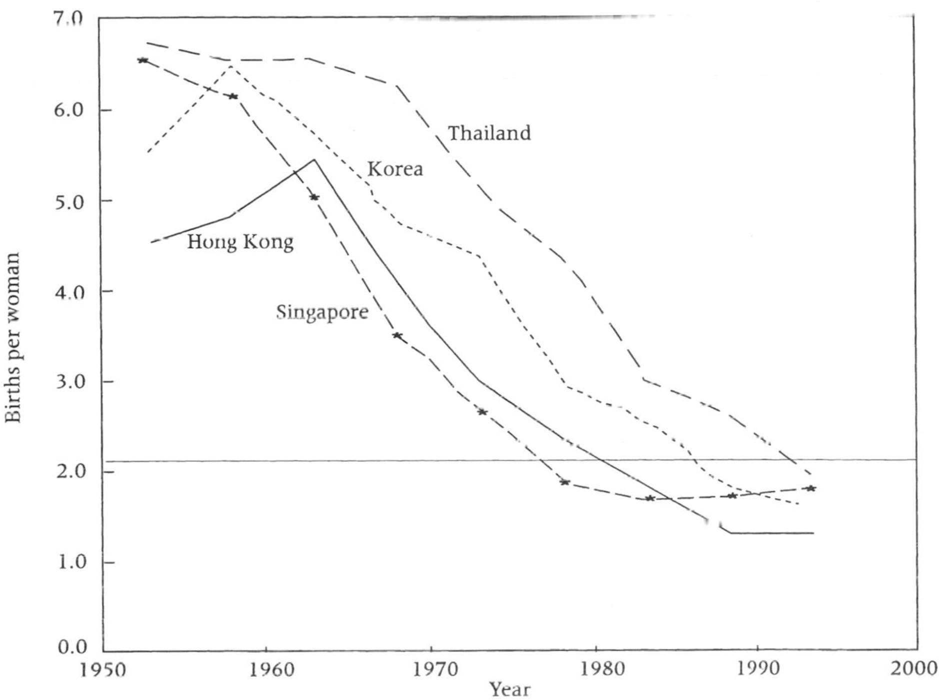

SOURCE: United Nations 1996.

development has been extremely rapid in recent decades. Steep declines since 1960 have left fertility in 1990–95 at 1.94 in Thailand, 1.79 in Singapore, 1.65 in Korea, and 1.32 in Hong Kong (see Figure 2). Outside Asia, fertility was below replacement only in the Bahamas, Barbados, and Cuba, but this list is expected to grow in the future according to the 1996 revision of the UN population projections (United Nations 1996).

Diverging trends in fertility and reproductive preferences

According to a 1989 survey in 12 European countries, average desired family size was 2.16 children per family (Lutz 1996; Eurobarometer 1991).[2] Individual countries clustered tightly around this average: Ireland (2.79) and Greece (2.42) had the highest preferences, and Germany (1.97) and Spain (1.94) the lowest (see Figure 3). Surprisingly, in every country the expressed preferences substantially exceed the observed rate of childbearing as measured by the total fertility rate (TFR). Average fertility in 1989 in the European Union

FIGURE 3 Observed fertility and desired family size for selected countries, ca. 1990

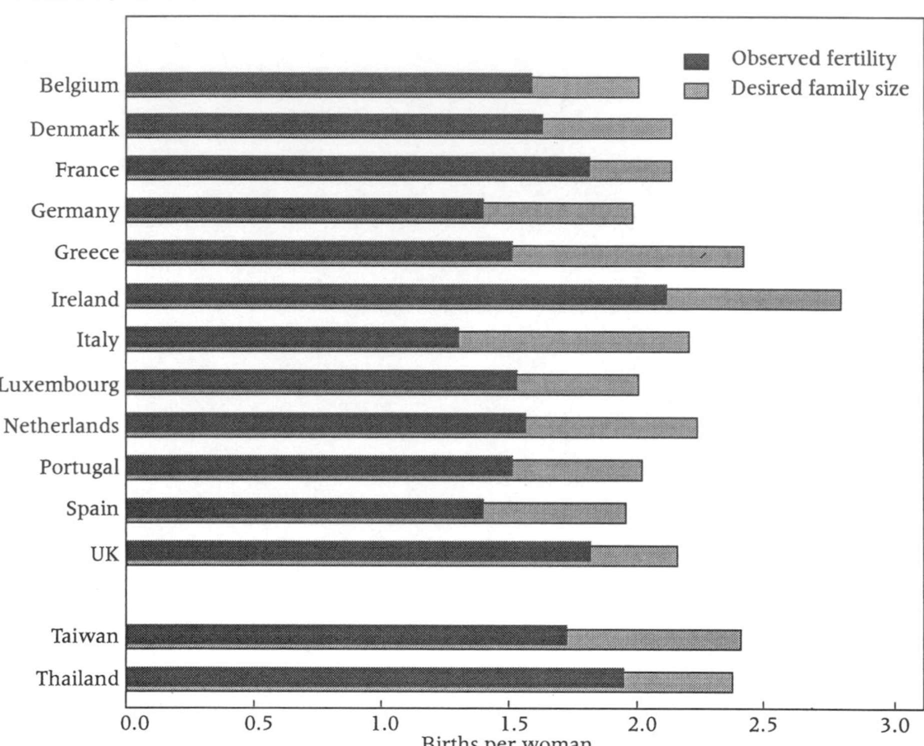

SOURCES: Coleman 1996; Knodel et al. 1996.

was 1.6 births per woman, fully 0.6 births below the average desired family size of 2.2. Similar differences between desired family size and TFR are observed in contemporary developing countries at the end of their fertility transitions; Figure 3 also includes recent estimates for Taiwan and Thailand.

These differences are notable because they are the opposite of what is typically found in the earlier phases of fertility transition, when observed fertility almost always exceeds preferences. The changes in these variables over time are clearly evident in the few countries, such as Thailand, where estimates of desired family size and the total fertility rate are available from a series of surveys covering most of the transition period (see Figure 4). In the late 1960s Thailand's fertility still stood at 6.1 births per woman, while desired family size was just 3.9 children. Since 1970 fertility has declined much more rapidly than preferences, and by the early 1990s the desired family size of 2.4 children exceeded the TFR of 1.9 by 0.5 births per woman. Over this 25-year period observed fertility dropped by 4.2 births per woman, which is more than twice the decline of 1.5 in desired family size over the same period. A broadly similar pattern is observed in Taiwan (Freedman et al. 1994).

FIGURE 4 Total fertility rate and desired family size, Thailand 1968–93

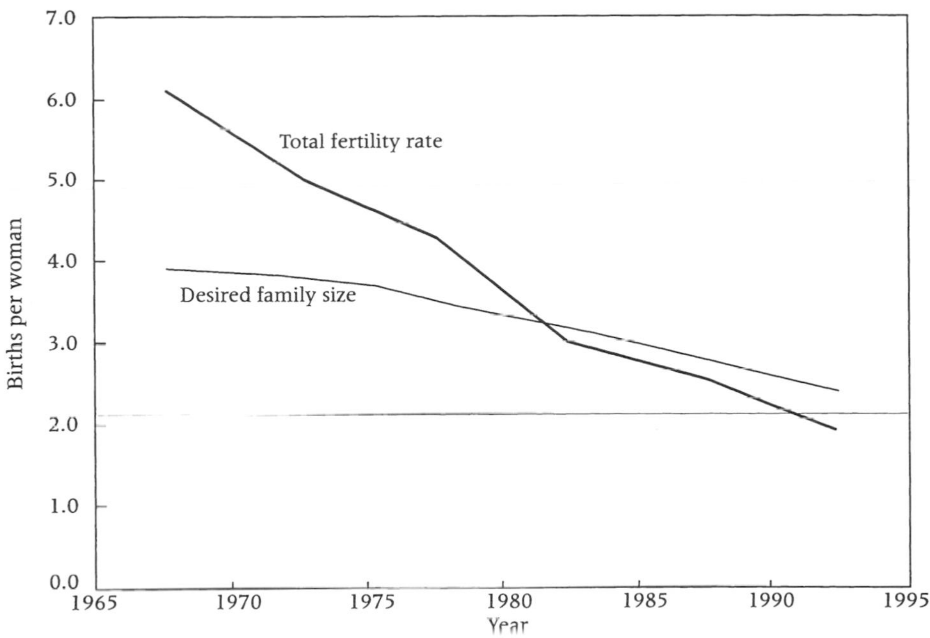

SOURCES: United Nations 1996; Knodel et al. 1996.

FIGURE 5 Relationship between total fertility rate and desired family size for 42 developing and 12 developed countries

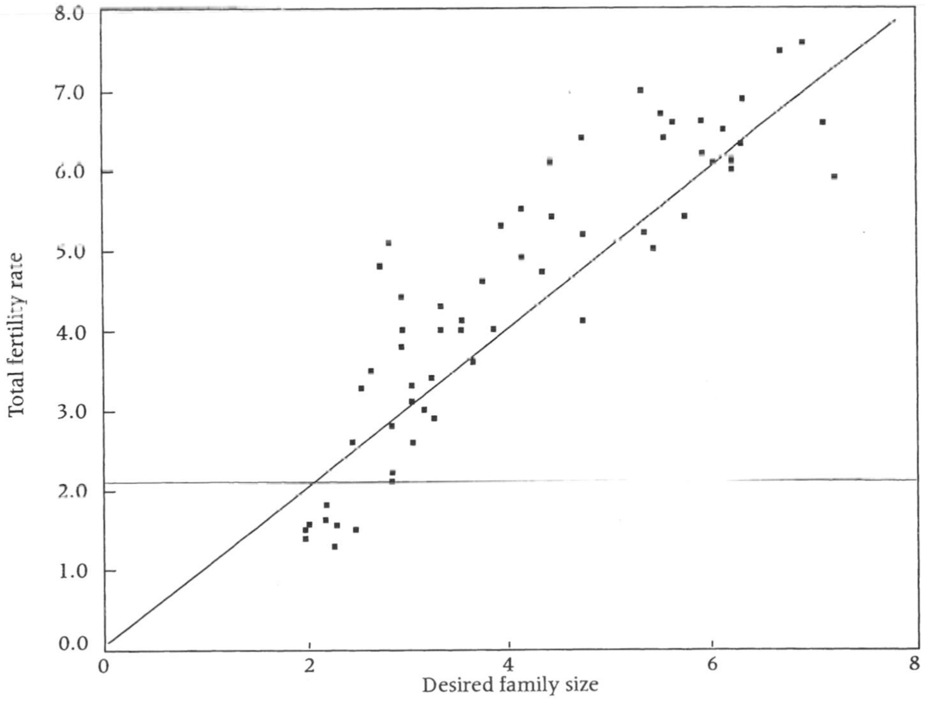

SOURCES: Coleman 1996; Westoff 1991; Westoff et al. 1987.

The trends over time observed in Thailand and Taiwan are consistent with cross-sectional evidence obtained from recent surveys in 42 developing and 12 developed countries (see Figure 5). In most countries in the early or middle stages of their transitions, the observed level of fertility exceeded desired family size, and in a few instances this excess reached as high as 2 births per woman. The reverse is true in countries at the end of the transition, where observed fertility was in every case lower than desired.

To explain these unexpected differences between actual and desired fertility, I now turn to a more detailed analysis of the demographic and behavioral processes that either enhance or depress fertility relative to desired family size.

Factors enhancing fertility relative to desired family size

The evidence reviewed in the preceding section demonstrated that during the early and midtransitional stages, observed fertility levels of populations typically exceed stated desired family sizes. Three distinct factors—unwanted fertility, child replacement, and sex preferences—can be identified as being responsible for this finding. (Measurement error no doubt can also be a significant factor, but it will not be discussed in detail.)

Unwanted fertility

In all countries where this subject has been examined, a significant proportion of women report bearing more children than they want. Detailed empirical evidence for unwanted childbearing in recent decades is available for a large number of developing countries from fertility surveys such as the DHS and WFS (Westoff 1991; Bankole and Westoff 1995). A recent analysis of levels and trends in unwanted childbearing in 20 developing countries estimated that on average 22 percent of fertility was unwanted around 1990 (Bongaarts 1997). The level of unwanted childbearing was found to vary systematically over the course of the fertility transition. In the most traditional pretransitional societies, preferences and fertility are often both high so that unwanted childbearing is relatively uncommon. However, with the onset of the fertility transition, unwanted fertility typically rises substantially. This rise is explained by a decline in desired family size, which leads to an increase in the proportion of women who are at risk of having more births than they wish. Resort to the practice of contraception and induced abortion is typically insufficiently rapid to avoid a rise in unwanted childbearing. Reasons for nonuse of contraception include lack of access to contraceptive services, fear of side effects, and opposition of husband or others. This incomplete control over the reproductive process leads to relatively high levels of unwanted fertility, usually exceeding one birth per woman on average in midtransitional societies. Finally, in the last part of the transition unwanted fertility declines again as couples are increasingly able to implement their preferences by practicing contraception effectively and/or by resorting to induced abortion.

Unfortunately, estimates of unwanted fertility are not readily available for developed countries, except the United States. A 1995 US survey found that 10.1 percent of births in the early 1990s were unwanted, down slightly from 12 percent in 1988 (Abma et al. 1997). Comparable estimates are not available for European countries, but Westoff et al. (1987) used an indirect procedure to estimate unwanted childbearing levels in six European countries circa 1981. The unwanted proportion of fertility ranged from 11.2 percent in France to 7.5 percent in the Netherlands. As in the United States, these proportions are presumably declining slowly over time as women are increasingly able to implement their reproductive preferences.

Unwanted childbearing is the main reason why observed fertility exceeds desired family size in many developing countries. This conclusion is based on a comparison of the wanted component of the TFR (WTFR) (i.e., the TFR from which unwanted births have been excluded) with the desired family size for 45 countries in Figure 6. This comparison shows that the wanted TFR is almost invariably somewhat below the desired family size, which is the reverse of the pattern observed in Figure 5. This finding implies that the unwanted component of the TFR was responsible for most of the excess of the TFR over desired family size in Figure 5. In the few developed countries where observed fertility was already below desired family size, the removal of unwanted births leads to a modestly larger discrepancy between observed and desired fertility.

The decline in unwanted fertility toward the end of the fertility transition explains in part why fertility drops more rapidly than the desired family size late in the transition. For example, in Thailand estimates from the 1975 WFS and the 1987 DHS are as follows (Westoff 1991):

	1975	1987
TFR	4.3	2.2
Wanted TFR	3.2	1.8
Unwanted TFR	1.1	0.4
Desired family size	3.7	2.8

Between 1975 and 1987 the unwanted TFR declined by more than half, from 1.1 to 0.4 births per woman. As a result the decline in the wanted TFR (from 3.2 to 1.8) is much less steep than for the TFR (from 4.3 to 2.2).

Clearly, a significant part of the excess of observed over preferred fertility found in midtransitional societies is attributable to substantial levels of unwanted childbearing. Under certain conditions two other factors,

FIGURE 6 Relationship between wanted total fertility rate and desired family size for 42 developing and 3 developed countries

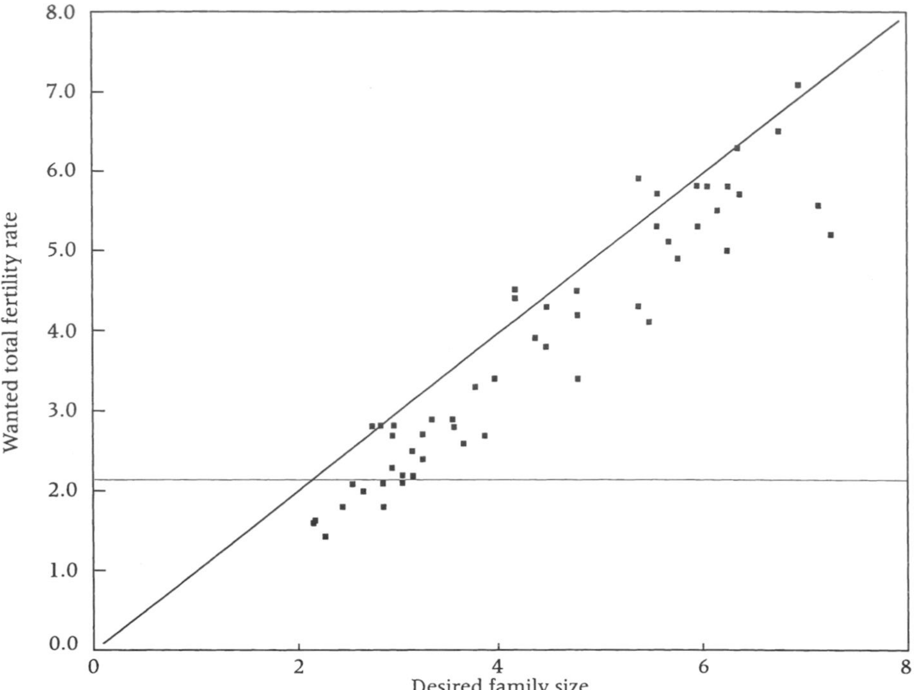

SOURCES: Coleman 1996; Westoff 1991; Westoff et al. 1987.

child mortality and compositional preferences, also play a role in elevating fertility. These are discussed next.

Replacement of deceased children

Despite the best efforts of many analysts, the impact of trends in child mortality on reproductive behavior remains incompletely understood (Montgomery and Cohen 1998).

Considerable effort has been devoted to identifying and measuring the specific societal and behavioral mechanisms through which mortality potentially affects fertility (Preston 1978; Lloyd and Ivanov 1988; Montgomery and Cohen 1998), but empirical support for several of these proposed mechanisms remains weak. There are two cases where the evidence is clear: the "lactation-interruption" effect (the death of an infant interrupts the anovulatory interval following a birth, so that the mother is exposed sooner to the risk of pregnancy than would have been the case had the child survived) and the "replacement" effect (parents replace children who have died in order to achieve their desired family size, which is expressed in surviving children). The lactation-interruption effect is largest in traditional societies with long durations of breastfeeding or postpartum abstinence and with limited use of contraception. The replacement effect is strongest in populations where the deliberate control of fertility is extensive, and it is therefore of greater interest than the lactation-interruption effect for present purposes. Although deliberate replacement is more prevalent in the later stages of the fertility transition, it is never complete and most studies find that only up to about half of dead children are replaced (Lloyd and Ivanov 1988).

When replacement occurs it increases the number of births a couple has without changing the desired family size, and it is therefore one of the reasons why the former might exceed the latter. While there is no doubt that replacement takes place in many families that experience the death of a child, it has only a small impact on fertility in late-transitional societies because few children die. In contemporary developed countries infant mortality averages 9 deaths per 1000 births (i.e., less than 1 percent). In such cases even complete replacement would raise fertility by only about 0.02 births per woman, which is small enough not to be of practical significance at the population level.

Sex preferences

When stating a preference for a family of a particular size, a couple may have a specific sex composition in mind (e.g., two sons or at least one son and one daughter). In such cases parents may continue to have births after they have reached their desired number of children if their preferred sex composition has not been achieved. The existence of sex preferences therefore leads to higher fertility than would be the case in their absence, except in societies where parents do not control their fertility.

Questions on the desired number of sons and daughters are not always included in surveys such as the DHS and WFS. However, evidence for sex preferences can be inferred from the effects of the sex composition of a woman's current family on the desire to continue childbearing. For example, Figure 7 plots the average proportion who want another child among women with two children, comparing women with two sons, women with a son and a daughter, and women with two daughters in different world regions.[3] Several conclusions can be drawn from this evidence. First, the desire for more births among women with two children varies widely among regions. It is highest in sub-Saharan Africa, intermediate in Asia and the Middle East, and lowest in Latin America. As expected, these differences are explained by regional differences in desired family size (Bankole and Westoff 1995). Second, son preference (as mea-

FIGURE 7 Desire for more children among women with 2 children, by region and family composition

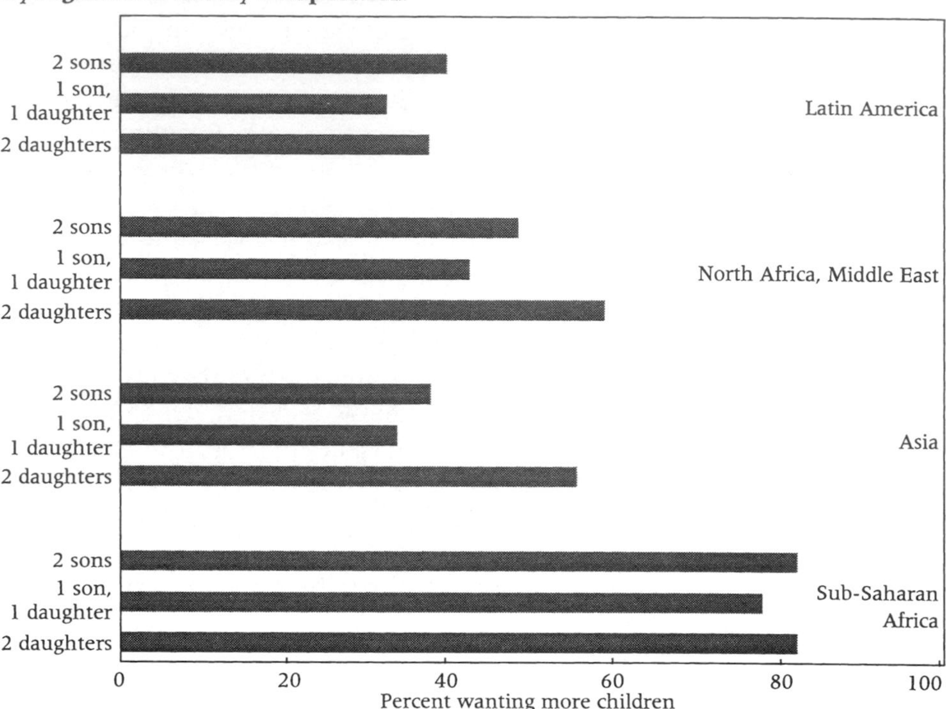

SOURCE: Arnold 1997.

sured by the ratio of the proportion wanting more births among women with two daughters to the proportion wanting more among women with two sons, 2D/2S) is highest in Asia and the Middle East and essentially nonexistent in sub-Saharan Africa and Latin America. In fact, in Latin America there is a slight tendency to prefer girls over boys. Among individual countries, son preference is highest in India, with a 2D/2S ratio of 2.6, and ratios exceeding 1.5 were found in Bangladesh, Nepal, and Turkey (Arnold 1997). Daughter preference is highest in Colombia and Trinidad and Tobago. Third, the U-shaped patterns observed in Figure 7 are evidence of a desire for balance in the number of boys and girls. This implies that even in the absence of son or daughter preference, women would rather have a family with at least one child of each sex than a family that consists solely of sons or daughters. As a result, among women with two children those with one son and one daughter are most likely to stop childbearing.

The fertility effect of these sex preferences in a particular society is not easily estimated because it depends on the structure of parental preferences for the sex composition and size of their families, on the way parents reconcile conflicting preferences for sex composition and size, on the degree to which these preferences are implemented by the effective use of birth control, and, in a few countries, on the extent of reliance on sex-selective abortion. In general, the fertility effect is small or nonexistent in countries with high fertility and low levels of contraceptive use. The impact rises over the course of the fertility transition as parents become increasingly effective in achieving their reproductive goals. A few recent studies provide quantitative estimates of the degree to which fertility is inflated because of son preferences: 8 percent in Bangladesh (Chowdhury and Bairagi 1990), 8.4 percent in India (Mutharayappa et al. 1997), and 13.5 percent in Korea (Park and Cho 1995). Estimates for states of India range from 4.5 percent in Uttar Pradesh (a state with a low level of contraceptive prevalence) to 24.6 percent in Himachal Pradesh (with one of the highest prevalence levels). These effects are large enough to have significant demographic consequences in post-transitional societies.

Factors reducing fertility relative to desired family size

As populations progress through the last stages of the transition, observed fertility typically moves from a level above desired family size to a level below it. Part of the explanation for this trend is the attenuation of the aforementioned three factors that inflate fertility during the early phases of the transition. In addition, three other factors—rising age at childbearing, involuntary infertility, and competing preferences—depress fertility relative to desired family size.

Rising age at childbearing

The total fertility rate is by far the most widely used indicator of aggregate period fertility and is therefore used throughout this chapter to measure levels and trends in the fertility of populations. Despite the apparent simplicity and wide availability of this indicator, it is a complex measure that is subject to misinterpretation. The main problem is that the fertility level observed in a given year or period is affected by ongoing changes in the timing of childbearing (Ryder 1959, 1980). The best-known example of this often unappreciated effect is the baby boom in the 1950s in the United States, which was partly attributable to a decline in women's mean age at childbearing following World War II. As successive cohorts started bearing children at younger ages, their births overlapped in the same time periods, thus boosting observed period fertility. The opposite effect is less familiar but of special interest for present purposes: increases in the age at childbearing deflate the TFR because births to successive cohorts are spread over a longer time period. The latter distortion has dominated in recent decades, since the age at onset of childbearing has risen in many late-transitional countries worldwide since the 1970s (Council of Europe 1996; Singh and Samara 1996). For example, as shown in Figure 8, sharp increases in the mean age at first birth have occurred in several countries of Europe and in the United States. Similar increases are observed for the mean ages at births of higher order. These trends imply that recent fertility (as measured by the TFR) in these countries has been lower than it would have been without this "tempo" effect.[4]

Although demographers have long been aware of the distortions caused by changes in the timing of childbearing, there is no agreed-upon methodology for removing tempo effects from observed total fertility rates. Ryder, who has written extensively on this subject, has proposed "translation" equations to calculate the period fertility measures from corresponding cohort measures when the timing of cohort fertility is changing (Ryder 1956, 1964, 1983). These procedures have not found wide acceptance for two main reasons. First, in his work on the translation issue Ryder assumes that the tempo and quantum of cohort fertility are the determinants of the TFR and other period fertility measures. However, extensive empirical analysis of this issue has demonstrated that this is not the case (Brass 1974; Page 1977; Foster 1990; Pullum 1980; Ní Bhrolcháin 1992). For example, Brass

FIGURE 8 Trend in mean age at first birth in selected populations, 1970–95

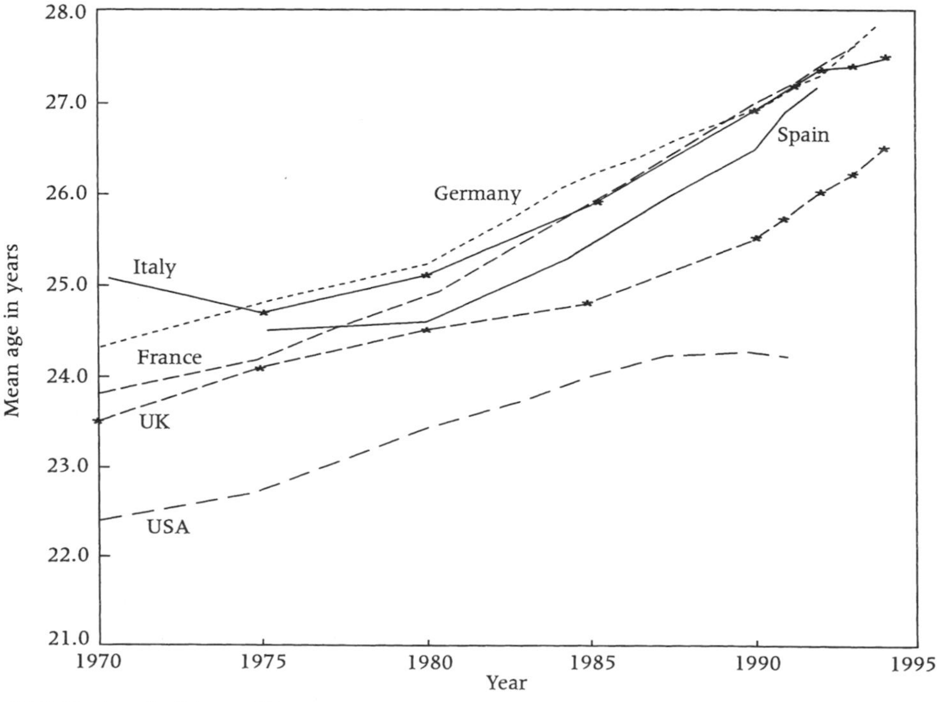

SOURCE: Council of Europe 1996.

(1974) concluded that cohort completed fertility revealed no significant feature that distinguishes it from time averages of period indexes. A review of this literature by Ní Bhrolcháin (1992) reached a similar conclusion. Second, the two dimensions of aggregate cohort fertility—quantum and tempo—are in practice not independent. When cohorts reduce their fertility they do so primarily by reducing childbearing at higher birth orders. As a result, the mean age at childbearing for all births to the cohort declines even if the timing of individual births does not change. In other words, a decline in the cohort quantum leads to changes in the cohort's mean age at childbearing that do not represent true tempo effects. Ignoring this effect—as Ryder does in much of his writing—therefore gives biased results except when cohort fertility is constant. Fortunately, this second problem can be solved by analyzing fertility trends separately for each birth order rather than for overall fertility. This option was actually mentioned by Ryder (1959), but for some reason he largely ignored order specificity in subsequent work on the translation problem.

An alternative approach to removing potential distortions from the period total fertility rates is through the application of life table procedures. Whelpton (1954) first proposed the calculation of revised total fertility rates using a life table based on age-parity-specific birth rates. This early work provided the foundation for further research in recent decades on alternative ways to standardize fertility measures—for example, not only by age and parity but also by duration since last birth (Henry 1980; Feeney and Yu 1987; Feeney et al. 1989; Ní Bhrolcháin 1987; Rallu and Toulemon 1994). Unfortunately, these life table procedures do not directly address the distorting effects of changes in the timing of childbearing. Tempo changes influence the age-specific fertility rates as well as age-parity-specific and age-duration-specific birth rates. The results from the life tables are therefore not free of tempo effects.

In a recent study Bongaarts and Feeney (1998) propose a new procedure for removing tempo effects from the TFR. The approach is an outgrowth of Ryder's original translation equation. The above objections to Ryder's approach are removed by assuming that fertility is strictly period driven and that cohorts have no independent explanatory power, and by applying adjustments to the order components of the total fertility rate rather than to the total fertility rate itself. Under these conditions, it is possible to estimate the adjusted (i.e., tempo-free) total fertility rate in any given year (or period) from the conventional TFR at each birth order with the following equation:

$$\mathrm{TFR}'_i = \mathrm{TFR}_i/(1 - m_i)\,,$$

where

TFR_i= the observed total fertility rate component for birth order i
TFR'_i= the adjusted total fertility rate component for birth order i
m_i= the annual rate of change in mean age of age-specific fertility schedule, birth order i.

In other words, by dividing the observed total fertility rate by $(1 - m)$ at any given birth order, one obtains the total fertility rate that would have been observed had there been no change in the timing of childbearing.

Summing results for different birth orders gives the overall tempo-free total fertility rate:

$$TFR' = \sum TFR'_i$$

According to these equations, an annual increase of one-tenth of a year in the mean age at childbearing ($m_i = 0.1$) reduces TFR_i by 10 percent below its tempo-free level (because $TFR_i = TFR'_i(1 - 0.1)$). Similarly, an annual decline in the mean age at a rate of just 0.1 years per year ($m_i = -0.1$) inflates TFR_i by 10 percent. Clearly, modest changes in the timing of childbearing at any birth order can produce substantial changes in observed fertility.

Estimates of the tempo-free TFR′ for the period 1985–89 for selected populations were obtained with the above procedure; the results of this exercise are summarized in Table 1. In each of the seven countries included in this table, the elimination of the tempo effect raised fertility (TFR′ > TFR); this is as expected from the rising age at childbearing in these populations. The adjustment for the tempo effect ranged from more than 0.35 births per woman in the Netherlands, France, and Taiwan to a low of 0.08 in the US. This low estimate for the US is attributable to the fact that the mean age at first birth stopped rising at the end of the 1980s (see Figure 8). For the seven countries as a whole, removal of the tempo effect led to an increase from the average observed TFR of 1.78 births per woman to an ad-

TABLE 1 Total fertility rate with and without adjustment for tempo effect, 1985–89

	TFR	TFR′ (adjusted)	Tempo effect
France	1.81	2.21	0.40
Netherlands	1.54	1.90	0.36
Norway	1.78	2.05	0.27
Sweden	1.90	2.00	0.10
UK	1.80	1.92	0.12
US	1.90	1.98	0.08
Taiwan	1.74	2.14	0.40
Average	1.78	2.03	0.25

SOURCE: See text.

justed TFR′ of 2.03 births per woman, which is close to the replacement level. In France and Taiwan the adjusted TFR′ actually exceeded replacement. In this set of populations the fertility-inhibiting effect of the rising age at childbearing is primarily responsible for the fact that observed fertility is below replacement.

Involuntary infertility

An individual who wishes to have a certain number of children may be unable to achieve his or her reproductive objective because of a number of involuntary factors. Involuntary childlessness can be the result of:

(a) Inability to find a suitable partner. This has historically been a key cause of relatively high levels of childlessness in Europe, as well as in selected populations elsewhere (e.g., Philippines).

(b) Union disruption. A union may end in divorce or with the death of a partner before any children have been born.

(c) Physiological sterility. A small proportion of otherwise healthy couples is unable to conceive or have offspring because of biological abnormalities in either partner. This proportion is thought to be relatively invariant among populations and rises with the age of the female partner from about 3 percent in her early 20s to about 20 percent in the late 30s and near 100 percent by age 50 (Bongaarts and Potter 1983).

(d) Disease-induced sterility. Sexually transmitted diseases such as untreated gonorrhea can lead to sterility. As a consequence, substantial levels of involuntary childlessness are found in societies where the prevalence of sexually transmitted diseases is high (Gray 1983; WHO 1995).

Among individuals who have already had a child the intention to have additional children may be frustrated for most of the same reasons that lead to involuntary childlessness. Further childbearing can be prevented by a divorce or death that ends the partnership, or by the onset of physiological or disease-induced sterility. The precise extent of involuntary family limitation is difficult to measure because it is not readily separated from voluntary limitation of childbearing. In general, involuntary infertility is greatest in populations with late ages at first union, high proportions never entering unions, high rates of divorce or widowhood, large desired family sizes, and high levels of prevalence of sexually transmitted diseases.

Competing preferences

In most fertility surveys small proportions of women report that they do not want any more children even though they have not yet attained their desired family size (Bongaarts 1991). The reasons for this apparent inconsistency are not entirely clear. One explanation could be that reproductive preferences are not measured accurately in standard fertility surveys. A plausible alternative explanation is that women do report their desired family size fairly accurately, but that competing preferences (e.g., for a career, income, freedom from child care responsibilities) cause some women to want to stop childbearing before they have reached their desired number of offspring. In that case, stated desired or ideal family size overestimates the current demand for children.

Discussion: Future prospects

The future course of fertility in countries where it is already at or below replacement is one of the most controversial issues in contemporary demography. One group of analysts points to the indisputable fact that fertility has dropped below replacement in virtually all countries that have reached the end of the transition. This is the case in Europe and North America, where fertility has been below replacement since the mid-1970s, as well as in the most-developed countries in the South, such as Hong Kong, Korea, Singapore, Taiwan, and Thailand. In a few instances fertility has leveled off above replacement (e.g., Argentina and Chile), but these are exceptions. According to this school of thought, replacement fertility is a theoretical threshold that has little or no meaning for individual couples building their families, and below-replacement fertility is expected to be the norm in post-transitional societies (Demeny 1997).

A contrary view is held by analysts who believe that the current low levels of post-transitional fertility are a temporary phenomenon and that concerns about imminent population declines caused by low fertility are misplaced in some countries (Le Bras 1991; Knodel et al. 1996). This perspective is supported by data on desired family size, which has remained near or above two children in all societies for which measures are available. In this view, the observed below-replacement fertility is largely attributable to ongoing shifts in the timing of childbearing. Once this rise ends—as it eventually must—the corresponding fertility-depressing effect stops, thus bringing fertility back up, presumably to near replacement.

These competing views are both partly valid, but incomplete. The actual situation is more complex and a full assessment requires a separate examination of trends in desired family size as well as in each of the six factors linking fertility to desired family size.

Desired family size. Whether desired family size remains at or drops below two is the most crucial issue determining post-transitional fertility. Conventional fertility theories are essentially silent on this topic. The empirical record suggests resistance to declines in desired family size below two children (typically couples want one boy and one girl), and for the moment it appears reasonable to assume that desired family size will level off at about two. However, in view of the high cost of children and the trend toward consumerism and individualism, it would not be surprising if desired family size did fall further (Lutz 1996; van de Kaa 1987). The levels of desired family size that will prevail when societies complete their transitions will no doubt vary systematically among populations because of differences in socioeconomic and cultural factors as well as social policies.

Unwanted fertility. In the later phases of the transition the rate of unwanted childbearing typically declines as a consequence of greater reliance on effective birth control among couples who want to avoid pregnancy (Bongaarts 1997). This trend is likely to persist and it will be aided by the expected availability of new contraceptive technology. New methods will make contraceptive use more convenient and safer, which should increase use and reduce contraceptive failure. Reliance on induced abortion probably will also rise as more convenient medical abortifacients are made accessible in more countries. As a result, couples' ability to limit fertility to desired levels will almost certainly improve in coming years, and unwanted childbearing will become correspondingly rarer. Exceptions to this trend might be found in a few societies where objections to induced abortion lead to restricted access to this procedure.

Child mortality. In recent decades sharp reductions in infant and child mortality have occurred worldwide, and further declines are expected in the future especially in those developing countries where mortality is still relatively high. In post-transitional societies typically only 1 or 2 percent of newborns die before reaching adulthood, and replacement births are therefore rare and only a minor factor in influencing fertility.

Gender preference. Son preference is still common in parts of Asia and the Middle East, but it will presumably decline as societies develop and increasingly treat boys and girls more equally. However, substantial son preference is still found in post-transitional populations including Taiwan, Korea, and China. The fertility impact of son preference is being eroded by sex-selective abortion, a relatively new practice that is growing rapidly in some Asian countries. Sex-selective abortion reduces the sex ratio at birth and lowers fertility. A preference for balanced sex composition (e.g., one son and one daughter) can have a separate fertility-enhancing effect if couples continue to have additional births in order to achieve their desired balance after they have reached their desired family size.

Rising age at childbearing. The fertility-depressing effect of this factor is present only as long as the age at childbearing keeps rising. In principle, this could be the case for decades, but eventually it will stop and at that time fertility will rise as the depressing effect is removed.

Involuntary family limitation and competing preferences. As societies move into the post-transitional phase, age at onset of childbearing and the proportion never entering into a marital union typically rise, as does the divorce rate. These trends raise the probability that individuals will be unable to achieve their desired family size. Until the causes of competing preferences are better understood it is difficult to forecast future trends in this factor.

The multiplicity of factors influencing fertility in post-transitional societies and the difficulty of projecting future trends in each factor make it virtually impossible to draw firm conclusions. As noted, the trend in desired family size is the most critical determinant of future fertility. If desired family size drops below two then it is likely that fertility will do the same. Even in societies where desired fertility remains at about two children, fertility can remain below replacement for a prolonged period if the combined effects of the fertility-depressing factors outweigh the combined effects of the fertility-enhancing factors. There is, however, one fairly robust conclusion that can be drawn from the above analysis: the total fertility rate is likely to rise in the not too distant future in countries where the age at childbearing is now rising rapidly. Once this upward trend stops and the age at childbearing stabilizes, the fertility-inhibiting effect of this rise is removed. Fertility will then rise closer to the desired level. This trend has apparently been responsible in part for the rise in fertility in the late 1980s in the United States (Bongaarts and Feeney 1998) and in Sweden (Hoem 1990). A similar pattern might well occur in other post-transitional societies, where observed fertility is currently depressed by a timing effect. Where this happens, further declines in population size will become less likely and population aging will be less rapid than would be the case without this upward adjustment.

Notes

1 The replacement TFR depends on the level of mortality. It equals about 2.1 births in populations with low mortality but it can exceed 2.5 when mortality is high.

2 The Eurobarometer surveys asked the following question of men and women in 12 countries of the European Community: "In [your country] today what do you think is the ideal number of children for a family like yours or the one you might have?" Estimates based on this question are close to but slightly higher than those obtained for the number of children ultimately expected in recent Fertility and Family Surveys, and they are significantly lower than those obtained for the average number of children considered ideal by respondents in the World Values Surveys (van de Kaa 1998).

3 Estimates presented in Figure 7 are based on country-specific data from 44 DHS surveys (Arnold 1997). Regional averages are unweighted. Countries included are: Botswana, Burkina Faso, Burundi, Cameroon, Central African Republic, Ghana, Kenya, Liberia, Madagascar, Malawi, Mali, Namibia, Niger, Nigeria, Rwanda, Senegal, Sudan, Togo, Uganda, Zambia, Zimbabwe, Bangladesh, Egypt, India, Indonesia, Jordan, Morocco, Nepal, Pakistan, Philippines, Sri Lanka, Thailand, Tunisia, Turkey, Bolivia, Brazil, Colombia, Dominican Republic, Ecuador, Guatemala, Mexico, Paraguay, Peru, and Trinidad and Tobago.

4 Tempo effects are caused by changes in women's mean ages at births of specific orders. The mean age of the fertility sched-

ule of all orders combined is not a reliable indicator of tempo distortions, because reductions in family sizes also affect this mean. This issue is discussed in greater detail in Bongaarts and Feeney 1998.

References

Abma, J., A. Chandra, W. Mosher, and L. Peterson. 1997. *Fertility, Family Planning and Women's Health: New Data from the 1995 National Survey of Family Growth.* National Center for Health Statistics. *Vital Health Statistics* 23 (19).

Arnold, Fred. 1997. "Gender preferences for children: Findings from the Demographic and Health Surveys," in *Proceedings of the XXIII IUSSP General Population Conference, Beijing.* Liège: IUSSP.

Bankole, Akinrinola and Charles Westoff. 1995. "Childbearing attitudes and intentions," *DHS Comparative Studies* No. 17. Calverton, MD: Macro International Inc.

Bongaarts, John. 1991. "The KAP-gap and the unmet need for contraception," *Population and Development Review* 17(2): 293–313.

———. 1997. "Trends in unwanted childbearing in the developing world," *Studies in Family Planning* 28(4): 267–277.

Bongaarts, John and Griffith Feeney. 1998. "On the tempo and quantum of fertility," *Population and Development Review* 24(2): 271–291.

Bongaarts, John and Robert G. Potter. 1983. *Fertility, Biology, and Behavior.* New York: Academic Press.

Brass, W. 1974. "Perspectives in population prediction: Illustrated by the statistics of England and Wales," *Journal of the Royal Statistical Society A,* 137: 55–72.

Caldwell, John C. 1982. *Theory of Fertility Decline.* New York: Academic Press.

Chowdhury, Mridul K. and Radheshyam Bairagi. 1990. "Son preference and fertility in Bangladesh," *Population and Development Review* 16(4): 749–757.

Coale, Ansley J. 1986. "Demographic effects of below-replacement fertility and their social implications," *Population and Development Review* 12 (Supp): 203–216.

Coleman, David. 1996. "New patterns and trends in European fertility: International and sub-national comparisons," in D. Coleman (ed.), *Europe's Population in the 1990s.* Oxford: Oxford University Press.

Council of Europe. 1996. *Recent Demographic Developments in Europe.* Belgium: Council of Europe Publishing.

Demeny, Paul. 1997. "Replacement-level fertility: The implausible endpoint of the demographic transition," in G. W. Jones, R. M. Douglas, J. C. Caldwell, and R. M. D'Souza (eds.), *The Continuing Demographic Transition.* Oxford: Clarendon Press.

Eurobarometer. 1991. "Desire for children," *Eurobarometer 32.*

Feeney, Griffith, Feng Wang, Mingkun Zhou, and Baoyu Xiao. 1989. "Recent fertility dynamics in China: Results from the 1987 One Percent Population Survey," *Population and Development Review* 15(2): 297–322.

Feeney, Griffith and Jingyuan Yu. 1987. "Period parity progression measures of fertility in China," *Population Studies* 41: 77–102.

Foster, Andrew. 1990. "Cohort analysis and demographic translation: A comparative study of recent trends in age specific fertility rates from Europe and North America," *Population Studies* 44: 287–315.

Freedman, Ronald and Bernard Berelson. 1974. "The human population," *Scientific American* 251(3): 31–39.

Freedman, Ronald, Ming-Cheng Chang, and Te-Hsiung Sun. 1994. "Taiwan's transition from high fertility to below-replacement levels," *Studies in Family Planning* 25(6): 317–331.

Gray, Ronald. 1983. "The impact of health and nutrition on natural fertility," in R. A. Bulatao and R. D. Lee (eds.), *Determinants of Fertility in Developing Countries,* Vol. 2. New York: Academic Press.

Henry, L. 1980. "Fertility of marriages: A new method of measurement," *Population Studies Translation Series*, No. 3. United Nations. Originally published 1953.

Heuser, Robert L. 1976. "Fertility tables for birth cohorts by color," DHEW Publication No. (HRA) 76-1152. Rockville, MD: National Center for Health Statistics.

Hoem, Jan M. 1990. "Social policy and recent fertility change in Sweden," *Population and Development Review* 16(4): 735–748.

Knodel, John Vipan Prachuabmoh Ruffolo, Pakamas Ratanalangkarn, and Kua Wongboonsin. 1996. "Reproductive preferences and fertility trends in post-transition Thailand," *Studies in Family Planning* 27(6): 307–318.

Le Bras, Hervé. 1991. *Marianne et les lapins: l'obsession démographique*. Paris: Olivier Orban.

Lloyd, Cynthia B. and Serguey Ivanov. 1988. "The effects of improved child survival on family planning practice and fertility," *Studies in Family Planning* 19(3): 141–161.

Lutz, Wolfgang. 1996. "Future reproductive behavior in industrialized countries," in W. Lutz (ed.), *The Future Population of the World: What Can We Assume Today?* London: Earthscan Publications.

Montgomery, Mark and Barney Cohen (eds.). 1998. *From Death to Birth: Mortality Decline and Reproductive Change*. Washington, DC: National Academy Press

Mutharayappa, Rangamuthia, Minja Kim Choe, Fred Arnold, and T. K. Roy. 1997. "Son preference and its effect on fertility in India." *National Family Health Survey Subject Reports No.* 3. East-West Center, Program on Population, Honolulu.

Ní Bhrolcháin, Máire. 1987. "Period parity progression ratios and birth intervals in England and Wales, 1941–1971: A synthetic life table analysis," *Population Studies* 41(1): 103–125.

———. 1992. "Period paramount? A critique of the cohort approach to fertility," *Population and Development Review* 18(4): 599–629.

Page, H. J. 1977. "Patterns underlying fertility schedules: A decomposition by both age and marriage duration," *Population Studies* 30: 85–106.

Park, Chai Bin and Nam-Hoon Cho. 1995. "Consequences of son preference in a low-fertility society: Imbalance of the sex ratio at birth in Korea," *Population and Development Review* 21(1): 59–84.

Preston, Samuel H. 1978. "Introduction," in S. H. Preston (ed.), *The Effects of Infant and Child Mortality on Fertility*. New York: Academic Press.

Pullum, T. W. 1980. "Separating age, period and cohort effects in white US fertility, 1920–70," *Social Science Research* 9: 225–244.

Rallu, Jean-Louis and Laurent Toulemon. 1994. "Period fertility measures: The construction of different indices and their application to France, 1946–89," *Population: An English Selection* 6: 59–94.

Ryder, Norman B. 1956. "Problems of trend determination during a transition in fertility," *Milbank Memorial Fund Quarterly* 34(1).

———. 1959. "An appraisal of fertility trends in the United States," in *Thirty Years of Research in Human Fertility: Retrospect and Prospect*. New York: Milbank Memorial Fund, pp. 38–49.

———. 1964. "The process of demographic translation," *Demography* 1: 74–82.

———. 1980. "Components of temporal variations in American fertility," in R. W. Hiorns (ed.), *Demographic Patterns in Developed Societies*. London: Taylor & Francis.

———. 1983. "Cohort and period measures of changing fertility," in R. A. Bulatao and R. D. Lee (eds.), *Determinants of Fertility in Developing Countries*, Vol. 2. New York: Academic Press.

———. 1986. "Observations on the history of cohort fertility in the United States," *Population and Development Review* 12(4): 617–643.

Singh, Susheela and Renee Samara. 1996. "Early marriage among women in developing countries," *International Family Planning Perspectives* 22(4): 148–157, 175.

United Nations. 1996. *World Population Prospects: The 1996 Revision. Annex I: Demographic Indicators*. New York.

Van de Kaa, Dirk. 1987. "Europe's second demographic transition," *Population Bulletin* 42(1): 1–57.

———. 1998. "Postmodern fertility preferences: From changing value orientation to new behavior," Working Papers in Demography, No. 74. Canberra: The Australian National University, Research School of Social Sciences.

Westoff, Charles F. 1991. "Reproductive preferences: A comparative view," *DHS Comparative Studies* No. 3. Columbia, MD: Macro International and Institute for Resource Development.

Westoff, Charles, Charles Hammerslough, and Luis Paul. 1987. "The potential impact of improvements in contraception on fertility and abortion in Western countries," *European Journal of Population* 3: 7–32.

Whelpton, Pascal K. 1954. *Cohort Fertility: Native White Women in the United States*. Princeton, NJ: Princeton University Press. [Reissued in 1973 by Kennikat Press, Port Washington, NY.]

World Health Organization. 1995. "Task Force on the Prevention and Management of Infertility. Tubal infertility: Serologic relationship to past chlamydial and gonococcal infection," *Sexually Transmitted Diseases* 22(2): 71–77.

Comment: Desired Family Size and the Future Course of Fertility

Massimo Livi Bacci

The current low fertility in Europe and the even lower levels in European Mediterranean countries—particularly Iberia and Italy—raise many questions. Why is fertility so low? Is there a minimum level below which it cannot fall? Has this threshold been reached already? Is low fertility a structural, permanent phenomenon or is it a transient one, dominated by a particular conjunction of economic, social, and cultural circumstances? Will recovery be brought about by the action of the invisible hand? What is the role of public policies? Have European societies developed a kind of "reproductive anorexia" or are they facing a temporary loss of appetite?

First, a general point concerning terminology. Demography suffers from an inflation of "transitions" used as a synonym for "change." We have a couple of demographic transitions and several isolated transitions: fertility transition and marriage transition; mortality transition with the attendant epidemiological transition, which is not unrelated to the health transition; and the mobility transition and the migration transition. The transition club is generous and hospitable: abortion, contraception, and nutrition are its occasional—if not permanent—guests. Hence a modest proposal: let us give to the expression "demographic transition" (which can be shortened to "the transition") the status economic historians have assigned to the expression "industrial revolution." In other words, let us reserve it to refer to an interrelated set of profound changes that have occurred only once in any given population, responding to the same paradigm, not always clearly recognizable because of the peculiarities of each society, and occurring at different times and with different durations: between the industrial revolution and the third quarter of the twentieth century in the rich countries, and after the 1940s (ending nobody knows when) in the poor ones. There is only one "demographic transition" in world history, although there have been many phases of deep and interrelated change. The acceptance of this modest proposal—thus reverting to the teaching of the old school—would simplify communication since everybody would understand what we are talking about when mentioning the "transition" or its components (fertility, marriage, migration, etc.). Expressions like pretransitional or post-transitional fertility (or mortality, etc.) would immediately convey a precise meaning.

Desired family size and the total fertility rate

John Bongaarts's chapter in this volume, on which I comment here, starts from one firm tenet. Couples express a "demand" for children that can be measured. For various reasons the couples' targets cannot be precisely attained, so that the expected or desired family size (DFS) is different from actual family size (as measured by the TFR): lower when fertility is high (in pretransitional societies or during most of the transitional process), but higher when fertility is low (typically in the late transitional or post-transitional phases). The reasons for divergence between DFS and TFR, when the former is lower than the latter, have been the object of many studies and debates. In Bongaarts's analysis, unwanted fertility—or the insufficient command over reproduction by women and men—together with the drive to replace unexpected deaths of children and dissatisfaction over the sex balance achieved among one's children, are the causes of TFR exceeding DFS, typical of developing societies.

Less clear are the reasons for the specular divergence in post-transitional societies (DFS higher than TFR), since couples are thought to have complete command of fertility. In low-fertility populations two factors explain why DFS exceeds TFR: one is involuntary infertility (inability to find a partner; termination of a partnership before the birth of a child because of death, separation, divorce; physiological sterility). The second is a kind of "residual factor" (defined by Bongaarts as "other constraints"), conceptually much less clear. Some women report that they want no more children although they have not yet attained their desired family size: they may do so for various reasons, but clearly experience has taught them that their aspirations were higher than their actual willingness to have more children. Maybe the first child cries too much at night and has proved to be difficult to handle; maybe pregnancy has been awkward; maybe the respondent is in a depressed state; maybe she would have answered the question differently had not she quarreled with her partner the day before. The residual factor summarizes the difficulty—or the inability—of surveys to measure expectations which are intimately linked with aspirations and desires that change with time and circumstances. As Bongaarts himself observes, "A plausible alternative explanation is that women do report their desired family size fairly accurately, but that competing preferences (e.g., for a career, income, freedom from child care responsibilities) cause some women to stop childbearing before they have reached their desired number of offspring. In that case, stated desired or ideal family size overestimates the current demand for children." I will return to this point later. Finally, another factor that may depress or raise period TFR over its "true" value is the "tempo" of fertility (well summarized by the trend in women's ages at childbearing). When the tempo accelerates (age at childbearing declines), TFR is above its "true" level; when the tempo slows (age at childbearing increases as has been happening in Europe during the last two or three decades), TFR falls below its "true" level.

Estimates of "involuntary infertility" could probably be based on the proportion of women childless at age 35 or 40 and may be thought of as an (exponential?) function of the mean age at childbearing. Among women born in the mid-1960s in north and central Italy, mean age at birth of the first child is close to 28 years, and the final proportion childless is estimated at 20 percent or more. Women who delay the first birth beyond age 30 face a risk of infertility or subfecundity that at this point increases rapidly with age. This applies also to women who want a second (or third) child but who delayed too long the birth of their previous child.

Is DFS a good index of the demand for children?

Is desired family size a good index of the demand for children? If so, it is worthwhile to try to understand the discrepancy between the actual number of children women bear and their stated preferences. Probably, in the long run, DFS (or similar measures) reflects the changes in demand fairly well. However, there are doubts that DFS is a good indicator of demand when fertility is very low. Indeed the suspicion is that stated preferences are heavily influenced by stereotypes and particularly by the model of the two-child family (a boy and a girl). This stereotype is pervasive and many surveyed individuals are "prisoners" of it. This would explain the fact that DFS very rarely falls below 2; the relative uniformity of DFS among countries; and the lack of differentials between cohorts or between social groups (e.g., with different levels of education).

If we take EFS (expected family size) as measured in the 13 European Fertility and Family Surveys, the value across age groups (20–24, 25–29, 30–34) is the same in four countries, varies at most by 2 tenths of a point in seven countries, and by 3 tenths and 6 tenths of a point in the other two. In only one case out of 39 (Polish women aged 20–24 in 1991) did EFS fall below 2. In the Eurobarometer survey of 1989 (the one used by Bongaarts) DFS falls between 2 and 2.3 in eight cases out of 12, and is below 2 in only one case. Greater variation (between 2.2 and 3) can be found for IFS (ideal family size) in the 19 developed countries of the World Values Survey, but for 14 out of 19 countries IFS remains in the narrow range of 2.2–2.6. Similarly homogeneous are preferences of women with different degrees of education or holding materialist/postmaterialist values.

It is also true that differential fertility has fallen considerably in the last decades, but variation in fertility across populations and cohorts appears to be by far larger than variation in preferences. Relative homogeneity of preferences may, of course, reflect a true homogeneity of demand. But it may also signal the inadequacy of these indicators to measure demand correctly.

Preferences and cohort fertility

In Bongaarts's analysis both DFS and TFR are intended as period measures. Hence the attempt to remove the "tempo" effect, a crucial step in determining the discrepancy between the two measures in low-fertility contexts. But suppose we compare cohort preferences with cohort outcomes: the tempo issue disappears as it is "incorporated" in each woman's stated preference.

Figure 1 compares the expected family size (derived from the Fertility and Family Surveys) for ages 25–29 (these are cohorts born roughly between 1960 and 1970, since the surveys were taken between 1989 and 1996)

FIGURE 1 Expected family size among women aged 25–29 years surveyed between 1989 and 1996 compared with TFR among women born 1960–65

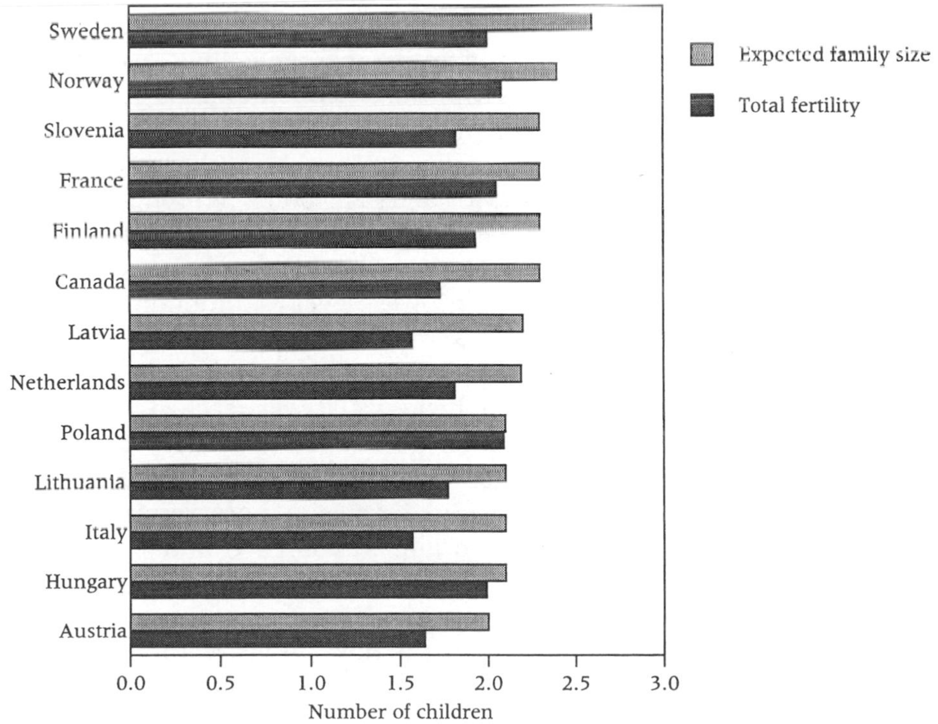

and estimated TFR of the cohort born in 1960–65. Admittedly, these are estimates and completed fertility may turn out to be different, so that the following considerations are subject to verification. Now, although the tempo effect is removed, EFS exceeds estimated TFR by an average of 0.44 points, or almost one-fourth of the mean TFR of 1.80 (similar results are reached using DFS and IFS instead of EFS). On the other hand, the correlation between the two measures is rather weak, thus raising doubts about whether expectations are a good approximation to the real demand for children. And expectations—much more than DFS or IFS—ought to get closer to cohort TFR in view of the experience that women have already accumulated.

Facing the future

Past experience as a guide

How low or high could fertility go (and remain) in the future—that is, a future not belonging to science fiction, but seen as a plausible extension of the present? Let us discard the answer "zero" as a possible minimum: true but a useless statement. In the north of Italy, cohorts born in the mid-1960s will end up with about 1.3 children, 3 tenths of a point below cohorts only ten years older; the decline has been precipitous and there is no theory to tell us when it will stop. However, another piece of evidence is interesting: in no sizable population has period TFR ever been lower than 0.8. In eastern Europe the stress of the transition from a socialist to a market economy has been traumatic and fertility has gone down everywhere. But nowhere has it gone below 1, with the exception of parts of Germany belonging to the former East Germany, where TFR fell to 0.8 in 1993–94. Now, in a year of stress (high unemployment, loss of security, etc.), women of all ages will change their behavior and "postpone" reproduction, and period TFR amplifies the negative effects. It is, however, implausible that the same stress will affect the entire life cycle of a cohort. So the very nature of period TFR justifies taking its lowest level as an empirical cohort minimum. This line of reasoning is symmetrical, and we could take the highest period TFR as an empirical maximum (in populations having completed their fertility transition). The highest TFR was reached, in western Europe, in the early 1960s, with values close to 3. But because in the early 1960s the "contraceptive revolution" had not been completed (in most countries contraception was illegal except for medical purposes; family planning programs were unheard of; abortion was still a criminal offense), a non-negligible proportion of births was unplanned. For this reason 2.5 can be taken as a possible "maximum" benchmark.

In the future of Europe—say for the next 30 years, the length of a generation—1.0 and 2.5 can be seen as minimum and maximum levels of "tempo-free" cohort fertility with widely diverging implications for long-term growth; probably these limits should be raised for North America. We have now witnessed more than 30 years of fertility decline, but the experience of the baby boom teaches that fertility can also go up. In ten countries where fertility showed an increase (Denmark, Sweden, Norway, England and Wales, Switzerland, France, Germany, Canada, United States, Australia) cohort TFR rose an average of 0.54 points.[1] The cohorts with minimum fertility were born, on average, in 1908 and those with the maximum in 1930. Since fertility control was not complete we may assume that the recovery of fertility was "dampened" by an increasing proportion of women who were reducing their "unwanted" births. Considering the central point (1.75) of the range (1.0 to 2.5), a variation between 1.4 and 2.1 would be consistent with the long-range fluctuations experienced in the past. Such variation could be expected for an array of countries, or a large region, while variation in individual countries could be even larger. The duration of the cycle—from high to low or vice versa—might approximate the intergenerational interval.

Substantive considerations

The preceding discussion addressed "mechanical" considerations concerning the potential amplitude of fertility cycles. But what about the forces that will drive fertility up or down? Fertility is the result of the interaction of biological, ideological, and material constraints and of thousands of years of evolution of our species. Humility when dealing with phenomena of this nature is the first imperative. I will mainly deal with the "material," or economic, aspects of the question, pointing to two main forces that affect the cost–benefit balance of procreation, the first quite general in nature, the second more specific.

Among the many factors that may be responsible for low fertility in Europe, one deserves greater attention than others: this is the "negative fertility drift" induced by current welfare systems. Children are doubtless a private good for the utility, satisfaction, and income that parents derive from them. But they are also a "public good": without them societies would stop functioning and, in a more narrow way, the services, income, and wealth that they produce are essential in providing health care, assistance, and pensions also to those who have chosen not to have children. In modern systems individuals may find it convenient (in purely economic terms) not to have children (or to have fewer children than the average). They will benefit from social protection in old age but will contribute only marginally to the cost of rearing children (mainly by paying for public education), who are also a public good. This inequitable system of transfers produces the "negative fertility drift." The negative drift is more pronounced in certain contexts than in others: if the give and take is calculated for the various age groups, Italians receive net transfers until age 17, and from age 59 on, while Americans receive net transfers until age 23 and from age 61 on.[2] Moreover, inequitable transfers have a much higher impact today than in the past. Indeed, in present-day Europe public expenditure amounts to about 50 percent of gross national product, and the way governments redistribute this 50 percent between generations greatly affects the relative cost of children. This was not so in the past: at the beginning of the twentieth century the proportion of GNP redistributed by the state was only 10 percent and around 1950 only 25 percent, and the potential effect on fertility of inequitable redistribution was much lower than today.[3] Correction of the distortions (where they exist) and attenuation of the negative fertility drift should be the main public policy task of governments in future decades.[4] These corrections imply a more equitable system of intergenerational transfers, and they imply that children be considered as public as well as private goods whose costs must be more equitably shared.

The second important force that may shape the course of future fertility is women's work. In the 1950s and 1960s women's employment in the nonprimary sector was lower than today, while the "mother and wife" lifetime role was widespread. Typically, gainfully employed women had fewer children than women outside the labor force. At the end of the twentieth century, even in societies that were latecomers to the benefits of development (Mediterranean Europe, for instance), women outside the labor force are a minority. Cultural as well as economic forces underlie this process. Societal adjustment has been more responsive to change in some societies than in others so that the burden of childrearing is probably lower in the north than in the south of Europe, where the transformation has taken place later. While 50 years ago childrearing competed with work, in the societies that are now being shaped employment may become a precondition for having children. Work provides the security, stability, and recognition needed when the decision to have a child is taken. "[I]n societies where fertility is below replacement,...higher status of women, and the policies necessary to bring about such a status, may in fact become preconditions for achieving and maintaining a level of fertility that is socially desired."[5] An empirical proof of the changing relation between fertility and work is the current positive association between employment rates and TFR in European countries (if the ex-socialist countries are excluded).[6] Higher employment rates are an indicator of the higher status of women that Chesnais indicates as a precondition for a socially desired level of fertility. This is a reversal of the inverse relation that prevailed decades ago. On the other hand, there is an inverse association (for the same countries) between the rates of women's unemployment and TFR. Unemployment is a powerful indicator of the lack of security, stability, and recognition that women in prosperous countries increasingly consider to be preconditions for having children. Many factors obscure this newly emerging relation, not least the fact that in many segments of society the traditional inverse relation between fertility and work survives because of delayed modernization.

The future course of fertility may be strongly affected by policies aimed at reversing the "negative fertility drift" of fiscal policies and by social and labor policies that will increase women's employment and security. These policies, we must add, work in tandem and may be integrated with one another.

Notes

1 Patrick Festy, *La fécondité des pays occidentaux de 1870 à 1970* (Paris: Presses universitaires de France, 1979).

2 For Italy, see Nicola Sartor, *Finanza pubblica e sviluppo demografico* (Torino: Fondazione Giovanni Agnelli, 1997). For the United States, personal communication from Ronald Lee.

3 Angus Maddison, *Monitoring the World Economy, 1820–1992* (Paris: Development Centre of the OECD, 1995).

4 Some comparative data on transfers to families and children in European countries can be found in Sheila B. Kamerman and Alfred J. Kahn, "Le politiche della famiglia nel secondo dopoguerra: la trasformazione degli impegni nazionali," *Polis* 12 (1998), no. 1; and J. Bradshaw, "La condivisione dei costi dei figli: i pacchetti di aiuti per i figli nei paesi dell'Unione Europea nel 1996," *Polis* 12 (1998), no. 1.

5 Jean Claude Chesnais, "Fertility, family, and social policy in Western Europe," *Population and Development Review* 22 (1996): 729–739; quotation from p. 738.

6 Massimo Livi Bacci, "The demographic transition: From where to where?" in *The African Population in the 21st Century: Third African Population Conference, Durban, South Africa, 6–10 December 1999* (Dakar: Union for African Population Studies, 1999).

Postmodern Fertility Preferences: From Changing Value Orientation to New Behavior

Dirk J. van de Kaa

"Aimez-vous Brahms?" The French novelist Françoise Sagan had the imagination to turn this simple question into the title of a book. Why would one ask of someone whether he or she liked Brahms? An obvious reason would be to see whether there could be a meeting of minds with that person. If someone likes a particular romantic composer, this admiration can probably be extended to a preference for romantic music more generally. It might even reveal a deep-seated romantic value orientation. The person could be imbued with a desire for adventure, might want to live dangerously, express emotions freely, and be greatly interested in the meaning of life. So, the answer to a single question may clarify whether one is dealing with a kindred spirit. It is, at any rate, reasonable to assume that the general cultural orientation of someone who likes Brahms may be different from that of someone who prefers the modern composer Erik Satie. Similarly, someone who prefers the "postmodern" composer John Cage to Satie and Brahms is likely to have yet another outlook on life.

In music, such terms as romantic and modern are well established. The term "postmodern" is also frequently used without raising eyebrows. The same is true for certain other fields of human endeavor such as literature, painting, and architecture. In the last of these, specific dates can even be attached to the shift from one approach to another, for example to modernism and postmodernism.

Even so, the use of the term postmodernism and of its various derivatives is not without problems. Bertens (1995), who analyzed the history of the idea of the postmodern, describes it as an "exasperating term" and elsewhere speaks of "a massive but also exhilarating confusion..." (p. 10). Since the late 1950s, he observes, the term "has been applied at different levels of conceptual abstraction to a wide range of objects and phenomena in what we used to call reality. Postmodernism, then, is several things at once." For example, depending on the artistic discipline, it is "either a radicalization of the self-reflexive moment in modernism, a turning away from narrative and representation, or an explicit return to narrative and representation. And sometimes it is both," writes Bertens (p. 5).

In several of the social sciences, and certainly in demography, the term postmodernism has not become part of the scientific discourse. People shy away from it, understandably find it difficult to deal with, or have the vague, intuitive notion that it is better to steer clear of such an ill-defined concept.

In this chapter I aim to explore without prejudice, and in an eclectic mode, whether the term postmodernism or one of its derivatives could usefully have a place in demographic studies and population analysis. My purview is Europe in the latter half of the twentieth century. My assumption is that, if the concept has a future in the scientific study of population, it will in all likelihood be in relation to the remarkable changes in demographic behavior observed in that region since the mid-1960s. The chapter will be speculative and frankly explorative.

Postmodernism: History and concepts

The term postmodernism has a long history. It seems to have been used as early as the 1870s. Bertens reports that the first book having the term in its title dates from 1926. At first it was used sparingly. It became more common in the 1950s and 1960s, while it suffused the 1980s and 1990s. At the same time its conceptual content changed. From a term coined to describe certain artistic strategies in poetry, and literature more generally, it has become an adjective denoting a specific approach to philosophy and a banner under which some seek to attack the ideological underpinnings of modern society.

Even though certain themes tend to recur in theorizing about the postmodern, there is no specific credo or articles of faith. Moreover, while postmodern thinking transcends the borders of disciplines and fields of human endeavor, its most pertinent theoretical propositions vary from area to area. Regarding scientific knowledge, Lyotard observed: "Scientific knowledge cannot know and make known that it is the true knowledge without resorting to the other, narrative, kind of knowledge, which from its point of view is no knowledge at all" (1984: 29). When directing his attention to society more generally, he wrote: "Simplifying to the extreme, I define postmodern as incredulity to metanarratives. This incredulity is undoubtedly a product of progress in the sciences..." (p. xxiv). Indeed, the rejection of grand narratives and theories is a recurrent element in postmodern thinking.

In Figure 1 I have attempted to present Bertens's stimulating historical analysis in a grossly simplified scheme, capable of clarifying the main conceptual dimensions of the term. It distinguishes three conceptual levels, as follows:

FIGURE 1 Conceptual dimensions of postmodernism

Level	Nature of the concept	Period of emergence	Main characteristics
1	Refers to anti-modernist artistic strategies	1950–60s	Questions the premises of modernism or seeks to undermine the idea of art itself
2	Denotes a certain cultural orientation	1960s	Refers to the radically democratic counterculture or "new sensibility" of the 1960s and rejects exclusivist liberal humanism
		1970s	Drawn into poststructuralist orbit, in two phases: a. deconstructionist approach, "language constitutes the world" (inspired by Derrida)
	Weltanschauung or *Zeitgeist*	1980s	b. "Knowledge is power" approach (inspired by Foucault), stresses hegemony of a single discursive system, importance of difference, pluralism, emancipation. Becomes a general cultural orientation, a spirit of the age.
3	Indicates a new historical era	1980–90s	Considers that around the mid-1960s, at least in Western societies, the era of postmodernity has begun

The purpose of this scheme is to argue that from a social sciences perspective, not all concepts and uses of the term postmodernism have the same relevance. While it may be valuable for demographers to know how strong the narrative element in their theories is (van de Kaa 1996), the use of postmodern in a sense that denies the representational function of language need not concern them. Similarly, while an awareness of the strategies in various disciplines in the arts seeking to overcome the constraints set by modernism in terms of representation, purity, autonomy, and intellectual content is relevant in social science research, the history of the precise usage of the term postmodernism in individual disciplines (dance, photography, architecture, history) is hardly pertinent. I would argue that postmodernism need only concern population scientists at two conceptual levels.

It is, first, pertinent to consider the possibility that our societies have experienced, or are experiencing, a major transformation that implies a shift from one historical period to the next. Such shifts have been recognized by historians for the past. One should expect them to continue to develop. In the sequence of historical periods the modern period would now seem to have come to an end. And since the term modern has already been usurped, the "youngest modernism," as von der Dunk has called it (1993: 66), could only be termed "postmodern."[1] There is much to be said for the idea that a new historical era, the era of postmodernity, has begun. Defining its precise nature is not so easy, however. There are furthermore, as we shall see, several counter arguments. The essential point is that postmodern theorizing per se plays virtually no role in considering this question. Central is the state of socioeconomic and cultural development in these societies. I am concerned simply with whether ideas and value orientations influenced by, and more or less clearly related to postmodern notions and thinking have, in a number of societies, diffused sufficiently widely to describe these societies as postmodern.

It is, second, valuable to consider whether the concept of postmodernity as indicative of a *Weltanschauung,* a way of looking at the world, can be helpful in explaining the remarkable value changes that have been documented for industrialized societies in the last few decades. Postmodernity would thus denote a value orientation that patterns and constrains behavior in a postmodern fashion. Used in this context, postmodernization would refer to a process of value change: the transformation from modern to postmodern value orientations. If it should prove possible to operationalize postmodernity as a general world view, as a specific value orientation (*Weltanschaung*), or as the spirit of an age (*Zeitgeist*), it could be an important instrument in explaining the sudden and spectacular demographic changes observed in nearly all European societies after the mid-1960s. It should again be noted that postmodern theorizing, as such, has only a limited role to play in considering this issue. The point is not whether people subscribe to some sort of postmodern credo, which in any case does not exist. The point is whether their outlook on the world has changed in such a way as to reflect postmodern concerns and notions.

An era of postmodernity?

Sketching the outlines of a period of postmodernity can, obviously, only succeed if it highlights the perceived contrasts with the modern era. The modern period is usually assumed to have begun at the end of the fifteenth century. It saw the demise of the feudal system, the development of nation-states and national economies, of capitalism, of the process of industrialization, of mass production, of mass education, and of certain countries building up worldwide empires. Urbanization became a general process. In the late modern period secularization began to change the belief system; liberal humanist and Marxist views dominated ideological positions. There existed a general belief in progress fueled by Enlightenment rationality in behavior and by the impact of scientific discoveries. In research and scholarship the search for the truth, for purity and timeless generalizations, was a central element. The necessity to achieve economic security through one's own efforts generated an "industrious" revolution. Nearly everyone participated in the labor force. The need to stimulate economic growth dominated thinking about the future. Some form of representational government became the standard for civilized societies. Ultimately, the state largely assumed the responsibilities for the social security of individuals traditionally vested in the family.

Those who argue that a new era has begun can marshal an impressive list of arguments. They may point out that the *metarécits*, the metanarratives, that legitimized and underpinned the modern period have lost their universality. The belief in progress, in the superiority of the white population, and in the value of the nation-state and its sovereignty have greatly diminished or disappeared. Christianity no longer is the religion uniting different peoples. Even the shortcomings of the traditional epistemological philosophy and of the search for "truths" have been amply demonstrated. Economic globalization has reduced the direct influence of governments on the welfare of their populations. The development of the welfare state freed individuals in large measure from the social control exercised by families and communities. Decolonization has led to a new economic order in the world. The superiority of Western civilization has ceased to be self-evident. The influx of migrants has made previously homogeneous societies multicultural. At the same time American and European mass culture is spreading over the globe. Consumerism is rife. A tremendous de-formalization has taken place. A great variety of images, life styles, and cultural symbols are produced by small groups and rapidly absorbed by others. The advent of the postindustrial information society has had a generation-specific impact: fragmentation, discontinuity, and incongruity are standard. The populations have become alienated from the political elites: yesterday's men are incapable of understanding the problems and desires of today's young women and men. Conflicts about ethical issues, the use of drugs, euthanasia, and abortion appear impossible to resolve now that the self-evident truth and value of certain moral positions have been questioned. Authority on such matters has evaporated. Culture can no longer serve to maintain the existing social order. In sum, the process of modernization so characteristic of the modern era has led to the era's inevitable demise. We have now entered a period without objective truths, in which people will continuously seek their identity in a self-reflexive way. They will give high priority to their well-being and self-expression, to instant gratification and play.

Equally, a range of criticisms can be leveled against the idea that a new era has begun. Let me mention a few. There is, first of all, no agreement on the date of its emergence. Some see it having emerged following the Enlightenment of the seventeenth and eighteenth centuries, others place it around 1875. Others again speak about the "last few decades," the 1980s and 1990s even. It seems to make much more sense, however, to date it about the mid-1960s and to associate it with the introduction of highly effective contraception and the sexual liberation that entailed; to relate it to the student revolts, the rapid expansion of social security systems, and the political changes of that time. It has also been argued that the modern period has by no means run its full course. Habermas's *Theorie des kommunikativen Handelns* (1985) does not stipulate, for example, that conflicts can only be resolved if all participants accept the existence and general validity of a specific set of societal values. Agreement on procedural issues would seem to be sufficient (van Reijen 1988). Bauman (1997: 3) sees postmodernity essentially as the "present version" of modernity. Others argue that one cannot possibly deny the existence of trans-cultural and amoral knowledge as a fact of life. Gellner, in particular, has made that argument. He abhors the cultural relativism to which postmodernistic philosophical thinking would seem to lead, and disagrees fundamentally with such an approach (Gellner 1992: 54). Moreover, if such trans-cultural knowledge did not exist, how could social order be maintained? The result would be a "de-moralization," a society in which people would no longer be responsible for their own actions. According to Himmelfarb (1995: 263) it could, alternatively, lead to a new sort of "moral correctness." Michon (1998), who recently assessed the relevance of postmodernism for the cognitive sciences, concludes that the gulf between the two cannot be bridged. In his view, the principles adhered to in postmodern thinking about science, and about the validity of its methods and findings, cannot possibly be shared by the cognitive sciences. It is, finally, evident that from a sociopolitical point of view the idea of a postmodern era is, if it has to encompass all postmodern strands of thought and theory, anathema to people on both the left and right of the political spectrum. While those of a liberal-humanist persuasion may well see diversity and pluralism within an otherwise capitalist society as quite acceptable and a logical extension of Enlightenment ideas, they do not accept postmodernist views on, for example, "the language game," self-reflexivity, or rationality.[2] Those on the left, most notably Marxists, reject the idea of a postmodern era that continues to be based on capitalist premises. They tend to accept the view that the autonomous, rationally acting human agent of liberal humanism is a fiction. And, while Bertens argued that the gulf between these different visions could easily be bridged if all were to see postmodernism as "the acknowledgement and acceptance of difference on the basis of an underlying sameness," we have not quite reached that situation (Bertens 1998: 38).

The idea that industrialized societies have witnessed numerous changes of great significance in the last few decades is quite generally accepted. However, support for the notion that a new, postmodern era has begun appears to decline with the precision and strictness with which the concept of postmodernity is formulated. If postmodernity is narrowly defined as relating to adherence to certain controversial (philosophical or socio-political) points of view, the conclusion that we live in a postmodern era is difficult to maintain. If it is broadly defined as accepting that we live in a world markedly different from that of modern times, a world that has seen a number of vague, postmodern notions about the role of the state, well-being, the linearity of societal progress, the need for solidarity, and the like diffuse to broad sections of the population, we do indeed live in the era of postmodernity. It is an era that, from a demographic perspective, offers great freedom to individuals and accepts diversity and unusual personal choices as a matter of course.

Postmodernity as a *Weltanschauung*

Perhaps the most essential tenet of postmodernism is that its key dynamic is cultural. The process of modernization, so the argument goes, has resulted in people being exposed to mass media, to a variety of cultural expressions, including those of a popular nature, and to many different types of behavior. This has made them understand the limitations of their own cultural traditions. It has made them reject formerly self-evident truths about religion, the social order, the rights and obligations of individuals, sexual behavior, gender roles, and so on. Through mass education, modernization has created a fertile ground for the development of groups and individuals whose views on society differ radically from those that long prevailed. They are intent on expressing them forcefully. And, at the cost of ever more insecurity, society has offered them ever more individual freedom (Bauman 1997: 124). Their postmodernistic outlook on the world questions the fundamentals of the meaning-giving system of modern societies (rational decisionmaking, work, stability in relationships, seeking progress). It is strongly influenced by philosophers such as Rorty and Lyotard, who insist that the role of language and discourse in these matters should be reconsidered. Consequently they share what Bertens (1995: 11) has described as "a deeply felt loss of faith in our ability to represent the real, in the widest sense. No matter whether...aesthetic, epistemological, moral, or political in nature...." Gibbins and Reimer, who wrote an interesting chapter on the topic, state the following (1995: 309): "The postmodern self is constructed in environments mediated by the mass media. But this postmodern self is an unfinished project: an identity is a role and a performance in the making, and public and private life are restless searches for self-knowledge and self-production for public consumption and recognition. Being incomplete, the self is restless, thus the postmodernist's search for identity is relentless." And elsewhere (p. 310): "Whereas modernists are committed to status and class segments, to means–end rationality and teleology, postmodernists are committed to the logic of the now and the immediate. At the heart of this distinction lies the belief that the modern self is being replaced by a more inner-directed postmodern self."

There is every reason to accept the idea that such a postmodern view of society and the self exists. In that sense, postmodernity can obviously be taken to represent a certain *Weltanschauung*. But how widely is that view held? I would, again, suggest that the more precise and strict the formulation of the concept is, the smaller the group of adherents will prove to be. If being postmodern means being demonstrably influenced by postmodernist thinking about people, about society and its meta-narratives, and giving high priority to well-being and cultural diversity, it is possibly such a widely held cultural orientation that for some countries it can be characterized as reflecting the *Zeitgeist*. After all, cultural orientations may shift without people being able to pinpoint the source of their new inspiration. If, alternatively, the requirement formulated is that postmodernists have to demonstrate a clear awareness and conscious acceptance of some of the more significant theoretical or philosophical principles of postmodernity, there would in any country only be a small minority of them. It would then be difficult to describe it as a *Weltanschauung* on its way to becoming a new, dominant world view.

Postmodernism and postmaterialism

An obvious point that will now have to be dealt with is the relationship between the concept of postmodernity and that of postmaterialism. the same or different? The latter concept owes much of its acceptance and use in the social sciences—and some would say also its notoriety—to the work of Inglehart. In a series of influential studies (1971, 1977, 1997) he has argued that as modernization progresses, the emphasis on survival and economic achievement as the top priority will give way to an emphasis on the quality of life. In his words: "the disciplined, self-denying, and achievement-oriented norms of industrial society are giving way to an increasingly broad latitude for individual choice of lifestyles and individual self-expression" (1997: 28). He characterizes that shift as one from "materialist" values (economic and physical security) to one of "postmaterialist" values (individual self-expression and quality of life). Materialist and postmaterialist orientations are measured with a survey instrument that may have 12 items. However, basically it asks respondents to make a choice of their first and second priority from among four items, formulated as follows (Inglehart 1997: 355):

1. Maintaining order in the nation
2. Giving people more say in important government decisions
3. Fighting rising prices
4. Protecting freedom of speech.

Respondents selecting 1 and 3 as their priorities are classified as materialists, those giving priority to 2 and 4 as postmaterialists. The prediction then formulated is that intergenerational value change in a postmaterialist direction will take place as standards of living increase and younger cohorts age. The theoretical underpinning rests on two key hypotheses, which Inglehart has formulated thus:

> 1. *A Scarcity Hypothesis.* An individual's priorities reflect the socioeconomic environment: one places the greatest subjective value on those things that are in relatively short supply.
>
> 2. *A Socialization Hypothesis.* The relationship between socioeconomic environment and value priorities is not one of immediate adjustment: a substantial time lag is involved because, to a large extent, one's basic values reflect the conditions that prevailed during one's preadult years. (1997: 33)

Evidently both postmodernism and postmaterialism are concerned with value change following, or emanating from, the process of modernization. What is the relation between these two approaches? What do they have in common? Where, if at all, do they differ? Should the theories, to use that term in a loose sense, be seen as being in competition with one another? Are they complementary? They certainly have in common that they seek to explain value changes as they occurred, by and large, in industrialized countries during the last few decades. They both see the well-known processes of secularization, urbanization, industrialization, economic development, occupational specialization, bureaucratization, individuation, steadily increasing entrepreneurial motivation, and mass education as the driving forces of these value changes. And both see the shift in value orientation further triggered or strengthened by institutional shortcomings. The authority of secondary groups (churches, labor unions, political parties, and the government) has eroded. They have reached the limits of their effectiveness. Hence their acceptability by the population at large is in question.

In his most recent publication, from which I quoted before, Inglehart appears to embrace the concept of postmodernization. He posits it as a wider concept than postmaterialization: "The shift from Materialist to Postmaterialist priorities is a core element of the Postmodernization process" (1997: 35). To quote a pertinent passage:

> In the past few decades, advanced industrial societies have reached an inflection point and begun moving on a new trajectory that might be called "Postmodernization."
>
> With Postmodernization, a new worldview is gradually replacing the outlook that has dominated industrializing societies since the Industrial Revolution.... It is transforming basic norms governing politics, work, religion, family,

> and sexual behavior. Thus, the process of economic development leads to two successive trajectories, Modernization and Postmodernization. Both of them are strongly linked with economic development, but Postmodernization represents a later stage of development that is linked with very different beliefs from those that characterize Modernization. These belief systems are not mere consequences of economic or social changes, but shape socioeconomic conditions and are shaped by them, in reciprocal fashion. (ibid.: 8)

I would not be surprised if those who identify themselves as convinced postmodernists would have difficulty accepting Inglehart's embrace. They may, first, object to the grand theorizing involved and to the assumption that people maintain their value orientations over a lifetime. Both would seem to go against the grain of postmodernistic thinking. They may argue, further, that Inglehart only embraced the concept after first having molded it to his own liking. It is evident, for example, that Inglehart has little patience with those who see cultural construction as the only factor shaping human experience. Among some of Inglehart's pertinent observations in this regard are the following: "There is an objective reality out there too..."; "External reality is crucial when it comes to the ultimate political resource, violence...", "There is a worldwide consensus among natural scientists that they are studying a reality that exists independently of their preconceptions..."; and "Postmodernization *does* seem to be inherently conducive to the emergence of democratic political institutions" (ibid.: 12–14; emphasis in original). The guise in which postmodernism appeals to Inglehart excludes its more extreme philosophical or theoretical manifestations.

The conclusion I draw from comparing and contrasting the two concepts, postmodernism and postmaterialism, is that again depending on the preciseness and strictness with which the first concept is defined, postmodernism can be seen either as encompassing postmaterialism or as a specific value orientation that goes well beyond it. In its first guise postmodernism has a bourgeois dimension. It represents a value orientation of recent vintage that quite ordinary people have now internalized. They assume it is shared by their families and friends, and they do not intend to shock or to be defiant when they express that cultural orientation. In the second guise it has retained an avant-garde dimension. It represents a value orientation held by people who are critical of contemporary society, who seek change and aim to be nonconformist in their behavior.

The application and operationalization of postmodernity

The discussion to this point leads me to the following conclusions regarding the relevance and applicability of the concept of postmodernity in demographic research. If one is interested in studying innovative demographic behavior, the behavior of a certain nonconformist elite or minority, or the diffusion process of a number of ideas originally held by a small vanguard, using a narrow definition would seem to be appropriate. The best research design then might be to identify a number of evidently postmodern philosophical and ideological positions and to investigate the demographic behavior of such "truly postmodern" individuals. In studies focusing on the relation between changes in demographic trends and changes in value orientation, in world view, at the macro level a broad definition would seem to be appropriate. In this bourgeois guise the concept of postmodern encompasses the postmaterialist dimension. It can then denote the characteristic traits of a new historical era that follows the modern era and that questions the meta-narratives of that era. It can also denote a contemporary world view that is, or may become, dominant in industrialized societies.

The postmodern era and the second demographic transition

It is characteristic of the concept of postmodernity that in many disciplines its use preceded its definition. It is frequently in hindsight that certain books, poems, or paintings have been recognized and labeled as postmodern. When in the mid-1980s Lesthaeghe and I developed the idea of the second demographic transition and related the demographic changes observed in Western Europe to changes in the value orientation of the population, we did not use the term postmodern to describe these changes (Lesthaeghe and van de Kaa 1986; van de Kaa 1987, 1988, abridged version published 1994; Lesthaeghe and Meekers 1986). But both of us referred to the ideas Inglehart had expounded in his book aptly titled *The Silent Revolution* (1977) and highlighted the profound attitudinal changes in the population. I noted, for example, that in the Netherlands the acceptance of divorce, abortion, and homosexuality had all increased spectacularly over a brief time span; evidently these changes were interrelated (1987: 8). Elsewhere, I wrote: "The strong emphasis on individualism requires people to search constantly for guiding and stabilizing orientations, for an individual life style and a personal identity. People are equal moral agents. This puts them under a great deal of strain and has clearly resulted in...value pluralism" (1988: 21). The shift toward greater "progressiveness" was described in some detail and it was linked to the materialist-postmaterialist dimensions identified by Inglehart. His approach was also used analytically (Lesthaeghe and Surkyn 1988). But to the best of my knowledge, the term postmodern was not part of the discourse at the time. It would now seem that it could well have been used to highlight the contention that the phenomena observed were so radically different that, from a demographic perspective, it seemed as if Western Europe had entered a new era. What demographic analysis drove forcefully home was that, almost simultaneously in all Western European countries, a series of trends showed a marked inflection in the mid-1960s. As time went by, other European or industrialized populations experienced similar demographic shifts.

That the changes in family formation and fertility were linked to socioeconomic development, to the process of modernization, was obvious. Lesthaeghe, who attempted to provide a general interpretation of the second transition, concludes, however, that "explanations solely relying on either the ideational changes or on structural economic factors are non-redundant, yet insufficient" (1991: 23). Hoffmann-Nowotny, who gave a careful description of the structural and ideational factors at work during the transition, presented a theoretical framework that he called the Structure/Culture Paradigm (1987, 1997). It incorporates two important shifts: the shift from *solidarité mécanique* to *solidarité organique* identified by Durkheim as basic to modernization, and the shift from *Gemeinschaft* to *Gesellschaft* distinguished by Tönnies as elementary in that process. It posits interdependency between structure (the position of societal units, i.e., individuals, families, etc.) and culture (values, norms, institutions, etc.). The outcome of societal modernization presents people with various dilemmas. Freedom and options increase, but choices have to be made taking into account societal expectations, individual interests, and personal resources (bounded rationality). Although appealing, this paradigm of the modernization process does not predict a point of inflection once the process has sufficiently advanced. Inglehart's concept of modernization owes more to Weber. By stressing as its two central dimensions the shift from (a) survival to well-being and (b) traditional authority to secular-rational authority, it is capable of predicting a nonlinear course of events. The approach also leaves more room for the impact of technological innovations. "Coherent cultural patterns exist," concludes Ingelhart, and "are linked with economic and technological development" (1997: 69). As I have argued earlier, the link with technological change is of particular significance in relation to the second demographic transition. The spread of efficient contraception undoubtedly helped to generate that transition (van de Kaa 1994: 105).

In fact, if one develops an overview of the demographic sequences constituting the second demographic transition, the facilitating role of efficient modern contraception is quite apparent. The introduction of highly efficient and effective means of contraception around the mid-1960s, in most countries supplemented at some stage by legislative changes allowing sterilization and/or making abortion available, increased considerably the demographic options of successive cohorts. It is, further, quite apparent that the choice made regarding family formation and fertility by a given cohort both limited and enriched the options of the next. "Mental" cohorts intent on increasing the freedom of choice of individuals, supportive of pluralistic ideas, and seeking gender equity and the emancipation of minority groups in the population exerted considerable influence on demographic preferences. The change in value orientations involved is well documented in the shift toward postmaterialism and, one must assume, in the postulated broader shift toward postmodernity. The demographic patterns resulting from the second demographic transition, I should like to argue, have to reflect the advent of the postmodern era. This leads to the hypothesis that countries which have moved farthest in a postmaterialist/postmodernist direction will also have advanced most in terms of the sequences of the second demographic transition.

The following overview of the sequences in the second demographic transition, based on observations for the period circa 1965–95, depicts a complex set of changes in trends (van de Kaa 1997):

(1) TFRs decline as a consequence of reductions in fertility at higher ages; higher-order birth rates decline.

(2) Avoidance of premarital pregnancies and "forced" marriages increases.

(3) Notwithstanding that, the mean age at first marriage continues to decline for a while.

(4) Childbearing within marriage is postponed, fertility among young women declines, and lower-order birth rates decline; these trends accentuate decline in period TFR.

(5) Judicial separation and divorce increase (when allowed).

(6) Postponement of marriage is largely replaced by premarital cohabitation and increased age at first marriage.

(7) Cohabitation becomes more popular; marriage is postponed until the woman is pregnant; increases occur in premarital births and in mean age at first birth.

(8) Legislation permitting sterilization and abortion further reduces unwanted fertility; fertility at youngest and oldest childbearing ages declines further.

(9) Cohabitation gains further support, and is frequently also preferred by the widowed and the divorced.

(10) Cohabitation is increasingly seen as an alternative to marriage; extramarital fertility increases.

(11) TFRs tend to stabilize at low levels.

(12) TFRs increase slightly where women who postponed births begin childbearing; lower-order birth rates increase at higher ages of childbearing.

(13) Not all postponed births can be made up in the years of childbearing remaining to women.

(14) Voluntary childlessness becomes increasingly significant.

(15) Cohort fertility appears to stabilize below replacement level.

Detailed studies of individual trends are valuable but are too narrowly focused to be of much use in attempting to gain a synoptic view of a complicated process of change. And, while the changes in individual trends may well have the same determinants, their sensitivity to change differs and clearly has both a regional and a sequential component. For example, extramarital fertility is unlikely to increase substantially before cohabitation is fairly generally accepted, and that will, if at all, be the case later in Catholic than in Protestant regions. It would seem that the overview allows one to overcome the disadvantages of dealing with each variable separately since it recognizes a marital and a fertility transition. I have devised a summary measure, based on the above scheme, for each of the two.

The measure of the stage of the marital transition is based on three standard demographic variables and one somewhat less frequently available, more specific variable.

(1) The period total first marriage rate of women below the age of 50: with the underlying assumption that the lower this rate is, the more important cohabitation and the postponement of marriage are likely to be;

(2) The mean age of women at first marriage: the older women are when they marry, the more advanced the marital transition;

(3) The total divorce rate, which is meant to measure the reduced stability of marriage; and,

(4) The prevalence of cohabitation.[3]

The fertility transition measure is based on four standard demographic indexes.

(1) The proportion of the TFR that can be ascribed to women aged 30 and older: meant to capture the characteristic aging of fertility;

(2) The proportion of all births born out of wedlock. The underlying assumption here again is that the higher the measure, the more advanced the transition;

(3) and (4) Two other measures are meant to reflect the level and change in the TFR. The period TFR for 1992 is used as an indication of the fertility level at the time of the World Values Surveys of the early 1990s (see below). The idea here is that the further the transition has progressed, the more the TFR will have recovered from the temporary effect of the postponement of births. The change in TFR between 1980 and 1995 is used as an indication of the degree of volatility in the societies concerned. The idea is that the farther the transition has run its course, the more stable the fertility level is likely to have become.

In each instance in the following analysis, the transition measure represents the mean of the standardized z-scores of the variables selected. The correlation matrix is shown in Table 1. The variables used in the construction of each of the summary indexes appear to be sufficiently independent to make the calculation of their mean z-score meaningful. The fertility and marriage indicators evidently capture different aspects of the demographic transition process, with the relationships having the expected signs. The

TABLE 1 Correlation matrix of demographic variables, postmaterialism, and subjective well-being

Variable	Period total first marriage rate	Mean age at first marriage	Cohabitation among women 25–29	Total divorce rate	Proportion of TFR to women 30+	Fertility change 1980–95	Total fertility rate 1992	Proportion extra-marital births	Fertility transition score	Marital transition score	Post-materialist score	Subjective well-being
Period total first marriage rate		–0.519**	–0.523**	0.124	–0.253	–0.089	0.164	–0.697**	–0.511**	0.016	–0.342	–0.510**
Mean age at first marriage	–0.519**		0.640**	–0.073	0.766**	–0.278	0.048	0.381	0.531**	0.534**	0.715**	0.790**
Cohabitation among women 25–29	–0.523**	0.640**		0.448*	0.448*	–0.533**	0.332	0.670**	0.552**	0.781**	0.421*	0.581**
Total divorce rate	0.124	–0.073	0.448*		–0.014	–0.745**	0.576**	0.275	0.055	0.716**	0.113	0.120
Proportion of TFR to women 30+	–0.253	0.767**	0.449*	–0.014		–0.451*	0.256	0.122	0.532**	0.476*	0.821**	0.837**
Fertility change 1980–95	–0.089	–0.278	–0.533**	–0.745**	–0.451*		–0.622**	–0.140	–0.121	–0.796**	–0.446*	–0.428*
Total fertility rate 1992	0.164	0.048	0.332	0.576**	0.256	–0.622**		0.313	0.550**	0.539**	0.055	0.243
Proportion extra-marital births	–0.697**	0.381	0.670**	0.275	0.122	–0.140	0.313		0.758**	0.337	0.051	0.408*
Fertility transition score	–0.511**	0.531**	0.552**	0.055	0.532**	–0.121	0.550**	0.758**		0.322	0.274	0.612**
Marital transition score	0.016	0.534**	0.781**	0.716**	0.476*	–0.796**	0.539**	0.337	0.322		0.453*	0.495**
Postmaterialist score	–0.342	0.715**	0.421*	0.113	0.821**	–0.446*	0.055	0.051	0.274	0.453*		0.814**
Subjective well-being	–0.510**	0.790**	0.581**	0.120	0.837**	–0.428*	0.243	0.408*	0.612**	0.495**	0.814**	

NOTE: See Appendix Table for list of countries.
** correlation is significant at the 0.01 level.
* correlation is significant at the 0.05 level
SOURCES: Council of Europe (1996); Monnier and Guibert-Lantoine (1995 and 1996); Coleman (1996); World Values Survey (1990–93); United Nations (1990, 1993); Carmichael (1995 and personal communication); Pool (1997, personal communication); Carmichael, Webster, and McDonald (1997); Australian Bureau of Statistics (1993); Statistics New Zealand (1996).

total divorce rate and the proportion of extramarital births have distinct positions in the marital and fertility transitions respectively. It is important to remember here that the divorce rate does not measure the dissolution of cohabiting unions. In some countries the number of such dissolutions is reportedly higher than the number of divorces (Manting 1994). One also has to recall that legal provisions may play an important part in both instances. Divorce may be very difficult to realize, while people are likely to hesitate having births outside marriage where the legal position of the children born is adversely affected.

Because postmodernity is assumed to encompass postmaterialism I first explore the relationship between the stages of the fertility and marital transitions and the level of postmaterialism as documented by Ingelhart through the World Value Surveys conducted around 1990. The Appendix Table gives the country scores on postmaterialism and subjective well-being as reported by Inglehart.[4] Table 1 illustrates that although there is a significant correlation between postmaterialism and several of the individual fertility and marital variables, the relation between postmaterialism and the overall fertility transition measure is weak and not significant. There is a negative correlation with fertility decline over the period 1980–95, while the level of postmaterialism clearly is not a good predictor of the current fertility level. The correlation between postmaterialism and the marital transition score is statistically significant. Apparently, postmaterialists cohabit, marry late, and have their children late.

Figures 2 and 3 show the regression of cohabitation and later ages at childbearing against the levels of postmaterialism as established by Inglehart. Although the level of postmaterialism was treated as the independent variable in the regressions, this does not imply the assumption of a one-sided causal relation. Figure 2 indicates that as regards later ages at childbearing, the industrialized countries can be divided in two distinct groups. In the countries of the former eastern bloc, "aging of fertility" has yet to begin. Their currently low levels of fertility are, therefore, most likely to some extent associated with the postponement of births. Once begun, the transition in that region may well occur rapidly. Rychtaříková (1999), for example, reports unusually rapid changes in the Czech Republic in the four years from 1992 to 1996. In the other industrialized countries the aging of fertility is well advanced. Very high proportions of children are being born to women over 30 in the Netherlands and, less surprisingly, Ireland. The other English-speaking countries (United States, Canada, Australia, New Zealand, and Britain) form a neat cluster. In the Southern European countries of Spain and Italy, the proportion of children born to women over 30 is comparable to that of some of the Nordic countries (Finland, Iceland, Norway, Denmark). The much lower fertility levels these countries currently experience are, thus, strongly related to the extremely low age-specific fertility rates below age 30.

FIGURE 2 Relationship between postmaterialism and fertility at later ages of childbearing

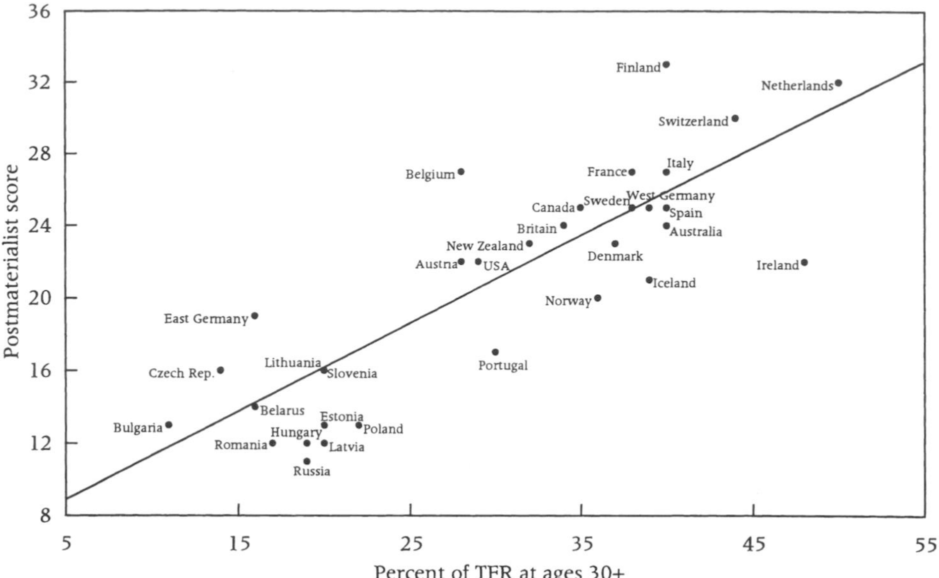

Figure 3, relating cohabitation to postmaterialism, is also instructive. The countries of Central and Eastern Europe again appear to constitute a separate group. The variation among the other countries is considerable. In three Nordic countries (Norway, Iceland, and Denmark) cohabitation is more popular than the level of postmaterialism would suggest. The opposite is the case in several other countries with a Protestant tradition (Finland, Netherlands). In countries with a Roman Catholic tradition such as Italy, Spain, Belgium, and Ireland, cohabitation remains below the level that acceptance of postmaterialist ideas would suggest.

The regional clustering observed in the scatter plots appears to coincide with long-standing cultural differences. East of an imaginary line running from Trieste in Italy to St. Petersburg in Russia, marriage and childbirth have always been much earlier than in Western Europe, for example. That cohabitation is more popular in traditionally Protestant than Catholic countries also indicates that the speed and impact of value change depend, at least in part, on the cultural setting encountered. Moreover, the generally unfavorable housing market in Central and Eastern Europe makes cohabitation prior to marriage less attractive.

The correlation between postmaterialism and subjective well-being is very high (R = .814). But given the extremely difficult economic situation that populations in the former eastern bloc countries faced in the early 1990s, I also briefly explored the relation between the fertility and marital

FIGURE 3 Relationship between postmaterialism and cohabitation

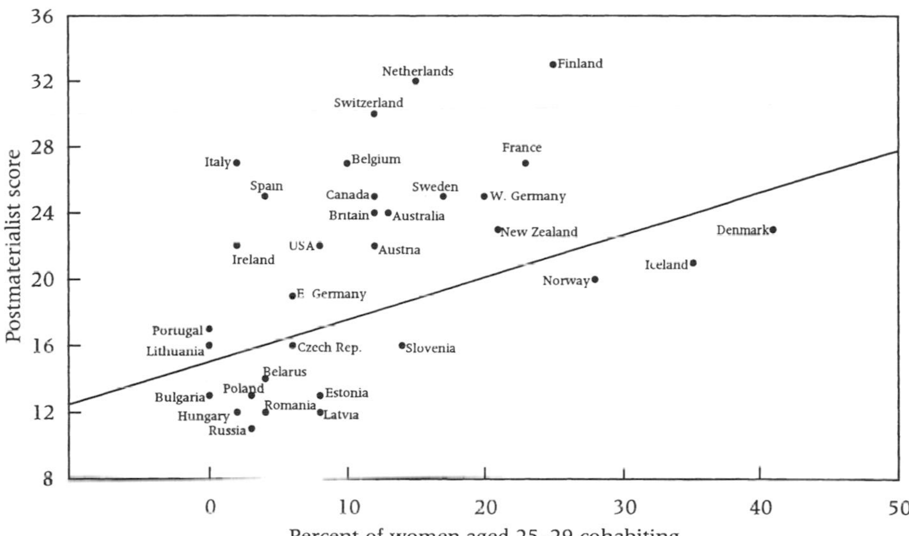

transition indexes and the subjective level of well-being in countries as reported in the World Values Surveys. The fertility transition score and the level of subjective well-being were found to be closely related (R = .612). The Central and Eastern European countries again constitute a separate group, the implied suggestion being that the low levels of fertility observed largely reflect the difficult socioeconomic circumstances encountered (see Katus and Zakharov 1997). The relation of subjective well-being with the marital transition mean standardized z-score is weaker (R = .495). The correlation is, however, still highly significant. As one would expect, fertility patterns appear to be more sensitive than marital patterns to conditions that obtain during a given period of time. In scatter plots applying the marital transition score (see Figure 5, for example) the three Southern European countries under consideration—Italy, Spain, and Portugal—lie fairly close together, which testifies to the enduring nature of cultural similarities and differences. Their marital transitions have not progressed as far as their fertility transitions (Sardon 1997). East Germany is an outlier in similar scatter diagrams, precisely because of the exceptionally low levels of marriage and divorce it experienced in the first few years after German reunification.

That subjective well-being is much more closely related than postmaterialism to the fertility and marital transitions is understandable. Subjective well-being is likely to depend directly, at least in part, on the demographic choices made. Nevertheless, it has sometimes been felt that the postmaterialist score was too sensitive to period fluctuations to serve as an indicator of deep-seated changes in value orientation. Inglehart himself has drawn attention to this and has further shown that this sensitivity affects all birth cohorts (1997: 136). A critical analysis of the materialist/postmaterialist dichotomy performed by Scarbrough (1995) yielded the same finding. Thus, if one seeks to obtain insight into the longer-term future, it would be desirable to develop a measure that incorporates elements of greater permanency.

Operationalizing postmodernity as a *Weltanschauung*

The "truly postmodern"

As I concluded above, in demographic research the concept of postmodernity as a *Weltanschauung* can be operationalized from two perspectives. The first would attempt to identify the (most likely still fairly small) groups of individuals having a very outspoken postmodernist value orientation: the "truly postmodern" who share a certain "structure of feeling" as Gibbins and Reimer characterize them (1995: 315). This is an approach one might apply in the study of voluntary childlessness, serial marriage, or some other uncommon form of demographic behavior. In such an effort, the operationalizing of postmodernism as undertaken by Gibbins and Reimer for the political sciences could be useful. Along the lines I highlighted earlier, they argue that "at the centre of the postmodern self is a value orientation which can collectively be called expressivism." By this they mean "a desire to actualize self-constructions or identities." This may be focused on clothing, possessions, and the like, but also on social self-expression, life style, emancipatory movements, and the like. According to Reimer and Gibbins two groups of postmodernists may be distinguished. "Instrumental postmodernists focus on private life and material goods; humanist postmodernists focus on the public world and social goods" (ibid.: 312–313). The first combine expressivism with instrumentalism, the second expressivism with humanism.

Gibbins and Reimer write that in the 12 European countries they studied, instrumental postmodernism was practically unrelated to the materialism/postmaterialism dichotomy. But in most countries humanist postmodernism showed a significant correlation with postmaterialism. Since this chapter focuses on "bourgeois postmodernism" and I do not immediately see the relevance of the measures devised for demographic behavior, I shall not explore the "truly postmodern" direction further. Moreover, the justification of the data manipulation performed escapes me.[5]

A measure of "bourgeois" postmodernity

The second approach to operationalizing postmodernity as a *Weltanschauung* clearly is to try to capture a much broader value orientation—that is, to explore whether the two dimensions that Inglehart has identified through factor analysis can be used. These two factors, it may be recalled, are traditional versus secular-rational authority, and survival versus well-being. Inglehart has further provided a list of 40 variables, grouped in five categories, that were found to have correlations above the .125 level with Materialist/Postmaterialist Values in the 1981 World Values Surveys (Inglehart 1997: 268–269).[6]

The list of variables under these categories certainly is representative of the broader shift toward postmodernity that I would like to capture and explore. Moreover, some of the variables are particularly relevant from the perspective of fertility preferences and demographic behavior more generally. Further information in this regard can be gleaned from an article by Lesthaeghe and Moors (1995). They used the pooled 1990 World Values Survey data of Belgium, France, Netherlands, and West Germany to describe the pattern of living arrangements, socioeconomic position, and values among young adults (aged 20–29) in these countries. Thirty variables were used to develop 11 scales. They cover such issues as religiosity, requirements for a successful marriage, gender roles, and socialization. Principal component analysis yielded three underlying value dimensions. Factor 1 is characterized by high religiosity and strict ethical standards. Factor 2 corresponds with right wing political convictions and aversion to emancipation and sexual minorities. Lesthaeghe and Moors report that the Materialist items on the Inglehart scale also correlate strongly with this factor. Factor 3, finally, describes conservatism regarding gender roles.

This leads to the conclusion that postmodernity is probably best ascertained by looking at attitudes regarding a fairly wide range of issues and not by considering whether an individual holds a particular view on a few specific points. It is a general world view that concerns us now. The aim is to capture a group that may never have heard of the concept of postmodernist but that, nevertheless, can be characterized as such.[7]

For present purposes I leave aside answers to survey questions about marriage, cohabitation, and family size—that is, to demographic questions per se. The type of postmodernity specified is, consequently, likely to be reflected most clearly in answers to questions about, for example:

—whether one should try to get the best out of life

—the approval of emancipatory movements (e.g., human rights or ecological movements)

—the degree of tolerance of the behavior of others (e.g., sexual freedom)

—the degree of support for female labor force participation

—the importance of personal freedom in comparison with equality.

The problem with resorting to survey questions of this sort is, however, that in most industrialized societies the process of postmodernization appears to be so far advanced that the proportions giving a postmodern

TABLE 2 Proportion of respondents with a specified value orientation agreeing with or approving of certain statements: World Values Surveys, 1990 round

Statement	Post-modernist	Mixed	Modernist	Total	Total observations
The meaning of life is that you try to get the best out of it	80	78	77	78	32,463
Having a job is the best way for a woman to be an independent person	74	67	65	68	32,582
Greater emphasis on the development of the individual is good	90	86	88	87	36,351
Do you approve of the human rights movement at home or abroad?	97	95	95	95	35,317

SOURCE: World Values Surveys 1990–93, Machine Readable Data File.

answer have largely lost their power to differentiate. Table 2, which is based on the World Values Surveys, illustrates this situation for a few questions that would otherwise have been potentially valuable for analytical purposes. The operationalization I have chosen in order to explore the issue further assumes that the measurement of postmaterialism provides a good guide to the placement of individual respondents on the survival versus well-being dimension. To ascertain the position of respondents on the traditional versus secular/rational authority dimension, I looked at two questions:

—how important is religion in your life?, and

—what would you think about a development toward greater respect for authority?

I felt that maintaining the postmaterialist/materialist dimension would ensure an element of continuity with the previous analysis. Moreover, in Inglehart's view postmaterialism is the core element of postmodernization. By bringing in the dimension of religiosity and respect for authority, I sought to reduce the sensitivity of postmaterialism to period fluctuations. I felt that one could further argue that those who answer that for them religion is unimportant and that more respect for authority would be a bad thing explicitly reject the meta-narratives that religion represents. I had, finally, noted that in their study Lesthaeghe and Moors identified religiosity (belief in God) as a powerful determinant of marital choices.

Classified as postmodern, then, were all respondents who would qualify as being postmaterialist on Inglehart's scale who replied that religion was not very, or not at all important in their lives, and/or that greater respect for authority would be a bad thing. Those who replied that religion was not very, or not at all important and/or that greater respect for authority would be a bad thing, and who showed a leaning toward postmaterialism by indicating at least one of the two postmaterialist items in Inglehart's scale as one of their priorities, were similarly classified as postmodern. The modern were identified as those who qualified as materialist on the Inglehart scale, replied that religion was very important in their lives, and/or that greater respect for authority would be a good thing. Those who showed a certain leaning toward materialism by indicating at least one of the two materialist items in the Inglehart battery as a priority, who replied that religion was very important in their lives, and/or that more respect for authority would be a good thing were also considered to be modern. All other respondents form the category mixed or undecided.[8]

The proportions postmodern and modern obtained by this procedure, and the size of the samples on which they are based, are given in the Appendix Table. They show a plausible pattern, but the variation from country to country is considerable. The amplitude is greater than I would have expected. In a large-scale international comparative survey program, one can never completely exclude the possibility that questions have been interpreted or have been put slightly differently in the participating countries. Nevertheless, postmodernity appears to be most extensive in Sweden (48 percent), Finland (48 percent), West Germany (43 percent), and the Netherlands (33 percent). Low fractions are found in most of the former eastern bloc countries (Russia 7 percent), in Ireland (8 percent), and, rather surprisingly, Iceland (11 percent). The pattern for the modern largely mirrors that for the postmodern. The association with age has the expected shape. Postmodernists constitute 19 percent of the 45–49-year-olds and 29 percent of those aged 20–24. And, while the modern constitute only 13 percent in the latter group, they form 25 percent of those aged 45–49.

The correlations between measures of postmodernity and the fertility and marital variables (see Table 3) show strong associations of postmodernity with the mean age of women at first marriage, the total first marriage rate for women, the proportion of cohabiting women, and the aging of fertility. The overall associations between the level of postmodernity and the state of the fertility and marital transitions in the 26 countries considered are shown as scatter diagrams in Figures 4 and 5.

The graphs are striking. The regression of postmodernity against the fertility transition score shows that the correlation (R = .202) is affected by no fewer than five outliers: West Germany, Finland, Sweden, Iceland, and Ireland. The latter two countries have low levels of postmodernity compared with the other Western and Northern European countries, while the level of postmodernity measured for the first three is unusually high, even for that part of Europe. Replying that religion is unimportant in one's life apparently is not difficult in these three societies. The remaining countries form a fairly tight cluster. But, interestingly enough, all Western and North-

TABLE 3 Correlation of demographic variables with postmodernism

Variable	Postmodern	Postmodern minus modern
Proportion with postmodern orientation		0.972**
Proportion postmodern minus proportion with modern orientation	0.972**	
Period total first marriage rate	–0.495**	–0.501**
Mean age at first marriage	0.637**	0.613**
Cohabitation among women 25–29	0.549**	0.603**
Total divorce rate	0.253	0.294
Proportion of TFR to women 30+	0.451*	0.363
Fertility change 1980–95	–0.370	–0.350
Total fertility rate 1992	–0.039	–0.059
Proportion extramarital births	0.307	0.343
Fertility transition score	0.202	0.172
Marital transition score	0.472*	0.504**
Postmaterialist score	0.662**	0.616**
Subjective well-being	0.541**	0.482*

** Correlation is significant at the 0.01 level.
* Correlation is significant at the 0.05 level.

ern European countries are situated above the regression line; the North American countries and those of Southern Europe lie below it.

The outlier position of Sweden, Finland, and West Germany is less marked in Figure 5, which shows the association between postmodernity

FIGURE 4 Relationship between postmodernity and the fertility transition score

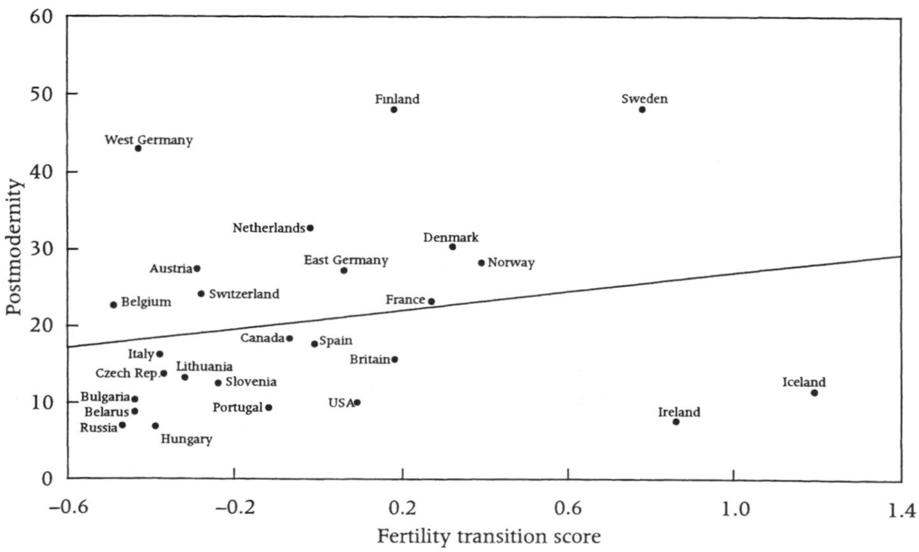

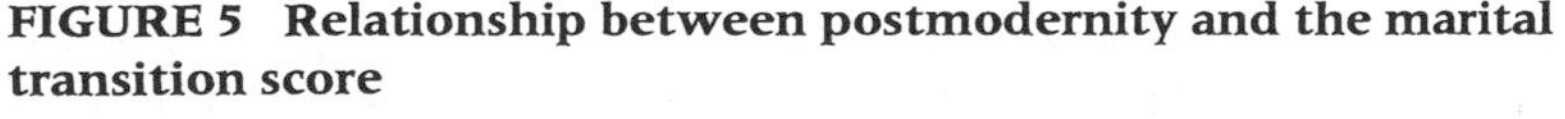

FIGURE 5 Relationship between postmodernity and the marital transition score

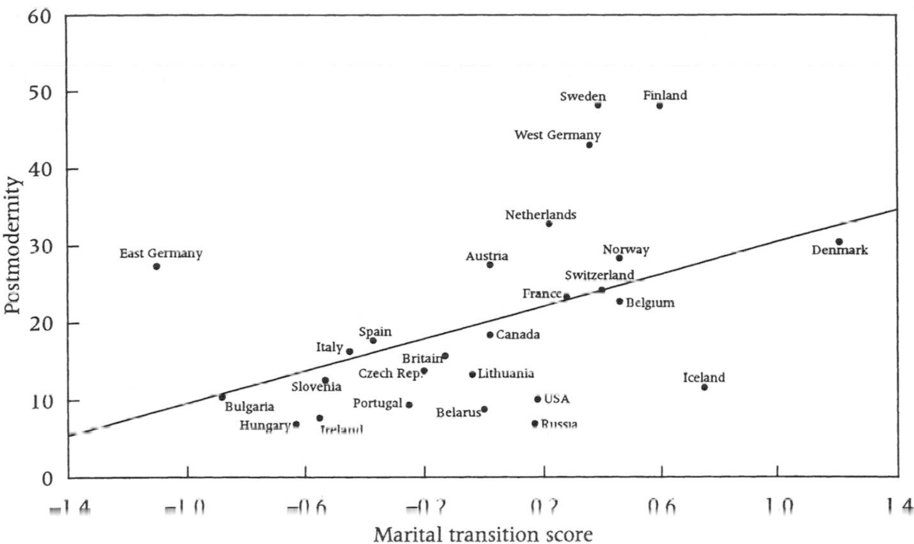

and the marital transition score (R = .472). The other European countries with a mainly Protestant tradition (Norway, Netherlands, and Denmark) fall in the upper right quadrant of the diagram. East Germany now shows up as an outlier because of its exceptional marriage and divorce figures in the first few years after the fall of the Berlin Wall. (Figure 5 refers to the early 1990s. This is no doubt a temporary phenomenon.) The grouping of the countries in the scatter diagram suggests that in several Central and Eastern European countries the era of postmodernity is still some way off. The cultural heritage of countries and the attendant institutional considerations give the marital transition a distinct regional flavor (Micheli 1996; Reher 1998).

Postmodernity as a value orientation and demographic attitudes

Values, attitudes, and behavior

The literature about the concept of values as used in the social sciences is extensive. The same can be said about the relation of values to attitudes and behavior. I will briefly indicate how the term "value orientation" is used in this chapter and how I see its relation to attitudes and behavior. Since the aim is to look at the possible relation between postmodernity as a value orientation and fertility preferences, there is no purpose in equating value with preference. It is similarly not a sensible strategy to posit a direct and one-sided relationship between values and attitudes. In line with the approach Inglehart has taken in the matter of postmaterialism, I start with the assumption that values cannot be observed directly. A value orientation, such as postmaterialism or postmodernity, will make its presence felt through the way it patterns and constrains attitudes. In a well-argued contribution van Deth and Scarbrough (1995) have pointed out that one must assume a reciprocal relationship between values and attitudes: "values will change as attitudes are changing, and attitudes are modified if values change. At the aggregate level, these individual-level changes may provide a clue to the understanding of processes of social and political change..." (p. 33). I follow these authors in the way they highlight two other aspects of values, namely: (a) that they indicate conceptions of the desirable, and (b) that they are used in moral discourse, with particular relevance to behavior. In this way value orientations derived from empirically observed patterns and constraints in attitudes serve as a heuristic device in understanding these attitudes, for example in their role as immediate antecedents to behavior.

Postmodernity and attitudes pertaining to fertility behavior

The World Values Surveys asked a number of questions that aimed to assess the attitudes of respondents toward a variety of issues. Some of those attitudes are quite interesting from a demographic perspective. Table 4 gives the reactions of the respondents classified as postmodernist and modernist to six questions.[9] Since the sample sizes of the World Values Surveys frequently are very small, no attempt has been made to distinguish between male and female respondents. It is evident that the differences in attitude between postmodernists and modernists as they emerge from Table 4 almost invariably go in the expected direction. Postmodernists do not as frequently agree that a child should grow up with two parents as do modernists, although, overall, there is a large measure of support for the idea that children need to grow up with both father and mother. As Kaufmann (1988) has earlier pointed out, the taboo on bringing children into the world if one is not willing to accept the responsibility of providing long-term care for them is still strong. It is an attitude bound to keep fertility levels low. On the whole, postmodernists do not feel that a woman needs a child. The differences between certain countries—Denmark versus the Netherlands and the other Nordic countries—are, at least at first sight, baffling. It could be that the Danes have interpreted the question in the sense that women have the right to have a child irrespective of their marital status or other considerations. It is, at any rate, evident that support for the idea that women may elect to be a single parent is exceptionally high in Denmark

TABLE 4 Proportion of respondents with a postmodernist or modernist value orientation who agree with or approve of certain statements: World Values Surveys, 1990s

Country	Agree that a child needs two parents		Agree that a woman needs a child		Agree that marriage is outdated		Approve of a woman as a single parent		Parents' own lives are a priority		Approve of abortion if couple does not want child	
	PM	M	PM	M	PM	M	PM	M	PM	M	PM	M
Austria	91	95	28	69	18	10	51	10	44	19	40	17
Belarus	n.a.	n.a.	96	98	23	12	53	44	25	24	72	63
Belgium	86	94	29	54	33	18	43	23	25	23	34	17
Britain	65	80	18	27	28	14	49	25	22	14	51	33
Bulgaria	92	96	74	94	16	7	68	40	42	19	89	72
Canada	71	85	16	33	23	8	53	23	23	17	56	12
Czech Rep.	99	99	86	89	13	9	29	18	27	22	42	29
Denmark	62	88	82	86	24	17	78	39	46	29	73	43
Finland	83	91	12	29	17	0	69	14	27	9	71	20
France	90	96	64	82	46	18	45	34	22	15	57	39
West Germany	91	100	27	74	25	6	34	9	48	15	43	9
East Germany	96	99	56	78	20	6	42	19	32	14	62	23
Hungary	97	99	100	95	22	12	59	32	38	27	79	61
Iceland	68	87	24	60	16	4	78	80	36	20	43	18
Ireland	70	86	24	28	25	7	46	15	27	12	17	7
Italy	90	98	48	78	31	8	57	29	17	6	49	15
Lithuania	94	94	87	93	14	9	69	47	59	50	61	37
Netherlands	65	89	4	28	36	8	63	16	27	13	47	9
Norway	80	90	18	29	14	7	35	15	12	6	57	28
Poland	100	98	73	83	29	5	18	17	36	18	25	20
Portugal	91	96	48	73	35	20	53	28	12	11	49	24
Russia	97	97	90	95	14	11	44	42	51	31	76	61
Slovenia	87	94	45	66	16	14	62	64	14	15	86	59
Spain	85	95	29	59	39	7	85	50	19	12	61	17
Sweden	81	94	15	24	16	5	30	10	16	15	58	31
Switzerland	n.a.	n.a.	20	46	20	7	51	27	23	12	n.a.	n.a.
United States	59	81	12	26	12	6	61	27	19	13	61	12

PM= postmodernist, M= modernist.
n.a. = not available.

and Iceland, but is even higher in Spain. The idea of a married couple seeking recourse to abortion is well accepted in Eastern Europe, where for a long time it was the most important means of fertility regulation, and in the Nordic countries, which tend to emphasize the free decision of women/couples in the matter. Agreement with the statement that marriage is an outdated institution is very limited. It is, however, without exception higher among the postmodern than the modern. The shift to emphasis on personal fulfillment is reflected in the degree of support for the idea that parents do not need to sacrifice their own well-being for the sake of their children. Although the responsibility toward children is obviously still taken quite seriously, frequently about a third of those classified as postmodern support this idea.

The general conclusion is that the "conception of the desirable" differs systematically between the two groups. Almost invariably the category "mixed"—which is not shown—takes an intermediate position. The differences between countries are quite marked.

Postmodernity and fertility preferences

Preferences and behavior: An illustration

Interest in fertility preferences obviously is based on the assumption that such preferences are related to fertility behavior. In surveys, questions on preferences are dealt with in different ways.[10]

I have no doubt that, from the perspective of forecasting demographic behavior, the most valuable information is that regarding the number of children respondents ultimately expect to have. In the Netherlands a number of birth cohorts have been asked that question on three successive occasions in the *Onderzoeken Gezinsvorming* of the Central Bureau of Statistics. This allows an assessment of both the consistency and the reliability of couples' expectations. De Graaf (1995), who has reported on the results of such an evaluation, concludes that the cohorts interviewed are rather stable in their expectations. If the data obtained in the 1982, 1988, and 1993 surveys are tabulated, it is evident that women born in 1950–54 have, as time went by, slightly reduced their childbearing expectations (see Table 5). But the average number of live births reported in 1993 (1.89) still comes remarkably close to the number expected in 1982 (2.02). And the fact that women adjust their estimates over time as they are confronted with divorce, death of a partner, or medical problems is quite understandable. Respondents were also asked to indicate how certain they were about their expectations. The proportions who were uncertain about whether or not to expect another child were usually below 10 percent. Moreover, with time the degree of uncertainty appears to have decreased (ibid.: 19).

TABLE 5 Average number of children per woman expected by and born to women of different birth cohorts in three successive surveys: Netherlands, 1982–93

Birth cohort	Year of interview	Number of children ultimately expected	Number of live-born children
1950–54	1982	2.02	1.35
	1988	1.96	1.74
	1993	1.97	1.89
1955–59	1982	2.00	0.48
	1988	1.97	1.22
	1993	2.00	1.71
1960–64	1982	1.99	0.04
	1988	1.93	0.45
	1993	2.11	1.09
1965–69	1988	1.82	0.06
	1993	2.11	0.33
1970–74	1993	2.13	0.04

SOURCE: De Graaf 1995: Staat 3.

Differentials in findings on preferred and ideal numbers of children

Given such results, it seemed worthwhile to tabulate data on expected family size for European countries from the Fertility and Family Surveys (FFS surveys) of the UN Economic Commission for Europe.[11] The FFS program is based on the voluntary cooperation of countries providing their own resources and, consequently, they are free to vary the questionnaire on the basis of their own requirements. The figures presented in Table 6 are therefore not fully comparable. They refer to the younger age groups of women in the process of family formation.

It appears that the expectations, hopes, and intentions of the younger age groups interviewed in the early 1990s were not, in general, markedly lower than those of their predecessors. The number of children ultimately wanted by women aged 25–29 years never drops below 2. But these expectations are not tempered as yet by experience. There is little doubt that the averages represent upper limits. From that perspective it seems likely that future levels of fertility will remain below replacement level in several countries. An interesting contrast is provided by Norway, Sweden, and, to a lesser extent, the Netherlands. The trend toward gender equity (McDonald 2000) may there have progressed sufficiently to make higher expectations realistic. The wishes and expectations of women do, in general, exceed those of men in the same age groups.

TABLE 6 Fertility preferences of young women in the early 1990s, by age group and level of education, FFS findings

Country	Year	No. of children wanted ultimately (25–29)	Percent wanting 2 children (20–24)	Percent wanting only one among women having 1 (25–29)	Wanted ultimately (U) and in the future (F) by level of education (25–29)[a]			
					ISCED 0–2		ISCED 5–6	
					U	F	U	F
Austria	1995/96	2.0	53	30	1.94	1.02	1.88	0.83
Canada	1995	2.3	48	21	2.26	0.78	2.42	2.09
Finland[b]	1989/90	2.3	45	20	2.5	1.0	2.4	1.9
France	1994	2.3	59	10	2.52	1.08	2.37	2.02
Latvia	1995	2.2	58	18	2.08	0.38	2.00	0.86
Lithuania	1994/95	2.1	51	20	3.29	0.57	2.10	1.19
Hungary	1992/93	2.1	61	22	2.35	0.35	2.12	1.24
Netherlands	1993	2.2	52	12	2.21	1.23	2.07	1.90
Norway[b,c]	1988/89	2.4	45	11	2.4	1.4	2.6	2.5
Poland	1991	2.1	39	15	2.35	0.35	1.40	0.69
Slovenia	1994/95	2.3	52	14	2.30	0.69	2.18	1.44
Spain[b]	1995	2.3	60	13	2.2	1.2	2.2	2.1
Sweden[b]	1992/93	2.6	58	7	2.6	0.9	2.4	1.7

NOTES: In FFS data read "expected" for France, Norway, and the Netherlands. For Finland, "How many do you hope to have?"; for Sweden, "How many do you believe you will have?"; and for Canada, "How many do you intend to have?"
[a]In the international standard classification of educational attainment, levels 0–2 are commonly grouped as "low" (elementary or less) and levels 5–6 as "high" (higher secondary and postsecondary).
[b]Figures by educational level provided with one decimal only.
[c]Norway did not use the customary age groups in the FFS, but rather the single years 23 and 28.
SOURCE: Fertility and Family Surveys, UN Economic Commission for Europe.

If distributional aspects are considered, a strong clustering on two children proves to be the normal pattern. From 40 to 60 percent of all 20–24-year-old women prefer or expect that number. The full tabulations reveal that relatively few of the younger women expect to have no children at all, while the corresponding figures for women aged 35–39 at the time of interview are also surprisingly low—much lower, no doubt, than one would expect on the basis of careful cohort estimates (Prioux 1993; Rowland in press). That beliefs and expectations about numbers of children may become more realistic with age is confirmed by the proportions of women ultimately expecting one child. The trend toward late childbearing characteristic of the second demographic transition is well illustrated by the FFS findings. Almost invariably women aged between 25 and 35 and having one child or no children do not consider their childbearing years to have passed. Among 25–29-year-old women having one child, not more than 7 to 30 percent see their families as completed.

The relation between level of education and fertility is well established. Women whose formal education is limited tend to have sexual relationships and children earlier than other women, while those whose formal level of education is high tend to have fewer children at later ages. With increasing levels of education in European populations this phenomenon would, ceteris paribus, lead to the inevitable conclusion of a further decline in fertility. However, analysis of the fertility surveys undertaken in the Netherlands since 1982 has revealed that the fertility differential associated with the level of education is narrowing (de Graaf 1995: 17). The fertility behavior of women having the three levels of formal education normally distinguished would seem to have converged. De Graaf notes that a similar finding has been reported for Great Britain by Cooper and Shaw. A few FFS findings on the matter are reported in Table 6. As regards the number of children ultimately expected, in contrast to the customary pattern among better-educated women in the older age groups, young educated women frequently expect to have more children than those with a low or intermediate level of education. But being better educated does not necessarily imply being a better judge of one's future behavior. If results of numbers of children expected to be born in the future are tabulated by level of education, it becomes obvious that, with a few notable exceptions, better-educated women expect many more future births than women with less education. The postponement of childbearing among the better educated is particularly marked in countries such as Canada, France, Norway, and the Netherlands. Thus, whether the educational differential will decline may to a large extent depend on the biological and social constraints better-educated women will encounter.

In a few of the countries participating in the FFS program, questions allowing the classification of respondents according to Inglehart's criteria of materialists, mixed, and postmaterialists have been asked during the interview. In view of the close relation between postmaterialism and postmodernism a few findings for selected age groups of women are presented in Table 7 for those countries that have provided such information for analysis.[12]

The figures may at first sight seem surprising. Female respondents aged 25–29 at the time of interview and classified as postmaterialists do not appear to want fewer children than those classified as materialist or, for that matter (although not shown in the table), those whose reactions were mixed. The difference in value orientation does not differentiate systematically as far as preferences are concerned. If attention is focused on children already born, a much clearer pattern emerges. Respondents classified as postmaterialists have almost always given birth to fewer children than those classified as materialists, particularly toward the end of the reproductive career. As has become clear already from the regression analysis, postmaterialist women begin that career later than materialists. To some extent this reflects an educational differential: postmaterialists tend to be better educated. Most likely it is also indicative of a difference in attitude

TABLE 7 Fertility preferences of women in the early 1990s by age group and materialist/postmaterialist value orientation, FFS findings

	Average number of children ultimately wanted, 25–29		Average number of children considered ideal, 25–29		Average number of children born, 30–34	
Country	Materialist	Post-materialist	Materialist	Post-materialist	Materialist	Post-materialist
Belgium	1.96	2.00	2.06	2.24	1.52	1.62
Finland	1.83	2.30	2.30	2.52	1.72	1.58
W. Germany	2.02	1.81	1.91	1.75	1.34	1.53
E. Germany	1.84	2.01	1.56	1.78	1.89	1.76
Hungary	2.08	2.05	2.11	2.52	1.89	1.63
Norway	2.57	2.29	2.58	2.52	2.01	1.48
Slovenia	2.15	2.40	2.15	2.40	1.83	1.48
Spain	2.14	2.18	2.02	2.12	1.63	1.26
Sweden	2.70	2.57	2.44	2.44	2.05	1.71
Switzerland[a]	2.50	2.45	2.26	2.49	1.46	1.09

[a]Provisional.
For notes see Table 6.

toward intimate relationships and the proper ages for marriage and childbearing. Postmaterialist women appear to overestimate the number of children they will ultimately have: the postponement is so substantial that catching up with the materialists will prove difficult.

That having children is, on the whole, viewed positively by postmaterialists is also evident from their ideals about family size: it may constitute an important element in their perception of well-being and self-realization. Young postmaterialists almost invariably report a higher average number of children as ideal for a family in the country they live in than do their materialist counterparts. One could postulate here that, as the process of postmodernization continues, postmaterialists might find it easier to combine childbearing with other activities and might then be able to match or exceed the numbers of children born to materialists. However, as yet support for that persuasive thesis is not strong. The differences in ideal family size from country to country are substantial. While figures well above replacement level are seen as ideal in the Nordic countries, for example, in Germany the average number of children considered ideal remains far lower.

Ideal and actual numbers of children as reported in the World Values Surveys

A question on ideal family size has also been asked in the World Values Surveys. The results of Fertility and Family Surveys and World Values Surveys by materialist/postmaterialist value orientation can therefore be looked at in conjunction. The most significant finding is again that in North America and Europe ideal family sizes exceed observed fertility levels substantially. Table 8 shows only three instances in which the overall average falls below 2.25 (postmaterialists in Norway, and both groups in East Germany). Averages above 3 are equally rare (materialists in Iceland and both groups in Ireland). The ideal family size still is 2 or 3 children. Comparison of the means calculated for both sexes combined for each age group (under 25, 25–34, 35–44, and 45+) confirms that the materialist/postmaterialist dichotomy does not lead to predictable or systematic differentials between age groups or countries.

TABLE 8 Average numbers of children considered ideal or born to respondents with specified value orientation, by age group, World Values Surveys

	Ideal number of children (all respondents)				Average number of children born			
					35–44		45+	
Country	Materialist	Post-materialist	Modern	Post-modern	Materialist	Post-materialist	Modern	Post-modern
Austria	2.51	2.36	2.63	2.30	2.04	1.74	2.16	1.84
Belarus	2.56	2.58	2.68	2.50	n.a.	n.a.	n.a.	n.a.
Belgium	2.52	2.74	2.59	2.67	1.86	1.58	2.11	1.76
Britain	2.54	2.69	2.69	2.61	2.14	1.92	1.98	2.21
Bulgaria	2.33	2.37	2.38	2.30	1.83	1.55	2.03	1.70
Canada	2.80	2.78	2.94	2.60	2.33	1.56	2.74	2.36
Czech Rep.	2.28	2.37	2.44	2.27	1.95	1.81	2.33	1.79
Denmark	2.63	2.63	2.79	2.55	n.a.	n.a.	n.a.	n.a.
Finland	2.88	2.66	3.13	2.63	2.33	2.21	2.77	1.95
France	2.72	2.78	2.77	2.62	2.76	1.78	2.20	2.15
W. Germany	2.42	2.45	2.61	2.36	1.91	1.35	2.28	1.77
E. Germany	2.18	2.15	2.25	2.02	1.68	1.91	2.17	1.76
Hungary	2.46	2.33	2.52	2.18	1.96	1.59	1.83	2.00
Iceland	3.01	2.88	3.17	2.88	2.37	2.17	2.97	2.33
Ireland	3.28	3.27	3.38	2.93	2.75	2.17	2.65	3.08
Italy	2.51	2.44	2.69	2.38	1.90	1.22	2.24	1.77
Lithuania	2.90	2.74	3.03	2.59	1.67	1.65	1.74	1.72
Netherlands	2.73	2.66	3.02	2.60	1.98	1.44	2.55	2.27
Norway	2.36	2.21	2.51	2.28	1.84	1.91	2.17	2.04
Portugal	2.48	2.36	2.52	2.30	2.06	1.85	2.23	2.37
Russia	2.65	2.66	2.67	2.56	1.85	1.67	1.87	1.74
Slovenia	2.50	2.38	2.59	2.35	2.00	1.60	2.04	1.91
Spain	2.53	2.40	2.62	2.33	2.08	1.67	2.49	2.43
Sweden	2.54	2.78	2.59	2.76	2.27	1.65	2.00	1.97
Switzerland	2.64	2.69	2.69	2.58	1.88	1.48	2.35	2.02
USA	2.75	2.64	2.77	2.43	2.13	1.24	2.60	2.27

NOTE: The number of postmaterialists in the survey samples in Hungary, Iceland, Belarus, Slovenia, and Bulgaria is less than 100. The base is also less than 100 in the case of materialists in Finland, modernists in Sweden and Finland, and postmodernists in Ireland, Hungary, Iceland, Belarus, and Bulgaria.
n.a. = not available.

Table 8 also indicates what respondents with postmodernist and modernist value orientations see as the ideal family size. In view of the small sizes of the samples, figures for the sexes have, again, been combined.[13] The overall mean ideal family size remains, of course, well above observed fertility levels. Averages between 2.5 and 2.7 children per family are common. The lowest value obtained is that of 2.02 for postmodernists in East Germany. What is striking is that the differences between postmodernists and modernists are much greater than between materialists and postmaterialists. In 10 out of 26 countries the postmodern ideal lies from 10 to 16 percentage points below that of modernists, while there are only two cases—Belgium and Sweden—in which the overall average of the postmodernists exceeds that of the modernists. Evidently, in terms of fertility preferences, the modernist/postmodernist divide discriminates more than the distinction between materialism and postmaterialism. The postmodernist preferences of younger age groups (<25 and 25–34) are rather high in several countries that are more advanced in the second demographic transition, such as Sweden, Norway, Iceland, West Germany, Switzerland, and Great Britain. There postmodernity has become the dominant *Weltanschauung*. Whether this is a highly significant finding is difficult to judge; there is, after all, quite a gap to bridge between a conception and a "conception of the desirable." But, at the very least, the finding suggests that postmodernity does not necessarily imply having a preference for very low fertility.

The World Values Surveys also contain a simple question on having children, as follows: "Have you had any children? If yes, how many?" In those countries for which the information appears acceptable, the FFS finding that postmaterialists/postmodernists have their children later, and ultimately have fewer, is confirmed. Tabulation of averages by broad age groups of women and by the postmodernist/modernist dimension shows striking differences in virtually all countries. To date, postmodernity is obviously associated with having children late and with having only a few.

Conclusions

My starting point has been that the term "postmodern" is bound to find its way into demographic literature, whether we want it or not.

Will it also contribute to the scientific study of population? That depends essentially on the way it is conceptualized. If, just as in anthropology or economics, for example, a number of demographers accept postmodernism as their ideology and analyze population issues from that perspective its impact would, I believe, be short lived. It could lead to some self-reflection among other scholars, as the "critical demographers" of the 1970s achieved, to heated discussions perhaps, but not a great deal more. Its impact will also be temporary if postmodernism is used as a simple, unspecified umbrella term to explain, or give a name to, the new demographic behavior in industrialized countries described by so many.[14] The term postmodern, or one of its derivatives, can only play a role in the scientific study of population if precise conceptualizations can be formulated.

Since postmodernity is an inherently elusive concept, such precision will be difficult to attain. I have argued in this chapter that three lines of approach appear possible. I found no data that enabled me to explore the usefulness or potential of the concept as an avant-garde value orientation. The way in which Gibbins and Reimer sketch the basic traits of a postmodernist does not augur well for a transparent conceptualization in those terms. For if a postmodernist is an "unfinished project," restlessly seeking and changing identity, "inner-directed," and "committed to the logic of the now and immediate," his or her demographic behavior is, almost by definition, impossible to specify or predict. Such a person's value orientation is likely to show little stability, and the choice of today will not be that of tomorrow. The group of people meeting the criteria of a "true" postmodernist undoubtedly is small. It would be foolish, however, to disregard them for that reason. In present-day society, new, unexpected, imaginative, shocking, and blatantly nonconformist behavior will be broadcast widely and may easily become trendsetting. New role models may be created through media exposure of celebrities from different walks of life. It may, thus, be worthwhile to investigate the possibilities further.

Better prospects and firmer ground can be found if postmodernity is conceptualized as a new historical era: the era of postmodernity. Potentially this has two important advantages. It could, first, strengthen the links between demography and theorizing in the social sciences more generally. It offers a second, stimulating opportunity to study demographic change as a complex, but well-integrated process and to understand it in its relation to much broader cultural and economic changes in society. In this chapter I have explored these possibilities. Postmodernity, I have argued, can be tied to postmaterialism, a concept that has now been used in sociology for a quarter of a century. In fact, the increase in the level of postmaterialism in the countries of the European Union has been carefully documented since 1970. Postmodernization should be seen as a broader concept than postmaterialism. It would encompass the latter concept, but would widen it and increase its stability over time. An increase in postmaterialism may thus be assumed to signify an increase in postmodernity. Hence my bold attempt to explore the relationship between the stage of the second demographic transition in the industrialized countries and their level of postmaterialism and "bourgeois" postmodernity.

The results are not incompatible with the idea that the second transition was fueled by these shifts in values, but are not particularly convincing either, unless one sees the later ages of childbearing and the increase in the age at first marriage as the central elements of the second demographic transition. There may be various reasons for doing so. The approach taken heretofore may have been too static. The transition reaches countries with different cultural heritages at different times and is, consequently, likely to differ in speed and impact. Moreover, macro-level univariate analysis has its limitations, and the relationships may not be linear. Further, it is likely that the attempt to develop summary measures for the stage of the fertility and marital transitions that appear to affect the industrialized countries in turn since the mid-1960s has not been optimal. That I had to rely on an existing data source to operationalize bourgeois postmodernity was an additional obstacle. The range in value orientation found is wider than I would have expected. No doubt, many improvements in conceptualization, measurement, and scaling can and must be made. But the notion that a broad change in value orientation is upon us, generated by the irresistible social and economic progress of our societies, is highly attractive. The notion also yields theoretical propositions that demographers can relate to easily and that can give guidance to our expectations. In fact, through its precise measurement of trends, demography is well positioned to contribute to the refining and testing of such propositions.

Another approach, the conceptualization of postmodernity as a world view, a *Weltanschauung,* has been explored with a certain measure of success. It has made the phrase "postmodern fertility preferences" more tangible. The review of existing data suggests that unlike value orientations and economic conditions, fertility preferences show little variation across industrialized societies. Moreover, the preferences of respondents with a postmaterialist or postmodernist value orientation at times appear to be higher than those of their materialist and modernist counterparts. Having children may well form part of a postmodern idea of self-fulfillment. But, at very low fertility levels the timing of births clearly becomes exceedingly important. The crucial factor that appears to determine completed family size of the groups discussed is not that they differ substantially in stated ideals, wishes, expectations, or preferences. Most likely postmodernists and postmaterialists have important competing preferences and priorities. They begin childbearing late: at every age they have below-average numbers of children born.

I would like to formulate two theoretical propositions underlying the shift to postmodernity. These are strongly inspired by the work of Inglehart. They rest on his most recent formulation as well as on other discussions that have taken place around the general theme of the genesis and diffusion of value change, and of new behavior. They are as follows:

1. *A needs hierarchy hypothesis.* As societies become more modern, the emphasis people place on higher-order needs will increase. They will seek self-expression and will focus on their own well-being and on actions they perceive as giving meaning to their lives.

2. *A socialization hypothesis.* The effects of specific forms of socialization, or of socialization in specific environments, will be traceable in society as birth cohorts pass through the age pyramid.

Taken in combination the two hypotheses lead to the following proposition about the effects of social, economic, and technological change on demographic change. As societies develop, the classical demographic transition will inevitably follow. At an advanced stage of development an inflection will occur. People's cultural representations will change. In demographic behavior bourgeois postmodernism will start to act as a consistency generator. A second demographic transition will inevitably follow. Demographic patterns currently observed across a wide range of industrialized countries should be interpreted in that perspective.

This chapter has concentrated on value changes and postmodernism in particular. My own preference for synthesis and for efforts to achieve a broader understanding of contemporary society has guided the exploration on which I have reported. I find the thought that I may have witnessed a change from one historical era to the next during my lifetime quite stimulating. I also believe that, at this stage of its development, more attempts at integration and synthesis would not harm demography. In fact, I have seen so many detailed model specifications regarding a specific issue, in a specific country, at a precise point in time, that I frequently find it difficult to be content with accumulation of knowledge achieved in that way. It should be understood, however, that I do not for one moment deny the importance of social and economic factors in the demographic processes that have unfolded since the mid-1960s. Nor do I think that analysis based on abstract meta-concepts can replace the customary, detailed analyses that tie well-defined measures of fertility or family formation to the emergence of specific views on gender roles or similar determinants. However, such analyses need to be complemented with bolder efforts.

Do you love postmodernism? It is a bit as with music. Ultimately the love for music should have precedence over the love for a particular composer or style of music. It is easy to love Johannes Brahms. Erik Satie is beautiful for those who have learned to appreciate his music. The same will be true for the work of Olivier Messiaen or John Cage. I love demography and accept the use of postmodern in it as long as it not a vague, unspecified umbrella term.

APPENDIX TABLE Summary demographic measures and social indicators used in this chapter

Country	Fertility transiton score[a]	Marital transition score[a]	Subjective well-being score[b]	Post-materialist score[b]	Percent post-modern[a]	Percent modern[a]	Sample size WVS
Australia	0.25	0.02	n.a.	24	n.a.	n.a.	n.a.
Austria	–0.28	0.03	59	22	27.3	19.7	1,383
Belarus	–0.43	0.01	–2	14	8.6	31.0	902
Belgium	–0.48	0.47	77	27	22.5	21.3	2,551
Britain	0.19	–0.12	75	24	15.5	26.2	1,436
Bulgaria	–0.43	–0.87	4	13	10.2	29.5	911
Canada	–0.06	0.03	69	25	18.2	24.0	1,650
Czech Rep.	–0.36	–0.19	32	16	13.6	21.5	1,382
Denmark	0.33	1.22	85	23	30.2	10.8	961
Estonia	0.11	–0.17	25	13	n.a.	n.a.	n.a.
Finland	0.19	0.61	76	33	47.9	4.9	468
France	0.28	0.29	67	27	23.1	21.6	901
W. Germany	–0.42	0.37	70	25	42.8	12.1	1,964
E. Germany	0.07	–1.09	57	19	27.1	16.1	1,276
Hungary	–0.38	–0.62	28	12	6.7	38.9	930
Iceland	1.20	0.76	89	21	11.4	22.4	675
Ireland	0.87	–0.54	80	22	7.5	47.2	990
Italy	–0.37	–0.44	66	27	16.1	25.7	1,945
Latvia	–0.15	0.31	10	12	n.a.	n.a.	n.a.
Lithuania	–0.31	–0.03	13	16	13.1	24.3	913
Netherlands	–0.01	0.23	85	32	32.6	19.0	986
New Zealand	0.46	–0.10	n.a.	23	n.a.	n.a.	n.a.
Norway	0.40	0.47	81	20	28.1	18.5	1,193
Poland	–0.20	–0.62	58	13	n.a.	n.a.	n.a.
Portugal	–0.11	–0.24	51	17	9.2	38.6	1097
Romania	–0.26	–0.25	20	12	n.a.	n.a	n.a.
Russia	–0.46	0.18	–1	11	6.8	34.9	1,751
Slovenia	–0.23	–0.52	23	16	12.4	30.6	913
Spain	0.00	–0.36	65	25	17.5	29.2	3,767
Sweden	0.79	0.40	86	25	48.0	6.8	977
Switzerland	–0.27	0.41	86	30	24.0	19.9	1,219
USA	0.10	0.19	77	22	9.9	43.1	1,756

[a]Proportions postmodern and modern calculated from World Values Surveys (WVS); for methods of calculation see text. [b]Source: Inglehart 1997 (Postmaterialist scores for Australia and New Zealand estimated).
n.a. = not available.

Notes

This chapter was drafted while I was Visiting Fellow in the Demography Program (Coordinator: Peter F. McDonald) in the Institute of Advanced Studies, Research School of Social Sciences, of the Australian National University in Canberra. Generous and expert research assistance was provided by Ann Evans, while Jacomien van Teunenbroek assisted greatly in the search for literature. I am very grateful to both of them. In the conceptual stage of the chapter I benefited from a presentation to the Demographic Speculators of the Program (Convenor: Geoffrey McNicoll). Special thanks for advice and comments are due to Erik Klijzing of the ECE Population Team, Michael Bracher, Gordon Carmichael, Adrian Hayes, Peter McDonald and Yves de Roo. I wish to thank the Advisory Group of the FFS program of comparative research for its permission, granted under identification number 39, to use the FFS data on which part of this study is based. I gratefully acknowledge the use of data from the World Values Surveys 1990–93, Machine Readable Data File, ICPSR No. I6160.

1 Cf. the statement by Lyotard: "A work can become modern only if it is first postmodern" (1993: 13).

2 One may, moreover, argue that to the degree that postmodernists identify the grand narratives of the Enlightenment as the pollutants of society that have ultimately led to fascism and nationalism, extreme materialism, and so on, they are also likely to reject postmodernism as a meta-narrative emanating from Enlightenment ideas.

3 Since cohabitation is not an event routinely recorded by statistical offices, indications of its signifcance in the different European societies in the early 1990s had to be obtained from survey data. The World Values Surveys allowed the calculation of a uniform measure: the proportion of cohabiting women aged 25–29. Supporting evidence was gleaned from the literature. Carmichael (1995) has provided a useful review of the information on consensual partnering in all more developed countries, while Prinz (1995) and Kiernan (1996) assessed the situation in various European populations.

4 Since Australia and New Zealand did not participate in the World Values Surveys program, the prevalence of postmaterialism in these two countries had to be estimated. This was achieved by comparing Australia's and New Zealand's scores on attitudes regarding abortion and divorce in the International Social Survey Programme with those of the three other English-speaking countries, Canada, Great Britain, and the United States, which participated in both international endeavors. See references in Evans and Kelley (1996).

5 Since to date surveys explicitly investigating the issue of postmodernism have not been undertaken, Gibbins and Reimer understandably tried to exploit existing data sets—the 1981 and 1990 European Values Survey—for their purposes. Two items were used to operationalize expressivism. In order to be classified in the expressive category, respondents had to consider individual development important. They were then given a score of 1. If they also shared a feeling of restlessness the score increased to 2. All others were assigned a score of 0. The humanist and instrumentalist dimensions were captured as follows. Those who claimed to believe either that most people can be trusted, or that an important aspect of a job is that it be useful to society, were classified as humanists (score of 1). Respondents were classified as instrumentalists if they believed either that an important aspect of a job is that it be well paid, or that placing less emphasis on money and material possessions in our way of life would be a bad thing (score of 1). The scores were then transformed into a three-point scale from 0 to 2 and mean scores on the instrumentalist and humanist scales were calculated.

6 These categories refer to: (1) norms concerning (a) respect for authority, (b) sexual and marital behavior, and (c) civil behavior; (2) religious norms, (3) norms concerning parent–child ties; (4) norms concerning (a) conventional and (b) unconventional political participation; and (5) norms concerning (a) control of business and industry, (b) Left–Right self-placement, and (c) confidence in authoritarian institutions.

7 If asked to give a concise description I would, in line with the earlier discussion, state the following. Bourgeois postmodernists have a strong postmaterialist leaning or orientation, aim at self-realization, value their personal freedom greatly, place well-being and the quality of life above material assets, and question meta-narratives in the sense of not adhering to the tenets of a religion and of wanting to determine their own life style and pattern of personal relations. Bourgeois postmodernists similarly do not accept authority without question, are tolerant of the behavior of others, seek to express themselves freely, support emancipatory (human rights, ecological, gender) movements, favor diversity, and look without prejudice at developments leading to multiculturalism.

8 Constructing a proper instrument to measure postmodernity would, obviously, require extensive testing and the development of an especially designed battery of questions.

9 These questions were formulated as follows: (1) If someone says a child needs a home

with both a father and a mother to grow up happily, would you tend to agree or disagree? (2) Do you think a woman has to have children in order to be fulfilled, or is this not necessary? (3) Do you agree or disagree with the following statement? Marriage is an outdated institution. (4) If a woman wants to have a child as a single parent but she doesn't want to have a stable relationship with a man, do you approve or disapprove? (5) Which of the following two statements best describes your views? Parents' duty is to do their best for their children even at the expense of their own well-being. Parents have a life of their own and should not be asked to sacrifice their own well-being for the sake of their children. (6) Do you approve or disapprove of abortion where a married couple do not want to have more children?

10 In surveys that do not have a clear demographic orientation, the question of preferences is usually dealt with in two ways. Respondents are asked to state what they consider to be the "ideal" number of children, while they may also be asked how many they personally "desire." If the orientation of the surveys is demographic, women are commonly further asked whether they are currently pregnant, whether that pregnancy was wanted and planned, whether they want to have a (an-other) child sometime, and how many children are "wanted" (sometimes "expected") in all. The Eurobarometer Surveys of the European Union and the World Values Surveys referred to earlier are surveys of the first type (Coleman 1996). The Fertility and Family Surveys (FFS) undertaken in the countries of the ECE region, and special fertility surveys undertaken in other individual countries, are of the second type.

11 In addition to the countries mentioned in either Table 6 or 7, based on the Fertility and Family Surveys, the United States and New Zealand are among the participants in the FFS program.

12 The classification followed Inglehart's algorithm for the four-item index (1997: 389). The results differ from the scores as contained in the Appendix Table.

13 This probably is not a serious matter. While at the individual level men's and women's expectations frequently differ, at the aggregate level they tend to be very close (Beets 1983).

14 See, e.g, Bodrova 1997; Carmichael 1995; Coleman 1996a, 1996b; Dorbritz and Höhn 1999; Hobcraft and Kiernan 1995; Hoem and Hoem 1992; Jain and McDonald 1997; Jensen 1997; Katus and Zaharov 1997; Klijzing and Macura 1997; Kuijsten 1996; Lapierre-Adamcyk, Pool, and Dharmalingam 1997; Lee and Casterline 1996; Macunovich and Easterlin 1990; Morgan 1996; Pinnelli and De Rose 1997; Roussel 1994; Rowland (in press); Santow and Bracher 1997; Sardon 1997.

References

Australian Bureau of Statistics. 1993. *Births Australia 1992.* Canberra: ABS.

Baudrillard, J. 1988. *Selected Writings.* Cambridge: Polity Press.

Bauman, Z. 1997. *Postmodernity and Its Discontents.* New York: New York University Press.

Baynes, K., J. Bohman, and T. McCarthy (eds.). 1987. *After Philosophy: End or Transformation?* Cambridge, MA: The MIT Press.

Beets, G. C. N. 1983. "Vruchtbaarheidsverwachtingen van Mannen en Vrouwen," *Maandstatistiek van de Bevolking* 31(2): 26–36.

Bertens, H. 1986. "The postmodern *Weltanschauung* and its relation with modernism: An introductory survey," in D. Fokkema and H. Bertens (eds.), *Approaching Postmodernism.* Amsterdam/Philadelphia: John Benjamins Publishing Company, pp. 9–51.

———. 1995. *The Idea of the Postmodern: A History.* London: Routledge.

———. 1998. "Postmodernism: The Enlightenment continued," *European Review* 6(1): 35–43.

Bodrova, V. 1997. "The ideal, desirable and expectable number of children in Russia, 1997," paper presented to the IUSSP General Conference, Beijing, 11–17 October.

Carmichael, G. A. 1995. "Consensual partnering in the more developed countries," *Journal of the Australian Population Association* 12 (1): 51–87.

Carmichael, G. A., A. Webster, and P. McDonald. 1997. "Divorce Australian style: A demographic analysis," *Journal of Divorce and Remarriage* 26(3/4): 3–37.

Casterline, J. B., R. D. Lee, and K. A. Foote (eds.). 1996. *Fertility in the United States. New Patterns, New Theories.* Suppl. to *Population and Development Review,* Vol. 22. New York: Population Council.

Coleman, D. (ed.). 1996a. *Europe's Population in the 1990s.* Oxford: Oxford University Press.

———. 1996b. "New patterns and trends in European fertility: International and sub-national comparisons," in D. Coleman (ed.), *Europe's Population in the 1990s.* Oxford: Oxford University Press, pp. 1–61.

Council of Europe. 1996. *Recent Demographic Developments in Europe 1996.* Strasbourg: Council of Europe Publishing.

De Graaf, A. 1995. "Vrouwen zijn Minder Onzeker over hun Kindertal," *Maandstatistiek van de Bevolking* (Netherlands Central Bureau of Statistics) (1): 14–20.

Derrida, J. 1978. *Writing and Difference.* London: Routledge and Kegan Paul.

Dorbritz, J. and C. Höhn. 1999. "The future of the family and future fertility trends in Germany," in *Below Replacement Fertility.* Special Issue, *Population Bulletin Nos. 40–41*. New York: United Nations, pp. 218–234.

Evans, M. D. R. and J. Kelley. 1996. "Divorce for couples with children: Attitudes in 22 nations," *World Wide Attitudes,* Vol. 1996-09-02: 1–7.

Foucault, M. 1980. *Power/Knowledge: Selected Interviews and Other Writings 1972–1977.* New York: Harvester Wheatsheaf.

Gellner, E. 1992. *Postmodernism, Reason and Religion.* London: Routledge.

Gibbins, J. R. and B. Reimer. 1995. "Postmodernism," in J. W. van Deth and E. Scarbrough (eds.), *The Impact of Values.* Oxford: Oxford University Press, pp. 301–330.

Habermas, J. 1985. *Theorie des Kommunikativen Handelns.* 2 Vols. Frankfurt a. M.: Suhrkamp.

Himmelfarb, G. 1995. *The De-moralization of Society: From Victorian Virtues to Modern Values.* New York: Knopf.

Hobcraft, J. and K. Kiernan. 1995. "Becoming a parent in Europe," in *Evolution or Revolution in European Population.* European Population Conference, Milan. Milan: FrancoAngeli, pp. 27–61.

Hoem, J. M. and B. Hoem. 1992. "The disruption of marital and non-marital unions in contemporary Sweden," in J. Trussell, R. Hankinson, and J. Tilton (eds.), *Demographic Application of Event History Analysis.* Oxford: Clarendon Press.

Hoffmann-Nowotny, H. J. 1987. "The future of the family," in *Plenaries, European Population Conference,* Jyväskylä, pp. 113–200.

———. 1997. "Fertility and new types of household and family formation in Europe: A theoretical analysis," manuscript.

Inglehart, R. 1971. "The silent revolution in Europe: Intergenerational change in post-industrial societies," *American Political Science Review* 65(4): 991–1017.

———. 1977. *The Silent Revolution: Changing Values and Political Styles among Western Publics.* Princeton: Princeton University Press.

———. 1997. *Modernization and Postmodernization: Cultural, Economic, and Political Change in 43 Societies.* Princeton: Princeton University Press.

Jain, S. K. and P. F. McDonald. 1997. "Fertility of Australian birth cohorts: Components and differentials," *Journal of the Australian Population Association* 14(1): 31–46.

Jensen, A-M. 1997. "New forms of reproductive and family behaviour in contemporary Europe: A review of recent findings," in *IUSSP General Conference, Beijing 1997,* Vol. 2. Liège: IUSSP, pp. 869–885.

Katus, K. and S. Zakharov. 1997. "Demographic adaptation to socioeconomic changes in the USSR successor states," paper presented at the IUSSP General Conference, Beijing, 11–17 October.

Kaufmann, F. X. 1988. "Familie und Modernität," in K. Lüscher, F. Schultheis, and M. Wehrspaun (eds.), *Die "Postmoderne Familie,"* Konstanzer Beiträge zur Socialwissenschaftlichen Forschung, Band 3, pp. 391–415.

Kelley, J. and M. D. R. Evans. 1996. "International differences in attitudes toward abortion," *World Wide Attitudes*, Vol. 1996-07-08: 1–6.

Kiernan, K. 1996. "Partnership behaviour in Europe: Recent trends and issues," in D. Coleman (ed.), *Europe's Population in the 1990s*. Oxford: Oxford University Press, pp. 62–91.

Klijzing, E. and M. Macura. 1997. "Cohabitation and extra-marital childbearing: Early FFS evidence," in *IUSSP General Conference, Beijing 1997*, Vol. 2. Liège: IUSSP, pp. 885–903.

Kuijsten, A. C. 1996. "Changing family patterns in Europe: A case of divergence?" *European Journal of Population* 12: 115–143.

Lapierre-Adamcyk, E., I. Pool, and A. Dharmalingam. 1997. "New forms of reproductive and family behaviour in the neo-Europes: Findings from the 'European Fertility and Family Survey' on Canada and New Zealand," paper presented at the IUSSP General Conference, Beijing, 11–17 October.

Lee, R. D. and J. B. Casterline. 1996. "Introduction," in J. B. Casterline, R. D. Lee, and K. A. Foote (eds.), *Fertility in the United States: New Patterns, New Theories*. Suppl. to Vol. 22 of *Population and Development Review*. New York: Population Council, pp. 1–15.

Lesthaeghe, R. 1991. "The second demographic transition in Western countries: An interpretation," Working Paper 1991-2, Interuniversity Programme in Demography, Brussels.

Lesthaeghe, R. and D. Meekers. 1986. "Value changes and the dimensions of familism in the European Community," *European Journal of Population* 2: 225–268.

Lesthaeghe, R. and G. Moors. 1995. "Living arrangements, socio-economic position, and values among young adults: A pattern description for Belgium, France, The Netherlands and West Germany, 1990," in H. van den Brekel and F. Deven (eds.), *Population and Family in the Low Countries 1994*. Dordrecht: Kluwer Academic Publishers, pp. 1–57.

Lesthaeghe, R. and J. Surkyn. 1988. "Cultural dynamics and economic theories of fertility change," *Population and Development Review* 14(1): 1–45.

Lesthaeghe, R. and D. J. van de Kaa. 1986. "Twee Demografische Transities?" (Two demographic transitions?), in D. J. van de Kaa and R. Lesthaeghe (eds.), *Bevolking: Groei en Krimp (Population: Growth and Decline)*. Deventer: Van Loghum Slaterus.

Lyotard, J-F. 1984. *The Postmodern Condition: A Report on Knowledge*. Minneapolis: University of Minnesota Press.

———. 1993. *The Postmodern Explained: Correspondence 1982–1985*. (Translation of *Le Postmoderne expliqué aux enfants*). Minneapolis: University of Minnesota Press.

Macunovich, D. J. and R. A. Easterlin. 1990. "How parents have coped: The effect of life cycle demographic decisions on the economic status of pre-school age children, 1964–87," *Population and Development Review* 16(2): 301–325.

McDonald, P. 2000. "Gender equity, social institutions and the future of fertility," *Journal of Population Research* 17(1): 1–17.

Micheli, G. A. 1996. "New patterns of family formation in Italy: Which tools for which interpretations?" *Genus* LII: 15–52.

Michon, J. A. 1998. "Cognitiewetenschappen en postmodernisme," in G. W. Muller and P. C. Muysken (eds.), *Vreemde Gasten: Deconstructie en Cognitie in de Geesteswetenschappen*. Amsterdam: Koninklijke Nederlandse Akademie van Wetenschappen, Vol. 4, pp. 33–61.

Monnier, A. and C. de Guibert-Lantoine. 1995. "The demographic situation of Europe and the developed countries overseas: An annual report," *Population: An English Selection* 7: 187–202.

Morgan, S. P. 1996. "Characteristic features of modern American fertility," in J. B. Casterline, R. D. Lee, and K. Foote (eds.), *Fertility in the United States: New Patterns, New Theories*, Suppl. to Vol. 22 of *Population and Development Review*. New York: Population Council, pp. 19–63.

Pinnelli, A. and A. De Rose. 1997. "Micro and macro determinants of family formation and dissolution," paper presented to the IUSSP General Conference, Beijing, 11–17 October.

Prioux, F. 1993. "L'infécondité en Europe," in A. Blum and J-L. Rallu (eds.), *European Population. II Demographic Dynamics.* Montrouge: John Libbey, pp. 231–255.

Prinz, C. 1995. *Cohabiting, Married or Single.* Aldershot: Avebury.

Reher, D. S. 1998. "Family ties in Western Europe: Persistent contrasts," *Population and Development Review* 24(2): 203–234.

Rorty, R. 1989. *Contingency, Irony, and Solidarity.* Cambridge: Cambridge University Press.

Roussel, L. 1994. "Fertility and the family," in *Proceedings European Population Conference, Geneva, 1993.* Vol. 1. Strasbourg: Council of Europe, pp. 35–110.

Rowland, D. R. (in press). "Cross-national trends in childlessness," in P. Dijkstra and D. Vaughan (eds.), *Ageing Without Children.*

Rychtaříková, J. 1999. "Is Eastern Europe experiencing a second demographic transition?" *Acta Universitas Carolinae, Geographica* 1: 19–44.

Sagan, F. 1959. *Aimez-vous Brahms?* Paris: R. Juilliard.

Santow, G. and M. Bracher. 1997. "Whither marriage? Trends, correlates, and interpretations," in *IUSSP General Conference, Beijing 1997,* Vol. 2. Liège: IUSSP, pp. 919–941.

Sardon, J-P. 1997. "L'évolution récente de la fécondité en Europe de sud," paper presented to the General Conference of the IUSSP, Beijing, 11–17 October.

Scarbrough, E. 1995. "Materialist-postmaterialist value orientations," in J. W. van Deth and E. Scarbrough (eds.), *The Impact of Values.* Oxford: Oxford University Press, pp. 124–159.

Statistics New Zealand. 1996. *Demographic Trends 1996.* Wellington: SNZ.

United Nations. 1990 and 1993. *Demographic Yearbook 1990* and *1993.* New York: United Nations.

Van de Kaa, D. J. 1987. "Europe's second demographic transition," *Population Bulletin* 42 (1). Washington, DC: Population Reference Bureau.

———. 1994. "The second demographic transition revisited: Theories and expectations," in G. C. N. Beets et al. (eds.), *Population and Family in the Low Countries 1993.* Lisse: Zwets and Zeitlinger, pp. 81–126.

———. 1997. "Options and sequences: Europe's demographic patterns," *Journal of the Australian Population Association* 14(1): 1–30.

Van Deth, J. W. and E. Scarbrough. 1995. "The concept of values," in J. W. van Deth and E. Scarbrough (eds.), *The Impact of Values.* Oxford: Oxford University Press, pp. 21–47.

Van Reijen, W. 1988. "Moderne en postmoderne filosofie: Habermas versus Lyotard," *Acta Politica* 2: 199–223.

Von der Dunk, H. W. 1993. "Bestaat er een 'Postmodernistische' Geschiedbeoefening?" in F. R. Ankersmit and A. K. Varga (eds.), *Akademische Beschouwingen over het Postmodernisme.* Amsterdam: Noord Hollandsche, pp. 65–70.

Comment: The Puzzling Persistence of Postmodern Fertility Preferences

CHRISTINE BACHRACH

DIRK VAN DE KAA explores whether, somewhere among the multiple meanings of the term "postmodernism," there are concepts that can help us better capture the ideational forces that have helped to shape the course of post-transitional fertility. This is a brave undertaking, because some inherent incongruities exist between postmodernism as expressed in many contexts (e.g., see the review by Rosenau 1992) and the concepts and approaches of demography. Van de Kaa explores three approaches to shaping postmodern themes into useful concepts: an avant-garde value orientation, a new historical era, and a new world view. He achieves some success in relating the latter two concepts to demographic questions.

However, his attempt to operationalize even these limited meanings using extant survey data proves fraught with difficulty, and arguably transforms the ideas of postmodernism into variables that would not be recognized or accepted by postmodernists. Van de Kaa rightly points out the potential for further theorizing and measurement development. It remains to be seen whether the need for precise conceptualization recognized by van de Kaa in order to produce measures useful to demography is compatible with the essence of postmodern ideas and thought. If it is not, the fruits of this exercise will be limited.

His chapter yields some important lessons nevertheless. One of these is that the value shifts that van de Kaa labels postmodern appear to be important for understanding the strategies people in most European countries use to mate, bear children, and rear them, and they are also important at present for understanding variations in the level and timing of fertility. On the other hand, they do not appear to be very important in understanding fertility *preferences*. I explore several questions in this commentary: (1) How do we think postmodernism should affect fertility preferences and fertility itself? (2) What might explain the persistence of fertility preferences at or above replacement where fertility itself has dropped below replacement, especially among those with postmodern value orientations? (3) What will the future bring?

Several caveats are in order. The focus of my comments (as well as of van de Kaa's analysis) is on Western industrialized countries. A valuable extension of this work would be to examine the relationships among value shifts, fertility preferences, and fertility in non-Western countries that have entered "post-transitional" periods of extremely low fertility. Also, as in van de Kaa's chapter, I advance arguments about the associations between values and fertility preferences at both the individual level and the country level. Although both are probably important, if we are ultimately trying to understand the fertility level in a given society, preferences and behavior at the aggregate level may be more predictive. We need better models for understanding the relationship of individual-level associations to broader mechanisms of societal change.

What are postmodern fertility preferences?

At the risk of doing disservice to van de Kaa's thoughtful development of the many concepts of postmodernism, I extract below a few themes that may be seen as features of a "postmodern worldview" or what van de Kaa refers to as "bourgeois" postmodernity—an inventory of values, attitudes, and orientations that capture the essence of the postmodern individual. They are:

—Self-realization
—Personal freedom; self-determination of lifestyle and personal relations
—Well-being and quality of life valued above material assets
—Questioning of meta-narratives and of traditional authority
—Toleration of and support for diversity.

How would these values, attitudes, and orientations be expected to influence fertility preferences? To the extent that such preferences reflect the influence of institutions that promote childbearing or support high fertility, the questioning of meta-narratives or authorities might lower fertility preferences by removing the influence of these institutional supports (Lesthaeghe and Surkyn 1988). To the extent that children reduce individual freedom, a high value placed on personal freedom, self-expression, and self-realization could certainly reduce fertility preferences. On the other hand, an emphasis on the quality and meaning of life, as well as on self-realization, might actually have a positive effect on fertility preferences, to the extent that children and parenthood are seen as important routes to personal fulfillment.

Beyond these effects on fertility preferences, postmodern values may influence fertility itself through mechanisms that have already been well described in research and theory on the transition to low fertility (e.g., Becker 1991; Bulatao and Lee 1983). Options other than parenthood, such as work and leisure activities, may be seen as alternative pathways to self-fulfillment, leading individuals to postpone childbearing or avoid it altogether. Reduced time spent in marriage or marriage-like relationships may depress actual fertility. An increased demand for child quality (which can be viewed as part and parcel of parents' quality of life) would increase the investment required for each child and make it less feasible to have many.

The overwhelming expectation here is that the postmodern world view would have a negative impact on fertility. Implications for fertility preferences are more ambiguous, although on balance a negative effect is also suggested. Table 1 extracts data on desired and ideal family size for countries that had high, medium, and low proportions of individuals espousing postmodern value orientations based on data from the World Values Surveys. Average ideal numbers of children are shown for individuals with postmodern and modern orientations within each of these countries. In most countries, postmodern individuals express lower average ideal family sizes than their modern counterparts in the same country. However, in Sweden, where modernists' average ideal is 2.6 children and postmodernists' is 2.8 children, the reverse is true. Thus, as van de Kaa points out, the idea that a postmodernist world view is associated with lower fertility preferences is mainly supported by the empirical evidence.

TABLE 1 Average number of children considered ideal by modern or postmodern value orientation, and average number of children wanted ultimately by women aged 25–29 in countries with high, medium, and low proportions of postmodern individuals

Proportions postmodern	Percent postmodern in country	Average number considered ideal		Average wanted ultimately
		Modern	Postmodern	
High				
Finland	48	3.13	2.63	2.3
Sweden	48	2.59	2.76	2.6
Medium				
Austria	27	2.63	2.30	2.0
France	23	2.77	2.62	2.3
Low				
Slovenia	12	2.59	2.35	2.3
Hungary	7	2.52	2.18	2.1

SOURCES: Data on percent postmodern and ideal family size from the 1990 World Values Surveys, presented in van de Kaa, this volume, Table 8 and Appendix Table; on number of children wanted ultimately from the Fertility and Family Surveys, ECE, as presented in van de Kaa, Table 6.

Why do fertility preferences remain at replacement levels?

At the same time, it is striking that fertility preferences have remained at levels well above the prevailing fertility rates,[1] both among individuals with postmodern value orientations and in countries where postmodern value orientations are strongly embraced. In Table 1, average ideal numbers are well above 2 children in all countries and in both groups of individuals. The average number of children "wanted ultimately" by women aged 25–29 years, also shown in the table, slips below replacement only in Austria. This is a more realistic measure of fertility preferences than ideal family size, because it is less likely to invite responses that disregard real-world constraints. Most significantly, wanted and ideal numbers of children tend to be as high or higher in countries with high proportions of postmodern individuals as they are in countries with low proportions postmodern. The "postmodern era" has clearly arrived in Finland and Sweden, but it has not brought low fertility preferences with it.

What can explain the persistence of fertility preferences at or above replacement levels in an era of below-replacement fertility? Several possible explanations can be advanced. First, our measures may be capturing aspects of fertility values that are insensitive to postmodern value shifts. Ideal family size may well be vulnerable to this criticism, but the number ultimately wanted should be less so, and this remains above replacement level among the most postmodern of countries. Still, measures of preferences, however defined, may not capture the tradeoffs that characterize fertility decisionmaking in modern society. We may need to develop measures of priorities that capture the value placed on childbearing relative to other investments. Such an approach was adopted in studies conducted by Moors and Palomba (1995: Table A.6.1); their results suggest that expressed priorities for childbearing are high even in countries with extremely low fertility.

Second, it could be that preferences are simply slow to change. There is a lag in how preferences respond to changing values and we may eventually see them drop. The most compelling evidence against this argument is that preferences are still high in countries that are far advanced in terms of ideational change.

Finally, even among individuals with the highest levels of postmodern values, the benefits of children as a means of self-expression may outweigh the negatives. In short, there may be a natural "floor" below which fertility preferences will not fall. One would expect a floor to fertility preferences if at least some of the benefits of having children were perceived as nonsubstitutable or imperfectly substitutable: for example, the experience of nurturing, the idea of being connected to future generations, or even the social status associated with being a parent. In their study of attitudes toward family issues, Moors and Palomba (1995: 259) conclude that Europeans view childbearing as a unique value: "Having children is considered a value in itself which cannot be compared with other life-values which concern sectors outside the family (like work, money, etc.) or other aspects of personal life (like free time, hobbies, relationship with a partner, etc.)."

Alternatively, one could argue for a floor to fertility preferences on evolutionary grounds. A simplistic evolutionary argument that individuals with subreplacement fertility preferences would be selected out of the gene pool over the course of evolution would founder on the fact that reproductive preferences probably played a minor role in human evolution. However, it is possible that modern-day fertility preferences are associated with a constellation of human traits (e.g., affiliation and nurturance) that *were* selected for in evolution, and as a result humankind today includes traits that make childbearing and childrearing central and appealing as means of self-expression. New research in the United States is providing suggestive evidence that there may be a genetic basis to fertility motivation (Miller et al. 1999).

But even if one accepts the idea that human beings are genetically predisposed to want children, fertility preferences could still easily drop below replacement if the predominant preference for two children were replaced with a preference for only one. In other words, there may well be a floor to fertility preferences, but it would not necessarily occur at replacement level.

The persistence of preferences for two or more children may be explained by other prevailing values, ideas, and norms. One such value might have to do with reducing uncertainty—not putting your eggs in one basket, so to speak. Recognizing that child outcomes vary partly as a function of in-born and environmental influences beyond parents' control, parents may feel that having only one child reduces their chances of having a child who satisfies their needs and expectations. The persistence of norms about what it takes to rear a high-quality child may also play a part: being a good parent may include giving your child a sibling. Evidence from studies of the costs and satisfactions of children suggests that, whereas values motivating a first birth emphasize family status, roles, and emotional rewards for the parent, values motivating second births are strongly associated with providing companionship for the first child (Fawcett 1983). Finally, modern societies still have differentiated ideas of gender. Preferring fewer than two children implies a willingness to have only a son or only a daughter. A preference for two or more children can incorporate having both.[2]

Inherent in these ideas is the notion that parenthood is something to be experienced fully and with investment in risk reduction and quality—ideas compatible with Inglehart's postmaterial worldview, if not with postmodernism itself. However, these ideas are themselves vulnerable to the forces of ideational change under certain conditions. That postmodernists are often ultimately unable to achieve their preferences for two children may trigger such ideational change. The greater prevalence of one-child families may lead to a reassessment of the costs and benefits of having or being an only child, and potentially to a reduction in fertility preferences.

What will the future bring?

Evidence suggests that a fundamental shift in values toward what van de Kaa and others have labeled postmodernism has been occurring and will continue to occur in industrialized societies. It is clear that, at least to this point, this value shift has not affected aggregate fertility preferences; but it has affected reproductive strategies—the way in which people fit childbearing into their lives. Because some of these strategies tend to fall short with respect to achieving fertility preferences, it has affected fertility itself.

But fundamental shifts in values tend to set up tensions, and the tension we see between actual and preferred fertility is indicative of broader tensions between what could be labeled family values and postmodern values. This tension stimulates answer-seeking processes that may lead to heated discussion of what is right and wrong behavior and to the search for models of behavior that resolve perceived value conflicts. The unfolding of these processes may alter the path of ideational, social, and institutional change in ways that have implications for future fertility.

One such value conflict is the conflict between the value for personal freedom and the value—still held by a large majority of people in most industrialized countries—that children need the stable presence of two parents in their lives (Inglehart 1997). In the United States, the proliferation of single-mother families (and especially single-mother families on welfare) prompted changes in policies relating to establishment of paternity, child support payment, and welfare programs. Conservative religious groups in the US during the 1980s launched a drive to promote abstinence among unmarried teenagers, a drive that is now showing some evidence of success (Ku et al. 1998; Bearman 1999). Pro-family groups have even challenged ideational change itself, as illustrated in an article in the publication *Focus on the Family* instructing parents in ways to steer their children away from a postmodern worldview (Arrington 1998).

Societal responses to tensions between family values and postmodern values are likely to be deeply colored by the political and cultural heritage of societies, as well as by current social and economic forces. One possible response is the establishment of new institutional supports that make it easier to satisfy both postmodern values and fertility preferences. As Sweden's experience suggests, this is a costly response, but one that can influence fertility. Another response may involve a reduction in fertility preferences to levels that are more compatible with postmodern realities, perhaps by elevating the desirability of the one-child family. Yet a third may include a partial retreat from or a recalibration of postmodern values, something that now seems to be happening to a limited extent in the United States. Even within the context of low fertility, variations in fertility levels and population growth rates implicit in these differential responses may have substantial demographic implications. As the long-term march of postmodern ideas continues, specific societal responses will play a significant role in shaping our demographic future.

Notes

1 As Bongaarts (this volume) demonstrates, prevailing TFRs are depressed by the tempo effects of delayed childbearing. However, TFRs adjusted for tempo effects remain below replacement for five out of the six Western countries for which adjustments are shown in Table 1 in his chapter. Thus, timing effects alone cannot account for the higher level of fertility preferences as compared to actual fertility.

2 This idea was contributed by Jean-Claude Chesnais during discussion at the Conference on Global Fertility Transition, Bellagio, Italy, 18–22 May 1998.

References

Arrington. Lael. 1998. "Hey Mom, what's a worldview?" *Focus on the Family* 22(4): 14.

Bearman, Peter. 1999. "Pledging the future: Virginity pledges and the transition to first intercourse," paper presented at the Annual Meeting of the American Sociological Association, Chicago.

Becker, Gary S. 1991. *A Treatise on the Family*. Enlarged edition. Cambridge, MA: Harvard University Press.

Bulatao, Rodolfo A. and Ronald D. Lee. (eds.) 1983. *Determinants of Fertility in Developing Countries*. 2 vols. New York: Academic Press.

Fawcett, James T. 1983. "Perceptions of the value of children: Satisfactions and costs," in Rodolfo A. Bulatao and Ronald D. Lee (eds.), *Determinants of Fertility in Developing Countries*. New York: Academic Press, pp. 429–457.

Inglehart, Ronald. 1997. *Modernization and Postmodernization: Cultural, Economic, and Political Change in 43 Societies*. Princeton: Princeton University Press.

Ku, Leighton, Freya L. Sonenstein, Scott Boggess, and Joseph H. Pleck. 1998. "Understanding changes in teenage men's sexual activity: 1979 to 1995," paper presented at the Annual Meeting of the Population Association of America, Chicago.

Lesthaeghe, Ron and Johan Surkyn. 1988. "Cultural dynamics and economic theories of fertility change," *Population and Development Review* 14(1): 1–45.

Miller, Warren B. et al. 1999. "Genetic influences on childbearing motivation: A theoretical framework and some empirical evidence," in L. J. Severy and W. B. Miller (eds.), *Advances in Population: Psychosocial Perspectives*, Vol III. London: Jessica Kingsley, pp. 53–102.

Moors, H. and R. Palomba. 1995. *Population, Family and Welfare: A Comparative Survey of European Attitudes*, Vol. I. Oxford: Clarendon Press.

Rosenau, P. M. 1992. *Post-Modernism and the Social Sciences: Insights, Inroads, and Intrusions*. Princeton: Princeton University Press.

AUTHORS

CHRISTINE BACHRACH is Chief of the Demographic and Behavioral Sciences Branch, Center for Population Research, National Institute of Child Health and Human Development.

JOHN BONGAARTS is Vice President, Policy Research Division, Population Council.

RODOLFO A. BULATAO is an Independent Consultant, Silver Spring, MD.

JOHN C. CALDWELL is Emeritus Professor of Demography, Australian National University, Canberra.

JOHN B. CASTERLINE is Senior Associate, Policy Research Division, Population Council.

JEAN-CLAUDE CHESNAIS is Senior Research Fellow, INED (Institut National d'Etudes Démographiques), Paris.

JOHN CLELAND is Professor of Medical Demography, London School of Hygiene and Tropical Medicine.

TOMAS FREJKA is International Consultant and Visiting Scholar, Max Planck Institute for Demographic Research, Rostock, Germany.

JOHN G. HAAGA is Director of Domestic Programs, Population Reference Bureau, Washington, DC.

CHARLES HIRSCHMAN is Boeing International Professor, Department of Sociology, University of Washington, Seattle.

MASSIMO LIVI BACCI is Professor of Demography, Faculty of Political Sciences, University of Florence.

KAREN OPPENHEIM MASON is Director of Gender and Development, The World Bank, Washington, DC.

GEOFFREY MCNICOLL is Senior Associate, Policy Research Division, Population Council.

HARRIET B. PRESSER is Distinguished University Professor and Director, Center on Population, Gender, and Social Inequality, Department of Sociology, University of Maryland.

LUIS ROSERO-BIXBY is Professor and Director, Centro Centroamericano de Población, Universidad de Costa Rica.

JOHN ROSS is Senior Fellow, The Futures Group International, Glastonbury, Connecticut.

AMY ONG TSUI is Professor, Department of Maternal and Child Health, and Director, Carolina Population Center, University of North Carolina at Chapel Hill.

DIRK J. VAN DE KAA is Emeritus Professor of Demography, University of Amsterdam.